HIV Medicine

HIV Medicine

Edited by Evan Maverick

hayle medical

New York

Hayle Medical,
750 Third Avenue, 9th Floor,
New York, NY 10017, USA

Visit us on the World Wide Web at:
www.haylemedical.com

ISBN: 978-1-63241-827-2

Cataloging-in-Publication Data

HIV medicine / edited by Evan Maverick.
p. cm.
Includes bibliographical references and index.
ISBN 978-1-63241-827-2
1. HIV infections. 2. HIV infections--Treatment. 3. HIV-positive persons. I. Maverick, Evan.
RC606.6 .H58 2020
616.979 2--dc23

Table of Contents

Preface

Every book is initially just a concept; it takes months of research and hard work to give it the final shape in which the readers receive it. In its early stages, this book also went through rigorous reviewing. The notable contributions made by experts from across the globe were first molded into patterned chapters and then arranged in a sensibly sequential manner to bring out the best results.

HIV or human immunodeficiency virus is the cause of HIV/AIDS. It is a retrovirus, which infects the human immune system, particularly the $CD4^+$ T cells, macrophages and dendritic cells. HIV is of two types- HIV-1 and HIV-2. HIV-1 is more infective and virulent. It causes the majority of HIV infections worldwide. HIV-2 is comparatively less pathogenic than HIV-1 and has lower transmission rates. However, both lead to AIDS in individuals and also mutate to develop drug resistance. Once HIV enters the body, it undergoes a period of rapid viral replication, which then reduces $CD4^+$ T cells. This results in a weakening of the immune system, thus allowing opportunistic infections to occur. The treatment of AIDS aims at slowing the progression of the disease, using antiretroviral therapy. This therapy consists of a combination of at least two classes of antiretroviral agents, non-nucleoside reverse transcriptase inhibitor and nucleoside analog reverse transcriptase inhibitors. This book covers in detail some existing theories and innovative concepts revolving around HIV medicine. Different approaches, evaluations, methodologies and advanced studies on HIV/AIDS and its management have been included herein. A number of latest researches have been included to keep the readers up-to-date with the global concepts in this area of study.

It has been my immense pleasure to be a part of this project and to contribute my years of learning in such a meaningful form. I would like to take this opportunity to thank all the people who have been associated with the completion of this book at any step.

Editor

1

Dual role of autophagy in HIV-1 replication and pathogenesis

M Scott Killian

Abstract

Autophagy, the major mechanism for degrading long-lived intracellular proteins and organelles, is essential for eukaryotic cell homeostasis. Autophagy also defends the cell against invasion by microorganisms and has important roles in innate and adaptive immunity. Increasingly evident is that HIV-1 replication is dependent on select components of autophagy. Fittingly, HIV-1 proteins are able to modulate autophagy to maximize virus production. At the same time, HIV-1 proteins appear to disrupt autophagy in uninfected cells, thereby contributing to CD4+ cell death and HIV-1 pathogenesis. These observations allow for new approaches for the treatment and possibly the prevention of HIV-1 infection. This review focuses on the relationship between autophagy and HIV-1 infection. Discussed is how autophagy plays dual roles in HIV-1 replication and HIV-1 disease progression.

Keywords: HIV, Autophagy, Innate immunity, T cells, Antiretroviral therapy, Pathogenesis

Introduction

Human immunodeficiency virus 1 (HIV-1) establishes a chronic infection that is characterized by persistent virus replication, a systemic decline in CD4+ T cell numbers, accumulating immunologic defects, and the eventual rise of AIDS-defining opportunistic infections and cancers [1]. It is increasingly evident [1] that autophagy, a proteolytic mechanism, plays roles in both HIV-1 replication and disease progression. This review discusses substantial findings from basic research and translational studies of autophagy and HIV-1. Emphasized is the relevance of (macro)autophagy to HIV-1 replication, anti-HIV-1 immune responses, and HIV-1 pathogenesis.

Overview of autophagy

Autophagy, first described many decades ago, has been popularized by recent advances in its cellular and molecular characterization [2]. Although other systems (e.g. microautophagy and chaperone-mediated autophagy) also transport cytoplasmic material to lysosomes, macroautophagy, hereafter referred to as autophagy, is the dominant mechanism for degrading long-lived proteins and organelles [3].

* Correspondence: scott.killian@ucsf.edu
Department of Medicine, University of California San Francisco, Box 1270, 513, Parnassus Avenue, San Francisco, CA 94143-1270, USA

Autophagy can be conceptualized as a three-stage process (Figure 1). Stage 1, the initiation of autophagy, is triggered by events that include nutrient starvation, cytokine signaling, and genomic stress. Many of these signals intersect with the mammalian target of rapamycin (mTOR) and act to reverse its inhibitory effects on autophagy [4]. Stage 2, autophagosome synthesis, involves the functions of more than 20 autophagy-related (ATG) genes (Table 1), two ubiquitin-like systems (Atg12-Atg5 and LC3-PE), and one lipid kinase signaling complex (PI3K/Beclin-1) [5]. Its end result is the formation of a double-membrane vesicle that contains cytosolic content. Stage 3, the proteolytic stage of autophagy, entails the fusion of mature autophagosomes with lysosomes [6]. Its coordination has recently been attributed to the function of the transcription factor EB (TFEB) [7]. The cytosolic contents are degraded by lysosomal acid hydrolases and then returned to the cytoplasm via channels in the autophagolysosomal membrane. Reactivation of mTOR terminates autophagy [8].

Measuring autophagy

Several methods are commonly used to measure autophagy (Table 2) [27]. One approach is to measure, by Western blot procedures, the intracellular levels of two variants of the MAP kinase light chain 3 (LC3) protein: LC3-I and LC3-II. LC3-I is lipidated to form LC3-II and

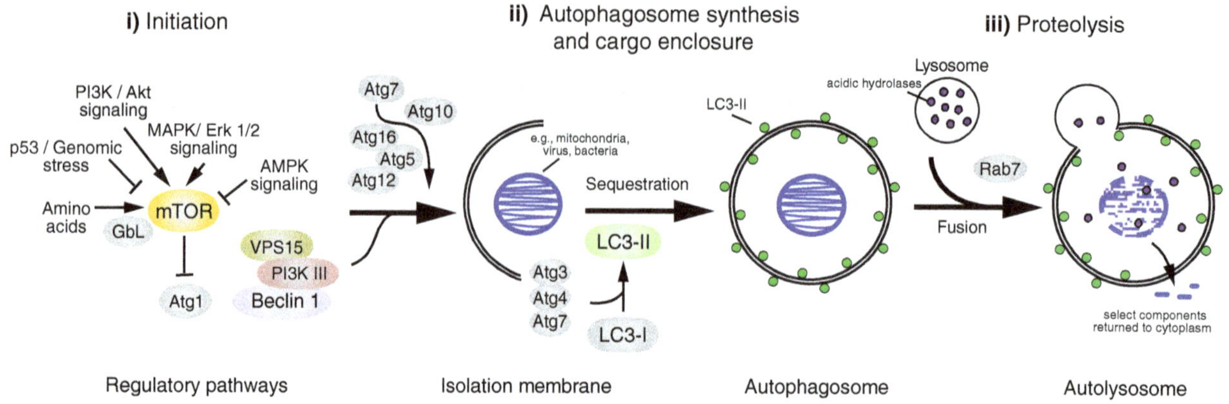

Figure 1 The 3 stages of autophagy. Illustrated are distinct stages in the process of autophagy. **i**) Autophagy is initiated by pathways that inactivate mTOR. **ii**) Autophagosome synthesis involves the coupling of LC3-II to the autophagosome membrane and the formation of double membrane vesicles that sequester cytoplasmic material. **iii**) The final stage of autophagy, proteolysis, entails the fusion of mature autophagosomes with lysosomes and the release of breakdown products into the cytoplasm.

then associates with the autophagosomal membrane upon the induction of autophagy. Thus, measurement of the ratio of LC3-II to LC3-I by Western blot methods is widely used to enumerate autophagic flux; the LC3-II/LC3-I ratio increases upon the induction of autophagy and autophagosome formation. Notably, there are three mammalian isoforms of LC3: LC3A, LC3B, and LC3C. LC3B-II is the only protein known to specifically localize to the autophagosome [28]. Another tactic is to visualize and enumerate autophagosomes by electron microscopy (Figure 2). The extraordinary magnification of intracellular constituents enabled by electron microscopy allows for the direct visualization of the double membrane autophagosome structures [29]. The use of LC3-GFP fusion proteins has been helpful for measuring autophagy, allowing for streamlined fluorescent microscopy procedures [30]. Finally, kinetic RT-PCR is regularly used to measure the relative levels of autophagy-related gene transcripts such as BECN1, the gene that encodes Beclin 1 (see Table 1).

Chemical compounds can also be useful for investigating the different stages of autophagy (see Figure 1). Rapamycin inhibits mTOR to induce autophagy [32]. 3-methyladenine (3-MA) inhibits class III phosphatidylinositol 3-kinase (PI3K) and thereby blocks autophagosome formation [33]. Bafilomycin A1 is a specific inhibitor of vacuolar H + ATPase that blocks the fusion between autophagosomes and lysosomes [34]. Thus, 3-MA and Bafilomycin A1 can be used to study the effects of inhibiting the early and late stages of autophagy respectively.

Studies of autophagy must be carefully evaluated with respect to the details of the assays employed and the interpretation of their results [27,28]. For example, punctate dots in fluorescent microscope images do not necessarily represent autophagosomes, as LC3 can form autophagy-independent aggregates within the cell [35]. In addition, the chemical compounds used to modify autophagic conditions, such as rapamycin, can be toxic to cells at relatively low concentrations [36]. Noteworthy is that prolonged 3-MA treatment in nutrient-rich medium is reported to promote autophagy flux in some cell lines [37]. Therefore, approaches to inhibit autophagy can actually have the opposite effect under certain conditions.

Autophagy and HIV-1 replication

As an obligate intracellular parasite, HIV-1 is dependent on its ability to evade intrinsic cellular defenses including xenophagy - the engulfment and destruction of intracellular microbes by autophagy (Figure 3) [38]. Discussed below are studies demonstrating that HIV-1 is able increase virus production by inducing autophagy and evading its proteolytic components.

Genetic studies

At least 35 genes (see Table 1) are involved in autophagy [3,38]. Several of these autophagy-associated genes have been linked with HIV-1 replication. Using small interfering RNA (siRNA) to knock down host genes in a HeLa-derived (epithelial) cell line, members of protein-conjugation pathways involved in autophagy (ATG7, ATG8, ATG12, and ATG16L2) and lysosomal-associated genes (CLN3, LapTM5) were found to be essential for HIV-1 replication [42]. Similarly, a recent study found that the knockdown of PIK3R4, ATG4A, ATG5, or ATG16 with short hairpin RNA (shRNA) led to the inhibition of HIV-1_{LAI} replication in SupT1 cells (T cell line) without having gross effects on the cell viability [43]. However, in separate studies, treatment of HIV-infected HeLa and H9 cells (a T cell line) with rapamycin to induce autophagy did not increase HIV-1 replication [39]. Thus, additional studies are needed to better determine the

Table 1 Major human autophagy-related genes and their functions

Stage of autophagy	Gene	Alternate name	Chromosome	Function in autophagy	References
Initiation of autophagy					
	mTOR		1p36.2	Negative regulator of autophagy.	[4]
	RPTOR		17q25.3	Acts to regulate mTOR.	[9]
	ULK1	ATG1	12q24.3	Components of ULK1 protein kinase complex.	[10]
	ATG13		11p11.2		[11]
	RB1CC1	FIP200	8q11.23		[12]
	C12orf44	ATG101	2q13.13		[11]
Autophagosome formation					
	ATG9A,B		2q35, 7q36	Components of ATG9-WIPI complex and Vps34-beclin1 class III PI3-kinase complex.	[3,13]
	WIPI	ATG18	17q24.2		[14]
	PIK3C3	VPS34	18q12.3		[3]
	PIK3R4	VPS15	3q22.1		
	BECN1	ATG6	17q21		[15]
	ATG14		14q22.3		[15]
	UVRAG	VPS38	11q13.5		[3,16]
	Rubicon	KIAA0226	3q29		
	AMBRA1		11p11		
	ATG2A, B		11q13, 14q32		[17,18]
	ATG12		5q22	Autophagosome formation; Atg12 conjugation. Atg7 and Atg10 are E1- and E2-like enzymes respectively.	[19]
	ATG5		6q21		[18]
	ATG16L	ATG16	2q37.1		[20]
	ATG7		3p25.3		[21]
	ATG10		5q14.1		[19]
	MAP1LC3B	ATG8	16q24.2	Autophagosome maturation; LC3/Atg8 conjugation.	[3]
	GABARAP	ATG8	17p13.1		[22]
	GABARAPL2	GATE16	16q22.1		
	ATG7		3p25.3		[21]
	ATG3		3q13.2		[23]
	ATG4		Xq22.3		[24]
Autophagosome-lysosome fusion and degradation					
	TFEB		6p21	Transcription factor that regulates Atg and lysosomal genes.	[7]
	RAB7		3q21	Mediates fusion between autophagosome and lysosome.	[25,26]

relationships between the select autophagy genes and HIV replication.

Studies of T cells

CD4+ T cells are the major targets of HIV-1 infection [1]. Zhou and Spector were the first to report that HIV-1 can down regulate autophagy in productively infected CD4+ T cells [44]. They found that Beclin 1 levels were substantially decreased in primary CD4+ T cells that were infected with HIV-1_{MN}, an X4 strain (i.e., using the CXCR4 co-receptor), in comparison to uninfected cells and to those treated with aldrithiol-2 (AT-2) inactivated HIV-1 [44]. In addition, LC3-II levels were reduced in the HIV-infected cells as measured by confocal microscopy and Western blot procedures [44]. The inhibition of autophagy in the HIV-infected cells was found to be reversible by nutrient starvation and rapamycin [44]. This finding suggests that the inhibitory effect of HIV-1 infection on autophagy in CD4+ T cells occurs upstream of mTOR and primarily acts to block the initiation stage of autophagy (see Figure 1). Others have observed that HIV-1 infection inhibits autophagy

Table 2 General methods for measuring autophagy*

Targeted component of autophagy	Procedure **
Direct enumeration and quantitation of autophagosomes. Visible as double-membrane vesicles.	Electron microscopy***
LC3-II to LC3-I ratio. Provides a measurement of autophagic flux with the LC3B-II/LC3B-I ratio concomitantly increasing with autophagosome numbers.	WB****
LC3 localization. Punctate spots visible by microscopy. Total intracellular levels may increase along with autophagosome numbers.	ICC, FC, transfection of LC3 reporter plasmid followed by fluorescent microscopy or FC
Quantitation of autophagy-associated gene expression levels, e.g., BECN1.	qPCR
Quantitation of autophagy-associated protein levels, e.g., Beclin-1.	WB, ELISA
Silencing of autophagy-associated genes.	RNAi
Manipulation of autophagic flux.	Use of rapamycin, bafilomycin A1, and 3-MA

* Because the process is highly conserved among eukaryotes, these methods are broadly applicable to studies of autophagy in humans and animal models [27,31].
** Western blot (WB), flow cytometry (FC), immunocytochemistry (ICC), quantitative PCR (qPCR), RNA interference (RNAi).
*** "Gold standard" method for quantifying the number of autophagosomes.
**** "Gold standard" method for quantitating autophagic flux. Some commercially available anti-human LC3 antibodies are cross-species reactive, allowing for studies with non-human primate cells (e.g. Anti-MAP1LC3B2, cat.no. AB2970, Millipore, Billerica, MA).

in the MOLT-4 CD4+ T cell line [45]. Infection of MOLT-4 cells with HIV-1_{NL4-3} (X4) or HIV-$1_{NL4-Ad8}$, an R5 variant (i.e., using the CCR5 co-receptor), caused reductions in the number of autophagosomes visible by transmission electron microscopy (TEM) and in the levels of LC3-II as measured in Western blots [45]. Notably, the LC3-I level was also reduced in the HIV-infected MOLT-4 cells, possibly reflecting the presence of a broad effect on transcription.

In contrast to the observations above, HIV-1 and HIV-2 infections have been recently reported to induce autophagy in Jurkat cells (a human T cell leukemia cell line) and primary CD4+ T cells [46]. HIV-1_{MN}- and HIV-2_{Rod}-infected Jurkat cells exhibited increased numbers of autophagosomes in electron micrographs and the increased expression of various autophagy-associated genes including ULK1, Atg4D, and BECN1. The inhibition of autophagy with 3-MA (concentration not stated) or through the siRNA-mediated knockdown of BECN1 resulted in decreased levels of HIV-1 RNA in the supernatants of HIV-1_{MN}-infected Jurkat cell cultures. Because 3-MA can be toxic to cells (e.g., when > [0.5 mM]) and the knockdown of BECN1 can slow cell growth [43], potentially reducing HIV replication in an autophagy-independent manner, it is important to note that the cell viability and proliferation was not adequately assessed in these studies. Also reported, primary CD4+ T cells infected with HIV-1 for 3 days were found to exhibit increased Beclin-1 levels in Western blots and increased LC3 immunofluorescence [46]. In light of the findings of decreased autophagy in HIV-infected primary CD4+ T cells by Zhou and Spector [44], the observations of increased autophagy in HIV-infected Jurkat cells [46] could be explained by the presence of inherent differences in autophagy between primary T cells and some immortalized cell-lines. The observations of increased Beclin-1 and LC3 levels in the later studies of HIV-1-infected primary CD4+ T cells [46] are most consistent with the effect of the exposure to HIV (see below) rather than the consequence of HIV infection, particularly as the percent of HIV-infected cells [2] was not established in those studies.

Importantly, HIV-1 also modifies autophagy in uninfected bystander CD4+ T cells. In a seminal paper, Espert et al. reported that the accumulation of autophagosomes and Beclin 1 in umbilical cord blood CD4+ T lymphocytes was similarly induced by i) HEK.293 cells transfected to express HIV-1 Env, ii) rapamycin, and iii) CEM T cells infected with HIV-1_{NL4-3} [47]. Autophagosomes did not accumulate in CD4+ T cells treated with the drugs 3-MA and AMD3100 (a CXCR4 antagonist). Also described in this study was that the Env-induced autophagy preceded apoptotic cell death (see Autophagy and HIV-1 disease progression). In follow-up studies, this group determined that the fusion activity of the HIV-1 envelope glycoprotein gp41 was primarily responsible for this effect [48] and that more than 30 candidate proteins are associated [49]. These proteins were largely involved in degradation processes, redox homeostasis, metabolism and cytoskeleton dynamics, and linked to mitochondrial functions. Espert et al. have more recently reported that R5 Env also induces autophagy and cell death in uninfected CD4+ T cell lines [45]. Thus, the effect of HIV-1 Env on autophagy in CD4+ T cells does not appear to be co-receptor specific. Env triggers a

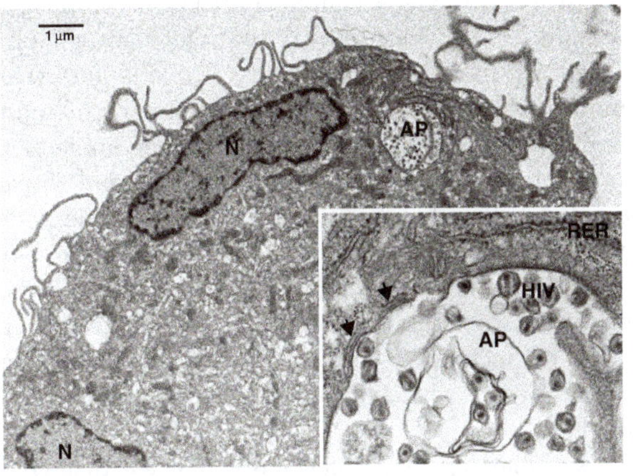

Figure 2 Example of an autophagosome in an HIV-infected cell. Shown is a transmission electron micrograph of an HIV-1_{SF33}-infected monocyte-derived macrophage (L Ackerman and MS Killian, unpublished data). At higher magnification, the HIV-1 particles (roughly 0.1 µm in diameter) are clearly visible within the autophagosomal structure (inset). Abbreviations: nucleus, N; autophagosome, AP; rough endoplasmic reticulum, RER. Arrows point to the multiple membranes surrounding the autophagosome.

broad decrease in protein synthesis that may act to induce autophagy by reducing levels of the inhibitory protein mTOR [49]. The contrasting observations of inhibited autophagy in HIV-1 infected CD4+ T cells and elevated autophagy in bystander CD4+ T cells suggest that productive infection can reverse the enhancing effect of HIV-1 Env on autophagy in uninfected CD4+ T cells.

Studies of macrophages

Macrophages are another important cellular reservoir of HIV-1 [50]. Two groups have reported similar findings regarding autophagy in HIV-infected monocyte-derived macrophages (MDM) [39,45]. In agreement with studies of HeLa cells [42], the induction of autophagy appears to be necessary for HIV-1 replication in MDM. The infection of MDM, upon exposure to HIV-infected cells, is associated with increased numbers of autophagosomes [45]. Interestingly, HIV was detected in the cells with moderate, but not high, numbers of autophagosomes [45]. HIV-infected MDM, cultured in the presence of 3-MA, exhibited substantial reductions in the production of both R5 and X4 viruses [45]. The siRNA-mediated knockdown of Beclin 1 and Atg7 also diminished virus production in HIV-1_{SF162}-infected MDM and U937 cells (a myelomonocytic cell line) [39]. Conversely, treatment of MDM, THP-1 (a myelomonocytic cell line), and U937 cells with rapamycin to induce autophagy increased HIV-1 production [39]. The late stages of autophagy (i.e., lysosome fusion and proteolysis) reduce

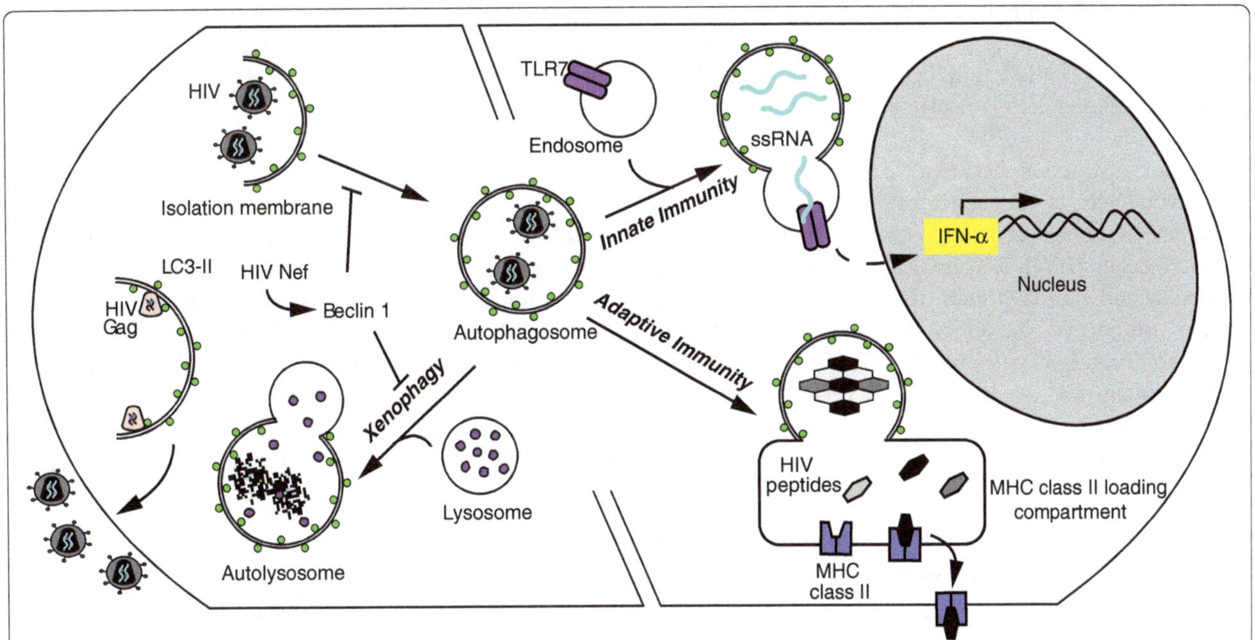

Figure 3 Autophagy in HIV-1 infection. Left) HIV-1 replication requires early autophagic events for its replication [39], perhaps because the autophagosomal membrane provides a scaffold for virion assembly. Incomplete, or fully formed virions that enter the cell via endocytosis [40], could be degraded by the autophagy (xenophagy) pathway. However, HIV-1 can inhibit the late stage of autophagy to avoid the digestion of virions within autolysosomes. Right) Autophagy is a crucial component of innate and adaptive immune responses to HIV-1 infection. Autophagy is required for the TLR7-mediated signaling of interferon-alpha (IFN-α) production by plasmacytoid dendritic cells (innate immunity) in response to HIV [41]. Autophagy also contributes to proteolytic processing for the presentation of HIV-1 peptides in the context of MHC class II (adaptive immunity).

HIV-1 production, as evidenced by the effects of bafilomycin A1 [39]. While most studies of macrophages indicate that HIV-1 promotes autophagosome formation and inhibits the late proteolytic stage of autophagy, decreased LC3-II levels in HIV-1-infected U937 cells have been reported [44]. Thus, the effects of HIV-1 on autophagy in monocytic cell lines can differ from those found in MDM.

Mechanisms enabling HIV-1 to subvert autophagy in macrophages have been elucidated [39]. Demonstrated is that HIV-1 Gag and Nef interact with the autophagy proteins LC3 and Beclin 1 respectively. The colocalization of Gag with LC3 suggests that autophagy plays a role in the biosynthesis, processing, or assembly of HIV-1 intermediates [39]. Alternatively, the Gag/LC3 colocalization could reflect the targeting of Gag for autophagic degradation. The association between Gag and LC3 appears to be unique to monocytic cells [39]. In binding protein complexes containing Beclin 1, Nef is able to inhibit the proteolytic stages of autophagy and thereby prevent the destruction of HIV-1 intermediates [39]. Thus, HIV-1 Nef acts as an "antiautophagic maturation factor" [39]. The Nef ^{174}DD^{175} motif that is needed for CD4 downmodulation [51] is required for its interaction with Beclin 1 [39]. Recently, Nef has also been shown to interact with immunity-associated GTPase family M (IRGM) to induce autophagy in macrophages [52]. These findings indicate that Nef can have the dual function of initiating autophagy and inhibiting its maturation. Unexplained is the normal replication and cytopathicity exhibited by some Nef-deleted HIV-1 isolates *in vitro* and *in vivo* [53,54].

Another distinction between CD4+ lymphocytic and monocytic cells is the effect of HIV-1 Env on autophagy in bystander cells. In contrast to its effect on CD4+ T cells, HIV-1 R5 and X4 Env, when expressed by transfected HEK.293 cells, do not trigger uninfected human monocytic leukemia THP1 cells, MDM, or U937 to undergo autophagy [45]. This distinction could explain the occurrence of CD4+ T cell losses amidst relatively stable monocyte levels in HIV-infected individuals [55].

HIV-1 Tat can have an indirect effect on autophagy in macrophages. In healthy macrophages, autophagy is induced by the pro-inflammatory cytokine interferon-gamma (IFN-γ) [56]. However, pretreatment of monocyte-derived macrophages with HIV-1 Tat, inhibits the stimulatory effect of IFN-γ on autophagy and impairs the antimicrobial functions of the cells [56]. The underlying mechanism involves the ability of Tat to block STAT1 phosphorylation [56]. In other studies, Tat has been found to inhibit autophagy in uninfected macrophages by increasing Akt, Src, and IL-10 production, leading to the silencing of STAT3 and inhibition of autophagy [57].

To summarize, the studies above indicate that HIV-1 proteins disrupt autophagy in HIV-infected and uninfected cells (Table 3). The effects of HIV-1 on autophagy are cell-type specific and could be associated with the observed differences in infectivity, virus replication kinetics, and cytopathicity among CD4+ cells of different hematopoietic lineages. In this regard, studies of cell-lines can be misleading with respect to the relationships between HIV and autophagy in primary cells.

Autophagy and anti-HIV-1 immune responses

Distinguishing features of progressive HIV-1 infection include impaired innate and adaptive immune responses and hyper-immune activation [1,61]. Autophagy is essential for the functionality of innate and adaptive immune responses (see Figure 3) and the maintenance of self-tolerance [38,62]. Thus, autophagy can play important roles in immune cell functions that have direct relevance to HIV-1 infection.

Innate immunity

Innate immune responses provide the earliest host defense against microbial invasion [63]. Cells of the innate immune system use pattern recognition receptors (e.g. Toll-like receptors [TLRs] and nucleotide-binding oligomerization domains [NODs]) to identify highly conserved pathogen-associated molecular patterns (PAMPs, e.g., unmethylated CpG motifs and viral single-stranded RNA) [64]. The cell types of the innate immune system

Table 3 Relationships between HIV-1 proteins and autophagy

HIV-1 protein	Relationship with autophagy	References
Gag	In macrophages: Gag colocalizes with LC3, perhaps to promote virion assembly.	[39,45]
Env	In bystander T cells and neuronal cells: Env induces autophagy and promotes autophagic T cell death.	[47,58]
Nef	Nef interacts with IRGM to induce autophagy. Nef also acts as an "antiautophagic maturation factor" and blocks the late proteolytic stage of autophagy.	[52,39]
Tat	In macrophages: Tat blocks IFN-γ-induced LC3 expression and inhibits autophagy.	[59]
	In bystander HUVEC*: Tat increases autophagy.	[60]

* Human umbilical vein endothelial cells.

that can exhibit direct anti-HIV-1 activity include plasmacytoid dendritic cells (pDCs), natural killer (NK) cells, and monocytes/macrophages. While pDCs are scarcely present in the blood (< 10 cells per μl), they are the major type-1 interferon (IFN-α) producing cells [65]. pDCs secrete large amounts of IFN-α in response to HIV-infected cells and thereby suppress HIV-1 replication in those cells [66]. The recognition of HIV-infected cells by pDCs appears to be primarily mediated by TLR7, a receptor for single-stranded RNA [67]. Importantly, the production of IFN-α by pDCs in response to TLR7 signaling is dependent on autophagy [68,69]. Furthermore, pDCs produce IFN-α in response to infectious or AT-2 inactivated HIV-1_{MN} through the induction of autophagy following TLR7 signaling [41]. NK cells are activated by pDCs responding to HIV-1 [70] and the ability of NK cells to lyse HIV-infected target cells is enhanced by IFN-α [71]. The activation of macrophages via innate biosensors to secrete anti-HIV cytokines such as the β-chemokines and the macrophage-derived anti-HIV factor (MDAF) [72] can require autophagy [73]. Consequently, autophagy is crucial for suppression of HIV-1 replication by the soluble factors and cytolytic functions of the innate immune system.

Adaptive immunity

In addition to their roles in innate immunity, dendritic cells (DCs) and macrophages promote adaptive immune responses by surveying proteins and secreting cytokines in response to pathogens [74]. In this regard, autophagy can contribute to the processing and presentation of viral peptides in the context of major histocompatibility complex (MHC) class I and II molecules. Autophagy has been observed to enhance the presentation of HSV-1 antigens on the MHC-I molecules of macrophages [75]. In contrast, the inhibition of autophagy in DCs by 3-MA prevents the presentation of HIV-1 antigens on MHC-II, but not cross-presentation on MHC-I to CD8+ T cells [76]. Also, treatment of DCs with 3-MA to inhibit autophagy results in reduced MHC-II expression and impairs antigen presentation of respiratory syncytial virus (RSV) [77]. In other studies, most Influenza A virus antigens were presented to CD4+ T cells by MHC-II on DCs without a requirement for autophagy [78]. These heterogeneous observations suggest that the contribution of autophagy to antigen presentation via MHC-I and II molecules could be pathogen and cell-type specific.

The cytokines produced by DCs and macrophages function to regulate autophagy in other immune cells by intersecting with pathways upstream of mTOR (see Figure 1) [62]. In general, Th1 cytokines (e.g. IFN-γ) upregulate autophagy, while Th2 cytokines (e.g. IL-4 and IL-13) abrogate this process [79,80]. Notably, an intense cytokine storm occurs during acute HIV-1 infection and large amounts of IFN-γ, TNF-α, and IL-10 are produced by T cells throughout the course of disease progression [81]. Thus, the cytokine response to HIV-1 infection can influence autophagy in distal cells and tissues and thereby have pathogenic consequences (see below).

Self-tolerance

The tight regulation of antiviral immune responses is necessary to prevent autoimmunity. The autophagic mechanisms used by DCs to direct adaptive immune responses (see above) are also used to promote self-tolerance. This function of autophagy is exemplified in murine models. Athymic mice implanted with $Atg5^{-/-}$ thymus tissue exhibit inflammation of the gut (colitis) and other organs, indicating that autophagy is crucial for thymic selection and self- tolerance [82]. Implicating a role for autophagy in human autoimmune disorders are findings that 1) polymorphisms in NOD2 and ATG16L1 are associated with susceptibility to the inflammatory gut disorder Crohn's disease [83], and 2) the interaction between the two proteins encoded by these genes is essential for normal autophagy in DCs [84,85]. The dysregulation of autophagy by viral proteins, perhaps due to Env-mediated effects on bystander CD4+ T regulatory cells, could contribute to aspects of autoimmunity observed in HIV-1 infection [86].

Autophagy and HIV-1 disease progression

As a general homeostasis mechanism, autophagy functions to maintain the health of cells and tissues. Aberrant autophagy has been implicated in a variety of neurodegenerative disorders, cancers, and autoimmune diseases [87]. Hence, the dysregulation of autophagy by HIV, as discussed below, could play a role in the broad pathology of HIV-1 infection (Table 4).

Persistent virus replication and CD4+ T cell loss

HIV-1 establishes a chronic viral infection with persistent virus replication that is the underlying cause of HIV-1 disease progression [1]. As discussed (see Autophagy and HIV-1 replication), HIV-1 subverts autophagy to promote virus replication in the infected cell. Also, the importance of autophagy in antiviral immunity was reviewed (see Autophagy and anti-HIV-1 immune responses). Because the primary targets of HIV-1 infection are CD4+ cells that play key roles in antiviral immunity, the dysregulation of autophagy in these cells further promotes the chronicity of HIV-1 infection. As described above, HIV-1 Env promotes hyper-autophagy in bystander CD4+ T lymphocytes. This effect is associated with increased apoptotic cell death and is proposed to be a major mechanism for CD4+ T cell loss [47]. During acute HIV-1-infection, massive losses of

CD4+ T cells occur in gastrointestinal tissues [92,93], perhaps due to the increased sensitivity of these cells to Env-mediated autophagic cell death. Conceivably, elite controllers of HIV-1 infection, who exhibit undetectable viral loads and maintain stable CD4+ T cell counts [94], differ in their regulation of autophagy. In this regard, the restriction of virus replication by xenophagy could be an important contributor to HIV-1 latency.

Opportunistic infections and cancers

The impairment of autophagy in cells of the innate and adaptive immune systems could facilitate the rise of opportunistic infections. Irregularities in the dendritic cell compartment become prevalent with progression to AIDS [1], including a decline in pDC number and function [79,95]. Thus, disruption of autophagy in dendritic cells as some studies suggest, could be an important contributor to HIV-1 disease progression. Monocyte-derived dendritic cells exposed to HIV-1 exhibit reduced LC3-II expression, decreased TLR responses, and impaired antigen presentation functions [76]. These inhibitory effects of HIV-1 on autophagy in DCs were mediated by Env-induced mTOR signaling [76]. Also, the interaction between HIV-1 Nef and Beclin-1 (discussed above) could inhibit autophagic pathways that protect against tumorigenesis [96]. Thus, by inhibiting autophagy-dependent mechanisms in DCs, HIV-1 could allow for opportunistic infections and cancers to evade innate and adaptive immune responses.

Neurodegenerative disease

The clearance of misfolded and aggregate proteins via autophagy plays a protective role against neurodegenerative disorders such as Huntington's and Parkinson's disease [97,98]. Defects in this housekeeping function of autophagy are linked with HIV-associated neurologic diseases. Autophagic markers are moderately increased in brain tissues of persons having HIV-encephalitis (HIVE) and HIV-associated dementia (HAD) in comparison to HIV-infected brains having no impairment [58,88]. HAD is associated with increased levels of a byproduct of CXCL12 (i.e., SDF-1), a chemokine that blocks neuronal autophagy [89,99]. Soluble factors in cultures of simian immunodeficiency virus (SIV)-infected microglia also inhibit neuronal autophagy [100].

Table 4 Roles of autophagy in HIV-1 infection, pathogenesis, and treatment

Topic	Observations	References
HIV-1 replication	In HeLa cells, autophagy-associated genes are necessary for HIV-1 replication.	[42]
	In CD4+ T cells, HIV-1 inhibits autophagy as evidenced by decreased autophagosome numbers and reduced levels of Beclin 1 and LC3 II.	[44]
HIV-1 pathogenesis	In macrophages, early nondegradative stages of autophagy promote HIV-1 replication. HIV-1 Gag interacts with LC3 to elevate these stages. The late proteolytic stages of autophagy inhibit HIV-1 replication. Nef interacts with Beclin 1 to inhibit these stages	[44,45]
	In bystander T cells, HIV-1 Env induces autophagy and the accumulation of Beclin1 in uninfected CD4+ T cells. This event leads to apoptosis.	[46,47]
	Bystander macrophages do not undergo Env-mediated autophagy. HIV-1 inhibits autophagy in bystander macrophage/monocytic cells through an Akt-dependent pathway.	[57]
	In dendritic cells, HIV-1 capture down-regulates autophagy and immunoamphisomes in monocyte-derived dendritic cells, impairing innate and adaptive immune responses. Plasmacytoid dendritic cells produce IFN-α in response to infectious or noninfectious HIV-1 through autophagy-dependent TLR7 signaling. This response could promote chronic immune activation.	[41,76]
	Neurotoxicity. The dysregulation of autophagy is a feature of neuroAIDS. The brains of persons with HIV-1 encephalitis exhibit increased levels of autophagic proteins and autophagosomes.	[88,89]
Treatment *	Antiretroviral therapy. HIV-1 protease inhibitors induce autophagy in cancer cells. Clinical concentrations of EFV induce autophagy and, in particular, mitophagy in hepatic cells. ddI treatment restores neuronal LC3 expression in the brains of FIV-infected animals.	[90,91]
	Vitamin D. It has been observed that HIV-infected individuals have reduced levels of the hormonally active form of vitamin D and that this compound has autophagy-dependent anti-HIV-1 effects on macrophages.	[36]

* Abbreviations: efavirenz, EFV; feline immunodeficiency virus, FIV; didanosine, ddI.

In other studies, the exposure of neuronal cells to HIV-1 gp120 resulted in increased Beclin 1, LC3-II and ATG5 levels [58]. This bystander effect of HIV-1 Env that increases autophagy in neuronal cells is similar to the one described above for CD4+ T cells (see Autophagy and HIV-1 replication).

In addition to Env, the HIV-1 transactivator protein, Tat, can also disrupt autophagy in the neurological system. Tat is detectable in the blood and cerebrospinal fluid of HIV-infected individuals [101] and has been shown to be cytotoxic to human brain microvascular endothelial cells [102]. Human umbilical vein endothelial cells (HUVEC), when exposed to cell culture medium conditioned by HeLa-Tat cells, exhibit increased levels of Nox4-dependent H_2O_2 production, endoplasmic reticulum (ER) stress, and autophagy [60]. Thus, circulating Tat may contribute to HIV-1 neuropathogenesis through an autophagy-dependent mechanism.

Cardiovascular disease and frailty

Receiving increasing attention is evidence that HIV-1-infected individuals age at a faster rate than others [103]. In this regard, autophagy may contribute to the increased rates of cardiovascular disease (CVD) and frailty observed in HIV-infected individuals. Hyper-autophagy has an important role in several types of cardiomyopathy by functioning as a death pathway [104]. CVD, particularly congestive heart failure, is strongly associated with a frailty phenotype (e.g., increased weakness, slowness, exhaustion, anergy, and weight loss) that becomes increasingly prevalent among older adults [105,106]. Independent of age, a strong inverse correlation exists between frailty and CD4+ T cell counts among HIV-infected individuals [107]. Thus, increased autophagic CD4+ T cell death due to Env-mediated effects [47] could potentially contribute to increased frailty. Also, autophagy influences longevity in eukaryotic organisms [108] and therefore aberrant autophagy could be an important frailty factor in the context of HIV-1 infection.

Implications for autophagy therapeutics

Irregular autophagy (e.g. Env-mediated hyper-autophagy), as a contributor to HIV-1 disease progression, could be therapeutically managed using a variety of pharmacologic agents (Table 5). Autophagy modifiers are being clinically evaluated for the treatment of Huntington's disease [109], renal cell carcinoma [110], aging [111], and other

Table 5 Pharmacologic modifiers of autophagy

Drug category	Drug or reagent	Mechanism	References
Inducers and enhancers of autophagy			
	Rapamycin*	Inhibits mTOR signaling.	[4]
	Carbamazepine	Inhibition of inositol monophosphatase.	[118]
	Lithium	Inhibition of inositol monophosphatase.	[119]
	Digoxin	Undetermined.	[120]
	Vitamin E	Increases phosphorylation of mTOR substrates.	[121]
	Verapamil	Reduces calcium flux into the cell.	[109]
	Clonidine	Reduces cyclic adenosine monophosphate (cAMP).	[109]
	Trehalose	mTOR independent mechanism.	[122]
	Tamoxifen	Increases the intracellular level of ceramide.	[123]
	Niclosamide	Inhibits mTOR signaling.	[124]
	Rottlerin	Inhibits mTOR signaling.	[124]
	Amiodarone	Inhibits mTOR signaling.	[124]
Inhibitors of autophagy			
	Chloroquine	Blocks the fusion of autophagosomes with lysosomes.	[125]
	Verteporfin	Inhibitor of autophagosome accumulation.	[126]
	3-Methyladenine*	Inhibitor of class III PI3K (Vps34).	[33]
	Bafilomycin A1*	Ion Channel Inhibitor; V-ATPase inhibitor.	[34]
	Wortmannin	PI3K inhibitor.	[127]
	LY294002	PI3K inhibitor.	[127]
	Leupeptin	Inhibitor of serine and cysteine proteases.	[128]
	Asparagine	Prevents transfer of autophaged material to lysosomes.	[129]

* Commonly used in basic research studies.

autophagy-related disorders [112]. Autophagy enhancing candidates include clonidine, minoxidil, verapamil, and STF-62247 [109,110]. Also, the protease inhibitors nelfinavir and saquinavir are under evaluation for their autophagy-enhancing activities [90,113]. In this regard, autophagy needs further study in HIV-infected subjects receiving protease inhibitors. Of note, very low concentrations of rapamycin (e.g., < 1 nM) can have anti-HIV-1 activity *in vitro* [114,115]. This finding makes rapamycin an attractive candidate for evaluation in the treatment of HIV-1 infection [116]. Moreover, recent evidence suggests that the autophagy promoting effects of vitamin D could be of therapeutic benefit to HIV-infected individuals [36]. Because HIV-1 can require autophagy for virus replication and this process becomes induced upon exposure to HIV, drugs that inhibit autophagy could potentially be used to lower HIV replication and to reduce hyper-autophagy levels. Candidate drugs include wortmannin and other PI3K inhibitors that are being evaluated for their potential clinical use as autophagy blockers [117].

In light of the contributions of autophagy to classical antigen presentation and innate pathogen sensory mechanisms, autophagy modifiers could also be helpful for an HIV-1 vaccine strategy. Indeed, the observation that rapamycin-enhanced autophagy increases antigen presentation by DCs and macrophages opens novel approaches for boosting adaptive immunity in immunocompromised individuals or in the context of vaccination [130]. Furthermore, the potential effects of exposure to HIV-1 proteins, such as gp120, on autophagy (see Table 3) should be evaluated in the context of vaccine studies.

Conclusions

Many questions remain pertaining to the relationship between autophagy and HIV-1 infection. Yet unknown is whether or not the ability of HIV-1 to promote autophagy in bystander CD4+ T cells renders those cells more susceptible to HIV-1 infection. Also unexplained are the differential effects of HIV-1 on autophagy in macrophages and CD4+ T cells. In addition to the need for further basic research, translational studies are needed to establish the magnitude of the effects of HIV-1 on autophagy in HIV-1 infected individuals. Moreover, few studies have evaluated autophagy in animal models of HIV infection.

In summary, the importance of autophagy in HIV-1 infection is becoming increasingly clear. Direct effects of HIV-1 on autophagy include the subversion of autophagy in HIV-infected cells and the induction of hyper-autophagy in bystander CD4+ T cells. Because HIV-1 targets key cytokine-producing and immunoregulatory cells, its disruption of autophagy in these cells can have broad pathogenic consequences. Indeed, autophagy appears to play a dual role in HIV-1 infection and disease progression.

Endnotes

[1] An April 2012 search of www.pubmed.gov using the terms "HIV AND autophagy" returned 55 entries in the database (Killian MS, independent observation).

[2] With typical procedures and HIV-1 stock concentrations (e.g. 1 μg/ml p24 equivalents), the frequency of productively HIV-infected primary CD4+ T cell blasts remains relatively low at day 3 post-infection e.g., generally less than 25% of the cells exhibit intracellular p24 or CD4 down-modulation (Killian MS, independent observation).

Competing interest

The author declares to have no competing interests.

Acknowledgements

This publication was made possible with support from the National Institutes of Health (P30 AI027763) and from the California HIV/AIDS Research Program (ID09-SF-058). I thank Dr. Jay Levy for his critical review of the manuscript.

References

1. Levy JA: *HIV and the pathogenesis of AIDS*. Washington, D.C: ASM Press; 2007.
2. Yang Z, Klionsky DJ: **Eaten alive: a history of macroautophagy.** *Nat Cell Biol* 2010, **12**:814–822.
3. Tanida I: **Autophagy basics.** *Microbiol Immunol* 2011, **55**:1–11.
4. Jung CH, Ro SH, Cao J, Otto NM, Kim DH: **mTOR regulation of autophagy.** *FEBS Lett* 2010, **584**:1287–1295.
5. Xie Z, Klionsky DJ: **Autophagosome formation: core machinery and adaptations.** *NatCell Biol* 2007, **9**:1102–1109.
6. Tong J, Yan X, Yu L: **The late stage of autophagy: cellular events and molecular regulation.** *Protein Cell* 2010, **1**:907–915.
7. Settembre C, Di Malta C, Polito VA, Garcia Arencibia M, Vetrini F, Erdin S, Erdin SU, Huynh T, Medina D, Colella P, *et al*: **TFEB links autophagy to lysosomal biogenesis.** *Science* 2011, **332**:1429–1433.
8. Yu L, McPhee CK, Zheng L, Mardones GA, Rong Y, Peng J, Mi N, Zhao Y, Liu Z, Wan F, *et al*: **Termination of autophagy and reformation of lysosomes regulated by mTOR.** *Nature* 2010, **465**:942–946.
9. Lee JW, Park S, Takahashi Y, Wang HG: **The association of AMPK with ULK1 regulates autophagy.** *PLoS One* 2010, **5**:e15394.
10. Hosokawa N, Hara T, Kaizuka T, Kishi C, Takamura A, Miura Y, Iemura S, Natsume T, Takehana K, Yamada N, *et al*: **Nutrient-dependent mTORC1 association with the ULK1-Atg13-FIP200 complex required for autophagy.** *Mol Biol Cell* 2009, **20**:1981–1991.
11. Hosokawa N, Sasaki T, Iemura S, Natsume T, Hara T, Mizushima N: **Atg101, a novel mammalian autophagy protein interacting with Atg13.** *Autophagy* 2009, **5**:973–979.
12. Hara T, Takamura A, Kishi C, Iemura S, Natsume T, Guan JL, Mizushima N: **FIP200, a ULK-interacting protein, is required for autophagosome formation in mammalian cells.** *J Cell Biol* 2008, **181**:497–510.
13. Webber JL, Tooze SA: **New insights into the function of Atg9.** *FEBS Lett* 2010, **584**:1319–1326.
14. Proikas-Cezanne T, Waddell S, Gaugel A, Frickey T, Lupas A, Nordheim A: **WIPI-1alpha (WIPI49), a member of the novel 7-bladed WIPI protein family, is aberrantly expressed in human cancer and is linked to starvation-induced autophagy.** *Oncogene* 2004, **23**:9314–9325.
15. Itakura E, Kishi C, Inoue K, Mizushima N: **Beclin 1 forms two distinct phosphatidylinositol 3-kinase complexes with mammalian Atg14 and UVRAG.** *Mol Biol Cell* 2008, **19**:5360–5372.
16. Weidberg H, Shvets E, Elazar Z: **Biogenesis and cargo selectivity of autophagosomes.** *Annu Rev Biochem* 2011, **80**:125–156.

17. Velikkakath AK, Nishimura T, Oita E, Ishihara N, Mizushima N: **Mammalian Atg2 proteins are essential for autophagosome formation and important for regulation of size and distribution of lipid droplets.** *Mol Biol Cell* 2012, **5**:896–909.
18. Mizushima N, Yamamoto A, Hatano M, Kobayashi Y, Kabeya Y, Suzuki K, Tokuhisa T, Ohsumi Y, Yoshimori T: **Dissection of autophagosome formation using Apg5-deficient mouse embryonic stem cells.** *J Cell Biol* 2001, **152**:657–668.
19. Geng J, Klionsky DJ: **The Atg8 and Atg12 ubiquitin-like conjugation systems inmacroautophagy. 'Protein modifications: beyond the usual suspects' reviewseries.** *EMBO Rep* 2008, **9**:859–864.
20. Itoh T, Fujita N, Kanno E, Yamamoto A, Yoshimori T, Fukuda M: **Golgi-resident small GTPase Rab33B interacts with Atg16L and modulates autophagosome formation.** *Mol Biol Cell* 2008, **19**:2916–2925.
21. Yuan W, Stromhaug PE, Dunn WA Jr: **Glucose-induced autophagy of peroxisomes in Pichia pastoris requires a unique E1-like protein.** *Mol Biol Cell* 1999, **10**:1353–1366.
22. Weidberg H, Shvets E, Shpilka T, Shimron F, Shinder V, Elazar Z: **LC3 and GATE-16/GABARAP subfamilies are both essential yet act differently in autophagosome biogenesis.** *EMBO J* 2010, **29**:1792–1802.
23. Tanida I, Tanida-Miyake E, Komatsu M, Ueno T, Kominami E: **Human Apg3p/Aut1p homologue is an authentic E2 enzyme for multiple substrates, GATE-16, GABARAP, and MAP-LC3, and facilitates the conjugation of hApg12p to hApg5p.** *J Biol Chem* 2002, **277**:13739–13744.
24. Hemelaar J, Lelyveld VS, Kessler BM, Ploegh HL: **A single protease, Apg4B, is specific for the autophagy-related ubiquitin-like proteins GATE-16, MAP1-LC3, GABARAP, and Apg8L.** *J Biol Chem* 2003, **278**:51841–51850.
25. Ganley IG, Wong PM, Gammoh N, Jiang X: **Distinct autophagosomal-lysosomal fusion mechanism revealed by thapsigargin-induced autophagy arrest.** *Mol Cell* 2011, **42**:731–743.
26. Yang Z, Klionsky DJ: **An overview of the molecular mechanism of autophagy.** *CurrTopMicrobiolImmunol* 2009, **335**:1–32.
27. Klionsky DJ, Abeliovich H, Agostinis P, Agrawal DK, Aliev G, Askew DS, Baba M, Baehrecke EH, Bahr BA, Ballabio A, *et al*: **Guidelines for the use and interpretation of assays for monitoring autophagy in higher eukaryotes.** *Autophagy* 2008, **4**:151–175.
28. Barth S, Glick D, Macleod KF: **Autophagy: assays and artifacts.** *J Pathol* 2010, **221**:117–124.
29. Yla-Anttila P, Vihinen H, Jokitalo E, Eskelinen EL: **Monitoring autophagy by electron microscopy in Mammalian cells.** *Methods Enzymol* 2009, **452**:143–164.
30. Mizushima N, Yamamoto A, Matsui M, Yoshimori T, Ohsumi Y: **In vivo analysis of autophagy in response to nutrient starvation using transgenic mice expressing a fluorescent autophagosome marker.** *Mol Biol Cell* 2004, **15**:1101–1111.
31. Mizushima N, Yoshimori T, Levine B: **Methods in mammalian autophagy research.** *Cell* 2010, **140**:313–326.
32. Raught B, Gingras AC, Sonenberg N: **The target of rapamycin (TOR) proteins.** *Proc Natl Acad Sci U S A* 2001, **98**:7037–7044.
33. Seglen PO, Gordon PB: **3-Methyladenine: specific inhibitor of autophagic/lysosomal protein degradation in isolated rat hepatocytes.** *ProcNatlAcadSciUSA* 1982, **79**:1889–1892.
34. Klionsky DJ, Elazar Z, Seglen PO, Rubinsztein DC: **Does bafilomycin A1 block the fusion of autophagosomes with lysosomes?** *Autophagy* 2008, **4**:849–950.
35. Kuma A, Matsui M, Mizushima N: **LC3, an autophagosome marker, can be incorporated into protein aggregates independent of autophagy: caution in the interpretation of LC3 localization.** *Autophagy* 2007, **3**:323–328.
36. Campbell GR, Spector SA: **Hormonally active vitamin D3 (1alpha,25-dihydroxycholecalciferol) triggers autophagy in human macrophages that inhibits HIV-1 infection.** *J Biol Chem* 2011, **286**:18890–18902.
37. Wu YT, Tan HL, Shui G, Bauvy C, Huang Q, Wenk MR, Ong CN, Codogno P, Shen HM: **Dual role of 3-methyladenine in modulation of autophagy via different temporal patterns of inhibition on class I and III phosphoinositide 3-kinase.** *J Biol Chem* 2010, **285**:10850–10861.
38. Levine B, Mizushima N, Virgin HW: **Autophagy in immunity and inflammation.** *Nature* 2011, **469**:323–335.
39. Kyei GB, Dinkins C, Davis AS, Roberts E, Singh SB, Dong C, Wu L, Kominami E, Ueno T, Yamamoto A, *et al*: **Autophagy pathway intersects with HIV-1 biosynthesis and regulates viral yields in macrophages.** *JCell Biol* 2009, **186**:255–268.
40. Uchil PD, Mothes W: **HIV Entry Revisited.** *Cell* 2009, **137**:402–404.
41. Zhou D, Kang KH, Spector SA: **Production of Interferon alpha by Human Immunodeficiency Virus Type 1 in Human Plasmacytoid Dendritic Cells Is Dependent on Induction of Autophagy.** *J Infect Dis* 2012, **205**:1258–1267.
42. Brass AL, Dykxhoorn DM, Benita Y, Yan N, Engelman A, Xavier RJ, Lieberman J, Elledge SJ: **Identification of host proteins required for HIV infection through a functional genomic screen.** *Science* 2008, **319**:921–926.
43. Eekels JJ, Sagnier S, Geerts D, Jeeninga RE, Biard-Piechaczyk M, Berkhout B: **Inhibition of HIV-1 replication with stable RNAi-mediated knockdown of autophagy factors.** *Virol J* 2012, **9**:69.
44. Zhou D, Spector SA: **Human immunodeficiency virus type-1 infection inhibits autophagy.** *AIDS* 2008, **22**:695–699.
45. Espert L, Varbanov M, Robert-Hebmann V, Sagnier S, Robbins I, Sanchez F, Lafont V, Biard-Piechaczyk M: **Differential role of autophagy in CD4 T cells and macrophages during X4 and R5 HIV-1 infection.** *PLoSONE* 2009, **4**: e5787.
46. Wang X, Gao Y, Tan J, Devadas K, Ragupathy V, Takeda K, Zhao J, Hewlett I: **HIV-1 and HIV-2 infections induce autophagy in Jurkat and CD4(+) T cells.** *Cell Signal* 2012, **24**:1414–1419.
47. Espert L, Denizot M, Grimaldi M, Robert-Hebmann V, Gay B, Varbanov M, Codogno P, Biard-Piechaczyk M: **Autophagy is involved in T cell death after binding of HIV-1 envelope proteins to CXCR4.** *JClinInvest* 2006, **116**:2161–2172.
48. Denizot M, Varbanov M, Espert L, Robert-Hebmann V, Sagnier S, Garcia E, Curriu M, Mamoun R, Blanco J, Biard-Piechaczyk M: **HIV-1 gp41 fusogenic function triggers autophagy in uninfected cells.** *Autophagy* 2008, **4**:998–1008.
49. Molina L, Grimaldi M, Robert-Hebmann V, Espert L, Varbanov M, Devaux C, Granier C, Biard-Piechaczyk M: **Proteomic analysis of the cellular responses induced in uninfected immune cells by cell-expressed X4 HIV-1 envelope.** *Proteomics* 2007, **7**:3116–3130.
50. Carter CA, Ehrlich LS: **Cell biology of HIV-1 infection of macrophages.** *AnnuRevMicrobiol* 2008, **62**:425–443.
51. Roeth JF, Collins KL: **Human immunodeficiency virus type 1 Nef: adapting to intracellular trafficking pathways.** *MicrobiolMolBiolRev* 2006, **70**:548–563.
52. Gregoire IP, Richetta C, Meyniel-Schicklin L, Borel S, Pradezynski F, Diaz O, Deloire A, Azocar O, Baguet J, Le Breton M, *et al*: **IRGM Is a Common Target of RNA Viruses that Subvert the Autophagy Network.** *PLoS Pathog* 2011, **7**:e1002422.
53. Gorry PR, McPhee DA, Verity E, Dyer WB, Wesselingh SL, Learmont J, Sullivan JS, Roche M, Zaunders JJ, Gabuzda D, *et al*: **Pathogenicity and immunogenicity of attenuated, nef-deleted HIV-1 strains in vivo.** *Retrovirology* 2007, **4**:66.
54. Terwilliger EF, Langhoff E, Gabuzda D, Zazopoulos E, Haseltine WA: **Allelic variation in the effects of the nef gene on replication of human immunodeficiency virus type 1.** *Proc Natl Acad Sci U S A* 1991, **88**:10971–10975.
55. Abel PM, McSharry C, Galloway E, Ross C, Severn A, Toner G, Gruer L, Wilkinson PC: **Heterogeneity of peripheral blood monocyte populations in human immunodeficiency virus-1 seropositive patients.** *FEMS Microbiol Immunol* 1992, **5**:317–323.
56. Li JC, Au KY, Fang JW, Yim HC, Chow KH, Ho PL, Lau AS: **HIV-1 trans-activator protein dysregulates IFN-gamma signaling and contributes to the suppression of autophagy induction.** *AIDS* 2011, **25**:15–25.
57. Van Grol J, Subauste C, Andrade RM, Fujinaga K, Nelson J, Subauste CS: **HIV-1 inhibits autophagy in bystander macrophage/monocytic cells through Src-Akt and STAT3.** *PLoS One* 2010, **5**:e11733.
58. Spector SA, Zhou D: **Autophagy: an overlooked mechanism of HIV-1 pathogenesis and neuroAIDS?** *Autophagy* 2008, **4**:704–706.
59. Au K, Li J, Yim H, Fang J, Lau A: **PP1-095 HIV Tat modulation of IFN-g-induced expression of autophagy-associated genes in primary human blood macrophages.** *Cytokine* 2009, **48**:46–90.
60. Wu RF, Ma Z, Liu Z, Terada LS: **Nox4-derived H2O2 mediates endoplasmic reticulum signaling through local Ras activation.** *Mol Cell Biol* 2010, **30**:3553–3568.
61. Killian MS, Levy JA: **HIV/AIDS: 30 years of progress and future challenges.** *Eur J Immunol* 2011, **41**:3401–3411.
62. Munz C: **Enhancing immunity through autophagy.** *Annu Rev Immunol* 2009, **27**:423–449.

63. Borrow P: **Innate immunity in acute HIV-1 infection.** *Curr Opin HIV AIDS* 2011, **6**:353–363.
64. Delgado M, Singh S, de Haro S, Master S, Ponpuak M, Dinkins C, Ornatowski W, Vergne I, Deretic V: **Autophagy and pattern recognition receptors in innate immunity.** *ImmunolRev* 2009, **227**:189–202.
65. Siegal FP, Kadowaki N, Shodell M, Fitzgerald-Bocarsly PA, Shah K, Ho S, Antonenko S, Liu YJ: **The nature of the principal type 1 interferon-producing cells in human blood.** *Science* 1999, **284**:1835–1837.
66. Schmidt B, Ashlock BM, Foster H, Fujimura SH, Levy JA: **HIV-infected cells are major inducers of plasmacytoid dendritic cell interferon production, maturation, and migration.** *Virology* 2005, **343**:256–266.
67. Heil F, Hemmi H, Hochrein H, Ampenberger F, Kirschning C, Akira S, Lipford G, Wagner H, Bauer S: **Species-specific recognition of single-stranded RNA via toll-like receptor 7 and 8.** *Science* 2004, **303**:1526–1529.
68. Lee HK, Lund JM, Ramanathan B, Mizushima N, Iwasaki A: **Autophagy-dependent viral recognition by plasmacytoid dendritic cells.** *Science* 2007, **315**:1398–1401.
69. Guiducci C, Ghirelli C, Marloie-Provost MA, Matray T, Coffman RL, Liu YJ, Barrat FJ, Soumelis V: **PI3K is critical for the nuclear translocation of IRF-7 and type I IFN production by human plasmacytoid predendritic cells in response to TLR activation.** *Journal of Experimental Medicine* 2008, **205**:315–322.
70. Alter G, Suscovich TJ, Teigen N, Meier A, Streeck H, Brander C, Altfeld M: **Single- stranded RNA derived from HIV-1 serves as a potent activator of NK cells.** *J Immunol* 2007, **178**:7658–7666.
71. Hervas-Stubbs S, Perez-Gracia JL, Rouzaut A, Sanmamed MF, Le Bon A, Melero I: **Direct effects of type I interferons on cells of the immune system.** *Clin Cancer Res* 2011, **17**:2619–2627.
72. Mikulak J, Gianolini M, Versmisse P, Pancino G, Lusso P, Verani A: **Biological and physical characterization of the X4 HIV-1 suppressive factor secreted by LPS stimulated human macrophages.** *Virology* 2009, **390**:37–44.
73. Sanjuan MA, Dillon CP, Tait SW, Moshiach S, Dorsey F, Connell S, Komatsu M, Tanaka K, Cleveland JL, Withoff S, Green DR: **Toll-like receptor signaling in macrophages links the autophagy pathway to phagocytosis.** *Nature* 2007, **450**:1253–1257.
74. Rossi M, Young JW: **Human dendritic cells: potent antigen-presenting cells at the crossroads of innate and adaptive immunity.** *J Immunol* 2005, **175**:1373–1381.
75. English L, Chemali M, Duron J, Rondeau C, Laplante A, Gingras D, Alexander D, Leib D, Norbury C, Lippe R, Desjardins M: **Autophagy enhances the presentation of endogenous viral antigens on MHC class I molecules during HSV-1 infection.** *NatImmunol* 2009, **10**:480–487.
76. Blanchet FP, Moris A, Nikolic DS, Lehmann M, Cardinaud S, Stalder R, Garcia E, Dinkins C, Leuba F, Wu L, *et al*: **Human immunodeficiency virus-1 inhibition of immunoamphisomes in dendritic cells impairs early innate and adaptive immune responses.** *Immunity* 2010, **32**:654–669.
77. Morris S, Swanson MS, Lieberman A, Reed M, Yue Z, Lindell DM, Lukacs NW: **Autophagy-Mediated Dendritic Cell Activation Is Essential for Innate Cytokine Production and APC Function with Respiratory Syncytial Virus Responses.** *J Immunol* 2011, **187**:3953–3961.
78. Comber JD, Robinson TM, Siciliano NA, Snook AE, Eisenlohr LC: **Functional macroautophagy induction by influenza A virus without a contribution to major histocompatibility complex class II-restricted presentation.** *J Virol* 2011, **85**:6453–6463.
79. Martinson JA, Roman-Gonzalez A, Tenorio AR, Montoya CJ, Gichinga CN, Rugeles MT, Tomai M, Krieg AM, Ghanekar S, Baum LL, Landay AL: **Dendritic cells from HIV-1 infected individuals are less responsive to toll-like receptor (TLR) ligands.** *Cell Immunol* 2007, **250**:75–84.
80. Harris J, Master SS, De Haro SA, Delgado M, Roberts EA, Hope JC, Keane J, Deretic V: **Th1-Th2 polarisation and autophagy in the control of intracellular mycobacteria by macrophages.** *Vet Immunol Immunopathol* 2009, **128**:37–43.
81. Norris PJ, Pappalardo BL, Custer B, Spotts G, Hecht FM, Busch MP: **Elevations in IL-10, TNF-alpha, and IFN-gamma from the earliest point of HIV Type 1 infection.** *AIDS Research and Human Retroviruses* 2006, **22**:757–762.
82. Nedjic J, Aichinger M, Emmerich J, Mizushima N, Klein L: **Autophagy in thymic epithelium shapes the T-cell repertoire and is essential for tolerance.** *Nature* 2008, **455**:396–400.
83. Massey DC, Parkes M: **Genome-wide association scanning highlights two autophagy genes, ATG16L1 and IRGM, as being significantly associated with Crohn's disease.** *Autophagy* 2007, **3**:649–651.
84. Cooney R, Baker J, Brain O, Danis B, Pichulik T, Allan P, Ferguson DJ, Campbell BJ, Jewell D, Simmons A: **NOD2 stimulation induces autophagy in dendritic cells influencing bacterial handling and antigen presentation.** *Nature Medicine* 2010, **16**:90–97.
85. Travassos LH, Carneiro LA, Ramjeet M, Hussey S, Kim YG, Magalhaes JG, Yuan L, Soares F, Chea E, Le Bourhis L, *et al*: **Nod1 and Nod2 direct autophagy by recruiting ATG16L1 to the plasma membrane at the site of bacterial entry.** *Nat Immunol* 2010, **11**:55–62.
86. Stratton R, Slapak G, Mahungu T: **Kinloch-de Loes S: Autoimmunity and HIV.** *CurrOpinInfectDis* 2009, **22**:49–56.
87. Mijaljica D, Prescott M, Devenish RJ: **Autophagy in disease.** *Methods Mol Biol* 2010, **648**:79–92.
88. Zhou D, Masliah E, Spector SA: **Autophagy is increased in postmortem brains of persons with HIV-1-associated encephalitis.** *J Infect Dis* 2011, **203**:1647–1657.
89. Zhu Y, Vergote D, Pardo C, Noorbakhsh F, McArthur JC, Hollenberg MD, Overall CM, Power C: **CXCR3 activation by lentivirus infection suppresses neuronal autophagy: neuroprotective effects of antiretroviral therapy.** *FASEB J* 2009, **9**:2928–2941.
90. McLean K, VanDeVen NA, Sorenson DR, Daudi S, Liu JR: **The HIV protease inhibitor saquinavir induces endoplasmic reticulum stress, autophagy, and apoptosis in ovarian cancer cells.** *GynecolOncol* 2009, **112**:623–630.
91. Gills JJ, Lopiccolo J, Dennis PA: **Nelfinavir, a new anti-cancer drug with pleiotropic effects and many paths to autophagy.** *Autophagy* 2008, **4**:107–109.
92. Veazey RS, DeMaria M, Chalifoux LV, Shvetz DE, Pauley DR, Knight HL, Rosenzweig M, Johnson RP, Desrosiers RC, Lackner AA: **Gastrointestinal tract as a major site ofCD4+ T cell depletion and viral replication in SIV infection.** *Science* 1998, **280**:427–431.
93. Brenchley JM, Schacker TW, Ruff LE, Price DA, Taylor JH, Beilman GJ, Nguyen PL, Khoruts A, Larson M, Haase AT, Douek DC: **CD4+ T cell depletion during all stages of HIV disease occurs predominantly in the gastrointestinal tract.** *Journal of Experimental Medicine* 2004, **200**:749–759.
94. Deeks SG, Walker BD: **Human immunodeficiency virus controllers: mechanisms of durable virus control in the absence of antiretroviral therapy.** *Immunity* 2007, **27**:406–416.
95. Killian MS, Fujimura SH, Hecht FM, Levy JA: **Similar changes in plasmacytoid dendritic cell and CD4 T-cell counts during primary HIV-1 infection and treatment.** *AIDS* 2006, **20**:1247–1252.
96. Edinger AL, Thompson CB: **Defective autophagy leads to cancer.** *Cancer Cell* 2003, **4**:422–424.
97. Garcia-Arencibia M, Hochfeld WE, Toh PP, Rubinsztein DC: **Autophagy, a guardian against neurodegeneration.** *Semin Cell Dev Biol* 2010, **21**:691–698.
98. Winslow AR, Rubinsztein DC: **The Parkinson disease protein alpha-synuclein inhibits autophagy.** *Autophagy* 2011, **7**:429–431.
99. Lipinski MM, Hoffman G, Ng A, Zhou W, Py BF, Hsu E, Liu X, Eisenberg J, Liu J, Blenis J, *et al*: **A genome-wide siRNA screen reveals multiple mTORC1 independent signaling pathways regulating autophagy under normal nutritional conditions.** *Dev Cell* 2010, **18**:1041–1052.
100. Alirezaei M, Kemball CC, Whitton JL: **Autophagy, inflammation and neurodegenerative disease.** *Eur J Neurosci* 2011, **33**:197–204.
101. Xiao H, Neuveut C, Tiffany HL, Benkirane M, Rich EA, Murphy PM, Jeang KT: **Selective CXCR4 antagonism by Tat: implications for in vivo expansion of coreceptor use by HIV-1.** *Proc Natl Acad Sci U S A* 2000, **97**:11466–11471.
102. Khan NA, Di Cello F, Nath A, Kim KS: **Human immunodeficiency virus type 1 tat-mediated cytotoxicity of human brain microvascular endothelial cells.** *J Neurovirol* 2003, **9**:584–593.
103. Effros RB, Fletcher CV, Gebo K, Halter JB, Hazzard WR, Horne FM, Huebner RE, Janoff EN, Justice AC, Kuritzkes D, *et al*: **Aging and infectious diseases: workshop on HIV infection and aging: what is known and future research directions.** *Clin Infect Dis* 2008, **47**:542–553.
104. Martinet W, Knaapen MW, Kockx MM, De Meyer GR: **Autophagy in cardiovascular disease.** *Trends MolMed* 2007, **13**:482–491.
105. Newman AB, Gottdiener JS, McBurnie MA, Hirsch CH, Kop WJ, Tracy R, Walston JD, Fried LP: **Associations of subclinical cardiovascular disease with frailty.** *J Gerontol A Biol Sci Med Sci* 2001, **56**:M158–M166.
106. Fried LP, Tangen CM, Walston J, Newman AB, Hirsch C, Gottdiener J, Seeman T, Tracy R, Kop WJ, Burke G, McBurnie MA: **Frailty in older adults: evidence for a phenotype.** *J Gerontol A Biol Sci Med Sci* 2001, **56**:M146–M156.
107. Desquilbet L, Margolick JB, Fried LP, Phair JP, Jamieson BD, Holloway M, Jacobson LP: **Relationship between a frailty-related phenotype and**

progressive deterioration of the immune system in HIV-infected men. *J Acquir Immune Defic Syndr* 2009, **50**:299–306.
108. Vellai T, Takacs-Vellai K, Sass M, Klionsky DJ: **The regulation of aging: does autophagy underlie longevity?** *Trends Cell Biol* 2009, **19**:487–494.
109. Williams A, Sarkar S, Cuddon P, Ttofi EK, Saiki S, Siddiqi FH, Jahreiss L, Fleming A, Pask D, Goldsmith P, *et al*: **Novel targets for Huntington's disease in an mTORindependent autophagy pathway.** *Nat Chem Biol* 2008, **4**:295–305.
110. Turcotte S, Chan DA, Sutphin PD, Hay MP, Denny WA, Giaccia AJ: **A molecule targeting VHL-deficient renal cell carcinoma that induces autophagy.** *Cancer Cell* 2008, **14**:90–102.
111. Bergamini E: **Autophagy: a cell repair mechanism that retards ageing and age-associated diseases and can be intensified pharmacologically.** *Mol Aspects Med* 2006, **27**:403–410.
112. Rubinsztein DC, Gestwicki JE, Murphy LO, Klionsky DJ: **Potential therapeutic applications of autophagy.** *Nat Rev Drug Discov* 2007, **6**:304–312.
113. Gills JJ, Lopiccolo J, Tsurutani J, Shoemaker RH, Best CJ, Abu-Asab MS, Borojerdi J, Warfel NA, Gardner ER, Danish M, *et al*: **Nelfinavir, A lead HIV protease inhibitor, is a broad-spectrum, anticancer agent that induces endoplasmic reticulum stress, autophagy, and apoptosis in vitro and in vivo.** *Clin Cancer Res* 2007, **13**:5183–5194.
114. Roy J, Paquette JS, Fortin JF, Tremblay MJ: **The immunosuppressant rapamycin represses human immunodeficiency virus type 1 replication.** *Antimicrob Agents Chemother* 2002, **46(11)**:3447–55. 2002, 46:3447–3455.
115. Heredia A, Amoroso A, Davis C, Le N, Reardon E, Dominique JK, Klingebiel E, Gallo RC, Redfield RR: **Rapamycin causes down-regulation of CCR5 and accumulation of anti-HIV beta-chemokines: an approach to suppress R5 strains of HIV-1.** *Proc Natl Acad Sci USA* 2003, **100**:10411–10416.
116. Donia M, McCubrey JA, Bendtzen K, Nicoletti F: **Potential use of rapamycin in HIV infection.** *Br J Clin Pharmacol* 2010, **70**:784–793.
117. Ng SS, Tsao MS, Nicklee T, Hedley DW: **Wortmannin inhibits pkb/akt phosphorylation and promotes gemcitabine antitumor activity in orthotopic human pancreatic cancer xenografts in immunodeficient mice.** *ClinCancer Res* 2001, **7**:3269–3275.
118. Hidvegi T, Ewing M, Hale P, Dippold C, Beckett C, Kemp C, Maurice N, Mukherjee A, Goldbach C, Watkins S, *et al*: **An autophagy-enhancing drug promotes degradation of mutant alpha1-antitrypsin Z and reduces hepatic fibrosis.** *Science* 2010, **329**:229–232.
119. Sarkar S, Floto RA, Berger Z, Imarisio S, Cordenier A, Pasco M, Cook LJ, Rubinsztein DC: **Lithium induces autophagy by inhibiting inositol monophosphatase.** *J Cell Biol* 2005, **170**:1101–1111.
120. Hundeshagen P, Hamacher-Brady A, Eils R, Brady NR: **Concurrent detection of autolysosome formation and lysosomal degradation by flow cytometry in a highcontent screen for inducers of autophagy.** *BMC Biol* 2011, **9**:38.
121. Underwood BR, Imarisio S, Fleming A, Rose C, Krishna G, Heard P, Quick M, Korolchuk VI, Renna M, Sarkar S, *et al*: **Antioxidants can inhibit basal autophagy and enhance neurodegeneration in models of polyglutamine disease.** *Hum Mol Genet* 2010, **19**:3413–3429.
122. Sarkar S, Davies JE, Huang Z, Tunnacliffe A, Rubinsztein DC: **Trehalose, a novel mTOR-independent autophagy enhancer, accelerates the clearance of mutant huntingtin and alpha-synuclein.** *JBiolChem* 2007, **282**:5641–5652.
123. Scarlatti F, Bauvy C, Ventruti A, Sala G, Cluzeaud F, Vandewalle A, Ghidoni R, Codogno P: **Ceramide-mediated macroautophagy involves inhibition of protein kinase B and up-regulation of beclin 1.** *J Biol Chem* 2004, **279**:18384–18391.
124. Balgi AD, Fonseca BD, Donohue E, Tsang TC, Lajoie P, Proud CG, Nabi IR, Roberge M: **Screen for chemical modulators of autophagy reveals novel therapeutic inhibitors of mTORC1 signaling.** *PLoS One* 2009, **4**:e7124.
125. Shintani T, Klionsky DJ: **Autophagy in health and disease: a double-edged sword.** *Science* 2004, **306**:990–995.
126. Donohue E, Tovey A, Vogl AW, Arns S, Sternberg E, Young RN, Roberge M: **Inhibition of autophagosome formation by the benzoporphyrin derivative verteporfin.** *J Biol Chem* 2011, **286**:7290–7300.
127. Blommaart EF, Krause U, Schellens JP, Vreeling-Sindelarova H, Meijer AJ: **The phosphatidylinositol 3-kinase inhibitors wortmannin and LY294002 inhibit autophagy in isolated rat hepatocytes.** *EurJBiochem* 1997, **243**:240–246.
128. Haspel J, Shaik RS, Ifedigbo E, Nakahira K, Dolinay T, Englert JA, Choi AM: **Characterization of macroautophagic flux in vivo using a leupeptin-based assay.** *Autophagy* 2011, **7**:629–642.
129. Hoyvik H, Gordon PB, Berg TO, Stromhaug PE, Seglen PO: **Inhibition of autophagic-lysosomal delivery and autophagic lactolysis by asparagine.** *J Cell Biol* 1991, **113**:1305–1312.
130. Jagannath C, Lindsey DR, Dhandayuthapani S, Xu Y, Hunter RL Jr, Eissa NT: **Autophagy enhances the efficacy of BCG vaccine by increasing peptide presentation in mouse dendritic cells.** *Nature Medicine* 2009, **15**:267–276.

2

Effects of highly active antiretroviral therapy and its adherence on herpes zoster incidence

Chenglong Liu[1*], Cuiwei Wang[1], Marshall J Glesby[2], Gypsyamber D'souza[3], Audrey French[4], Howard Minkoff[5], Toby Maurer[6], Roksana Karim[7] and Mary Young[1]

Abstract

Background: Herpes zoster (HZ) is common among HIV-infected individuals, but the impacts of highly active antiretroviral therapy (HAART) and HAART adherence on HZ risk have not been well studied.

Methods: The effects of HAART and HAART adherence on HZ incidence were evaluated by comparing HIV-infected women on HAART (HAART use group) with the HIV-infected women remaining HAART naïve (HAART naïve group) in the Women's Interagency HIV Study (WIHS). A 1:1 matching with propensity score for predicting HAART initiation was conducted to balance background covariates at index visit, including HIV disease stage. Kaplan-Meier method was used to compare the risk of HZ development between the matched pairs. Cox proportional hazard models were used to assess the effects of HAART and HAART adherence on HZ incidence.

Results: Through propensity score matching, 389 pairs of participants were identified and they contributed 3,909 person years after matching. The background covariates were similar between the matched pairs at the index visit. The participants had a mean age around 39 years old, and about 61% of them were Black and 22% were Latina. No significant difference in HZ risk was observed between the HAART use group and the HAART naïve group during the first year of follow-up in any analyses. In the univariate analysis, the HAART use group had marginally lower HZ risk (Hazard Ratio (HR): 0.72; 95% Confidence Interval (CI): 0.48-1.1) over the entire follow-up period. However, women with a HAART adherence level of ≥95% had significantly lower HZ risk (HR: 0.54; 95% CI: 0.31, 0.94) compared to the HAART naïve women. The association remained significant after adjusting for quality of life score and acyclovir use, but it attenuated and was no longer statistically significant after adjusting for an intermediate variable, either CD4+ T cell counts or HIV viral load.

Conclusions: Among adult women, we observed a significant preventive effect of long-term HAART use on HZ incidence when a HAART adherence level of ≥95% was attained, and this effect was mediated through reduction of HIV viral load and improvement of CD4+ T cell counts.

Keywords: HAART, Adherence, Herpes zoster, Incidence, Propensity score

* Correspondence: cl278@georgetown.edu
[1]Department of Medicine, Georgetown University, 2115 Wisconsin Avenue NW, Suite 130, Washington, DC 20007, USA

Background

Highly active antiretroviral therapy (HAART) has been demonstrated to be very effective in decreasing the incidence of opportunistic infections, acquired immunodeficiency syndrome (AIDS) and death among HIV-infected patients. However, previous studies showed that the incidence of herpes zoster (HZ) is less likely than those of other opportunistic infections to be reduced by HAART as it still occurs at a relatively high rate in the HAART era [1-3].

According to studies conducted so far, the effect of HAART on HZ incidence may differ depending on how long HAART has been used. Martinez et al. first reported a high HZ incidence in patients with AIDS soon after initiation of therapy with protease inhibitors [4]. Later, many other studies confirmed their observation as part of an immune reconstitution inflammatory syndrome [5-15]. It was proposed that this transient increase of HZ risk may be associated with immunodysregulation rather than profound immunesuppression. However, other studies showed no association of HZ incidence with recent HAART initiation [2,16].

The long-term effect of HAART on HZ incidence has also been inconsistent across studies. One study reported that the HZ incidence did not change between the pre-HAART era and the HAART era, and that being on HAART was associated with a high risk of HZ [16]. Furthermore, there are anecdotal reports of failure of antiretroviral therapy to control HZ complications, such as varicella zoster retinitis [17]. However, many other studies showed a protective effect of HAART on the incidence of HZ [18-21] and its complications [16,22]. Unfortunately, most of these studies did not take into account HAART adherence, which might partially explain the inconsistent results observed.

The objective of our study was to examine the effects of HAART and HAART adherence on HZ incidence by comparing HIV-infected women on HAART as a group (HAART use group) or stratified by HAART adherence level, with the matched HIV-infected HAART naive women (HAART naïve group) using longitudinal data from the Women's Interagency HIV Study (WIHS).

Methods

Study population

The WIHS was initiated in 1993/1994 and expanded in 2001/2002 to examine the natural and treated history of HIV disease among women. The study design of the WIHS is detailed elsewhere [23,24]. Briefly, 2,813 HIV-infected and 953 high risk HIV-negative women were recruited from six study sites (Chicago, Los Angeles, San Francisco, Washington D.C., Brooklyn and the Bronx) in the United States. Women visit a study site every 6 months. During each visit, structured interviews are performed to collect data on socio-demographical characteristics, sexual behaviors, substance use, health care utilization, antiretroviral therapy, treatments of comorbidities and different disease outcomes. In addition, physical and obstetric/gynecologic examinations are performed and biological specimens are collected. The local institutional review board at each site has approved the study protocol, and all women have given their written informed consents. For this study, our analyses were restricted to the HIV-infected participants only.

Propensity score matching

Unlike in randomized clinical trials, use of therapy in observational studies is not based upon random assignment. Thus, unbalanced distributions of background covariates may bias estimated treatment effects. To account for this, a propensity score matching method was used in our analysis. This method approaches more closely a randomized clinical trial by balancing background covariates via matching propensity score, which is the probability of HAART initiation in our study. The propensity score was calculated for each subject at each of her visits before starting HAART using a logistic regression model, with potential confounders for HAART initiation as predictors, including age, race, education, AIDS status, CD4+ and CD8+ T cell counts, HIV viral load and quality of life score. Each HAART user was matched at the last visit before her HAART initiation to a visit of a HAART naïve participant with similar propensity score (±0.1%). For any HAART naïve participant already selected as a control, the rest of her visits were removed from the matching pool to ensure 1:1 matching ratio. Participants who had HZ history on or before the matched visits were also removed from the analysis. The matched visits are the index visits after which all follow-up occurs in this analysis.

Study variables

We used a longitudinal cohort design to assess the impact of HAART use and its adherence on HZ incidence. In the WIHS, questions about HZ occurrence were asked from visit 1 (October 1994) to visit 30 (April 2009). At WIHS study enrollment, participants were asked "Has a health care provider ever told you that you had shingles (herpes zoster)?" At follow up visits, participants were asked "Since your last visit, has a health care provider told you that you had shingles (herpes zoster)?" The study outcome was time to first HZ event from the index visit and participants were censored at the last study visit, death, or loss to follow up. As a participant usually had difficulty in recalling exact date of a HZ event, we used a visit date as the HZ event date when HZ was first reported at that visit, in our calculation of time to first HZ event. The exposure variables were HAART use group (yes/no) and HAART adherence level. The definition of HAART in the WIHS was guided by the DHHS/Kaiser Panel guidelines [25]. The HAART use group was defined as the matched HAART using women, while the HAART naïve group was defined as the matched women who never initiated HAART during the follow-up. HAART adherence level was self-reported and at each visit participants were asked the extent to which they took antiretrovirals as prescribed over the past 6 months. Participants categorized their level of adherence into one of five categories: 100% of the time, 95-99% of the time, 75-94% of the time, <75% of the time, and have not taken any prescribed medications. In WIHS, a shortened version of MOS-HIV developed by Bozzette et al. was adopted to measure QOL and its summary score was used [26]. The score ranged from 0–100, with higher score indicating better QOL. Time varying covariates were selected based on causal diagram analysis of factors that might affect HZ incidence; CD4+ T cell counts, CD8+ T cell counts and HIV viral load were potential intermediate variables, while quality of life score and acyclovir use since the last study visit were potential confounders.

Statistical analysis

Descriptive statistics such as mean and proportions were used to assess distributions of background covariates before and after propensity score matching. Kaplan-Meier method was used to describe HZ free curves during study follow up. Cox proportional hazards models were used to estimate associations of risk factors with time to first HZ event from the index visit, as reflected by hazard ratios (HR) and their corresponding 95% confidence intervals (CI). The underlying proportional hazard assumption in the Cox models was assessed for each covariate, and we found the assumption was satisfied, with the smallest P value being 0.2959. Values of time varying variables at the last study visit were excluded from analyses to avoid temporal ambiguity. For example, acyclovir use that was reported at the visit at which HZ was first reported was not counted as acyclovir use prior to HZ since the drug may have been prescribed to treat HZ. Univariate associations were first evaluated and only variables significant in univariate analysis were included in multivariate models. For short-term HAART effect, the study was assumed to end one year after the index visit. For long-term HAART effect, the participants were followed from the index visits to either their first HZ event or censored events such as death, loss to follow up or at the last visit (visit 30). To assess the effect of HAART use on HZ incidence, we assumed that a woman who initiated HAART will continue on HAART, which is similar to an intent-to-treatment analysis in a clinical trial. To assess the effect of HAART adherence on HZ incidence, time varying HAART adherence level was used as exposure variable, which is similar to the as-treated analysis in a clinical trial. To examine whether HAART exerts its effect via immune recovery, we purposely added into the multivariate models an intermediate variable between HAART use and HZ incidence, along with an exposure variable and potential confounders. All statistical analyses were carried out using SAS 9.2 (SAS Inc, Carey, NC).

Results

Trends in HAART use and HZ incidence in the WIHS

2,813 HIV-infected WIHS women were followed from the WIHS enrollment until visit 30 (2009) and contributed 22,658 person years. Figure 1 shows trends in HAART use and HZ incidence among these women during this period. HZ incidence decreased substantially during the first few years and it declined steadily thereafter, coincident with an increase in the proportion of HIV-infected women taking HAART.

Propensity score matching and participant characteristics balancing

Characteristics of all HAART using women (2053) and all HAART naïve women (760) at the WIHS enrollment, and characteristics of the subsets of these women who were matched by propensity score at the index visit are presented in Table 1. At the WIHS enrollment, distributions of age, race, AIDS diagnosis, HIV viral load, CD4+ and CD8+ cell counts were significantly different between HAART use and HAART naïve women. However, after propensity score matching, all background covariates of the 389 matched pairs were well balanced at the index visit.

Comparison of HZ free curves between the HAART use group and HAART naïve group

During the follow up, the 389 matched pairs contributed 3,909 person years and reported 109 HZ events. The HAART use group had a median follow-up time of 6.9 years (interquartile range (IQR: 25th percentile to 75th percentile): 3.5-11 years) and an average HZ incidence of 25 (95% confidence interval(CI): 20–32) per 1000 person years. The HAART naïve group had a median follow-up time of 1.5 years (IQR: 0.7-3.8 years) and an average HZ incidence of 35 (95% CI: 26–48) per 1000 person years Figure 2 describes the cumulative probability of remaining HZ free (i.e. not developing HZ) for the HAART use group and the HAART naïve group. During the first year of follow up, HZ-free survival was similar. However, with additional follow-up, the difference started showing up. Overall, the HAART naïve group had marginally lower HZ-free survival (i.e. a higher incidence of HZ) over time than the HAART use group ($P = 0.113$).

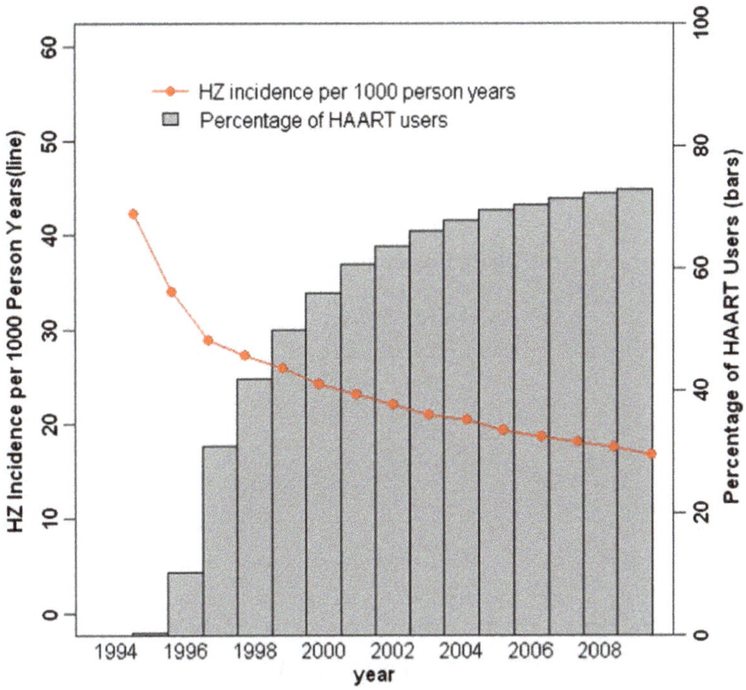

Figure 1 Trends in percentage of HAART users and herpes zoster Incidence among HIV-infected women in the WIHS.

Table 1 Characteristics comparison before and after matching

Covariates	Before matching at WIHS[b] enrollment			After matching at index visit		
	All HAART[c] use women (N = 2053)	All HAART naïve women (N = 760)	p-Value	Matched HAART use women (N = 389)	Matched HAART naïve women (N = 389)	p-Value
Age, mean (SD[a])	35 (7.9)	37 (7.6)	*<.0001*	39.7 (8.7)	39.4 (8.2)	0.57
Race, N (%)			*0.015*			0.81
White, non-hispanic	308 (15.0)	122 (16.1)		57 (14.7)	52 (13.4)	
Black, non-hispanic	1119 (54.5)	451 (59.3)		233 (59.9)	246 (63.2)	
Hispanic	560 (27.3)	162 (21.3)		88 (22.6)	80 (20.6)	
Other	66 (3.2)	25 (3.3)		11 (2.8)	11 (2.8)	
Education, N (%)			0.086			0.64
Less than high school	759 (37.1)	304 (40.1)		148 (38.1)	158 (40.6)	
Completed high school	612 (29.9)	237 (31.2)		126 (32.4)	127 (32.7)	
Some college and above	677 (33.1)	218 (28.7)		115 (29.6)	104 (26.7)	
AIDS, N (%)	407 (19.8)	308 (43.08)	*<.0001*	135 (34.7)	138 (35.5)	0.82
CD4+ cell counts, mean (SD)	430 (291.7)	398 (365.3)	*<.0001*	372.6 (248.1)	358.7 (279.2)	0.47
CD8+ cell counts, mean (SD)	899.7 (464.1)	792.2 (597.3)	*<.0001*	847.2 (519.3)	806.8 (521.4)	0.28
log10 (Viral load), mean (SD)	3.9 (1.1)	4.4 (1.2)	*<.0001*	3.9 (1.1)	4.1 (1.2)	0.14
Quality of life score, mean (SD)	64.8 (20.4)	57.4 (21.2)	0.18	63.8 (21.5)	62.4 (22.2)	0.35

[a]standard deviation; [b]WIHS: Women's Interagency HIV Study; [c]HAART: highly active anti-retroviral therapy.

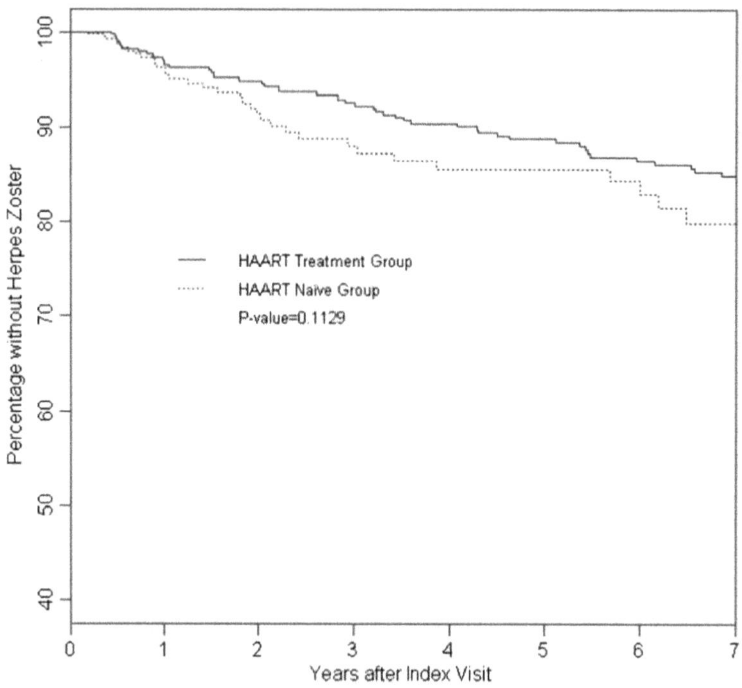

Figure 2 Percentage without herpes zoster for HAART treatment and HAART naïve group.

Short-term Effect of HAART on HZ incidence

During the first year of follow up, the HAART use group and the HAART naïve group reported 13 (incidence rate: 49 per 1000 person years; 95% CI (29, 82)) and 12 (incidence rate: 47 per 1000 person years, 95% CI (27, 81)) HZ events respectively. In the univariate analysis, compared to the HAART naïve group, neither the HAART use group (HR: 0.88; 95% CI: 0.39-1.99) nor women with a HAART adherence level of ≥95% (HR: 1.20; 95% CI: 0.42-3.11) had significantly different risk of HZ incidence.

Long-term Effects of HAART on HZ incidence

Effects of long-term HAART use and HAART adherence on HZ incidence are described in Table 2. In univariate analysis, the HAART use group had a marginally lower HZ incidence (HR: 0.72; 95% CI: 0.48-1.09) compared to the matched HAART naïve group. However, women with a HAART adherence level of ≥95% had significantly lower HZ incidence (HR: 0.54; 95% CI: 0.31-0.94) than HAART naïve individuals, while women with lower HAART adherence levels (less than 95%) or HAART discontinuation had similar HZ risk to that of the HAART naïve group. Higher CD4+ T cell counts (per 100 increase; HR: 0.85; 95% CI: 0.77-0.93) was significantly associated with lower HZ incidence while higher HIV viral load (per $\log_{10}$ increase; HR: 1.55; 95% CI: 1.30-1.84) was significantly related to higher HZ incidence. After adjusting for QOL score and acyclovir use, a HAART adherence level of ≥95% remained significantly associated with lower HZ incidence. However, after adding an intermediate variable - either CD4+ T cell count or HIV viral load, along with QOL score and acyclovir use, the association of a HAART adherence level of ≥95% with HZ incidence attenuated and was no longer statistically significant.

Discussion

Though the mechanisms by which HAART exerts its effect on HZ incidence are not yet clear, accumulating evidence suggests that HAART might have different effects on HZ incidence depending on how long HAART has been used. Many studies demonstrated that HZ occurs at a high level shortly after initiation of HAART [4-15], which might reflect dysregulated immune responses against pre-existing varicella zoster antigens at the beginning of immune restoration, rather than profound immunosuppression [4,27]. However, like a few other observational studies [2,16], we did not observe such a phenomenon in this study. Possible reasons for this discrepancy might include: (1). HAART users in our study had higher CD4+ T cell counts (372 cells/μl) before starting HAART; (2). In this short term analysis, our study might not have sufficient power to detect minor difference in HZ incidence due to relatively small sample size and rarity of HZ events; (3). Participants were followed every 6 months and the exact dates of HAART initiation could not be determined.

Table 2 Long-term effect of haart[a] use on herpes zoster incidence

Variable	Univariate HR[b] (CI[c])	Multivariate[1] HR (CI)	Multivariate[2] HR (CI)	Multivariate[3] HR (CI)
HAART use group:				
No	1.00			
Yes	0.72(0.48–1.09)			
HAART use adherence since last visit[c]				
>95%	0.54*(0.31–0.94)	0.56*(0.32–0.99)	0.61(0.33–1.11)	0.76(0.41–1.38)
75%–95%	0.32(0.09–1.05)	0.31(0.09–1.03)	0.30(0.09–1.03)	0.34(0.10–1.14)
0 < adherence <75%	1.70(0.70–4.14)	1.38(0.53–3.63)	1.25(0.46–3.41)	1.23(0.46–3.31)
HAART users, but did not use HAART since last visit	0.95(0.52–1.72)	0.87(0.47–1.62)	0.77(0.39–1.52)	0.65(0.33–1.27)
No HAART users	1.00	1.00	1.00	1.00
Current CD4+ cell counts (per100 cell increase)[d]	0.85***(0.77–0.93)		0.86***(0.78–0.94)	
Current CD8+ cell counts (per 100 cell increase)[d]	0.96(0.90–1.01)			
HIV viral load (per Log 10)[d]	1.55***(1.30–1.84)			1.59***(1.31–1.93)
Quality of life score[d]	0.98**(0.97–0.99)	0.99*(0.98–0.99)	0.98*(0.97–0.99)	0.98*(0.97–0.99)
Used acyclovir since last visit[d]:				
No	1.00	1.00	1.00	1.00
Yes	1.88*(1.04–3.18)	1.68(0.88–3.22)	1.52(0.75–3.10)	1.56(0.79–3.08)

[a]HAART: highly active antiretroviral therapy; [b]hazard ratio; [c]95% confident interval; [d]time dependent variables ***$p < 0.001$; **$0.001 \le p < 0.01$; *$0.01 \le p < 0.05$; [1]after adjusting for quality of life and acyclovir use; [2]after adjusting for quality of life, acyclovir use and CD4+ T cell counts; [3]after adjusting for quality of life, acyclovir use and HIV viral load.

Since HAART became available in 1996, a steady decrease in HZ incidence over time has been observed among HIV-infected women in the WIHS coincident with their increasing access to HAART. Like many other studies [18-21,28], ours showed a protective effect of long-term HAART use on HZ incidence. However, a statistically significant effect was achieved only when a HAART adherence level of ≥95% was attained. Thus, a further examination of the role of HAART adherence level might shed light on the lack of associations between HAART use and HZ incidence as reported by some earlier studies as no such information was reported [16]. In addition, we found that the long-term effect of HAART on HZ incidence was mainly mediated through its effects in reducing HIV viral load and improving host immune status. Enhanced immune status and decreased shedding of varicella zoster virus antigen by HAART [29] might explain the protective effect of HAART on HZ incidence as observed in our study.

In this study, we found that acyclovir use was surprisingly associated with higher HZ incidence in univariate analysis. Possible explanation for this lies in that prior acyclovir use might be an indication of other herpes infections that were closely related to HZ incidence due to common cause - immunosuppression by HIV infection, rather than be used to prevent occurrence of HZ [30,31]. In addition, lower overall QOL was also associated with higher incidence of herpes zoster, which is consistent with the role of psychological stress in the development of HZ [32].

Our study had some advantages over previous studies. First, we used a propensity score matching method to balance background covariates. In this way, the indication bias for HAART initiation was dramatically decreased. Second, previous studies focused on HAART use but did not take into account HAART adherence level. Our study showed the protective effect of HAART use was most clear when a ≥95% HAART adherence level was attained, suggesting that HAART adherence level should always be considered in future similar studies. However, some limitations of our study should also be mentioned. First, self-reported HZ was not documented by a health professional; however, a previous study has ascribed high validity to self-reports of HZ [33], suggesting that HZ misclassification in our study was likely to be very low. Second, we used self-reported HAART adherence as an exposure variable. However, this concern might be mitigated by the fact that the relationships between the WIHS participants and their interviewers have been built on trust and respect over many years, and previous WIHS research has shown that self-reported medication use is consistent with objective measures of HIV outcomes, such as CD4+ T-cell count, HIV viral load, and self-reported physical functioning [34]. Lastly, our study only included women, and the results might not be generalizable to men.

Conclusion

We have shown that individuals highly adherent to HAART regimes had a significantly lower incidence of HZ than similar individuals who were not as adherent to HAART, underscoring the importance of high HAART adherence level in the clinical management of HIV-infected individuals, in addition to its role in decreasing HIV disease progression and HIV transmission.

Abbreviations

HAART: Highly active antiretroviral therapy; HZ: Herpes zoster; HR: Hazard ratio; CI: Confidence interval; IQR: Inter-quartile range; HIV: Human immunodeficiency virus; AIDS: Acquired immune deficiency syndrome; WIHS: Women's Interagency HIV Study.

Competing interests

Dr. Glesby had consultancy relationship with Gilead Sciences and Pfizer. All other authors declare that they have no competing interests.

Authors' contributions

(Please use initials to refer to each author's contribution): CL was responsible for study design, data interpretation and manuscript writing. CW participated in study design and statistical analysis. MJG, GD, AF, HM, TM, and RK participated in drafting and improving manuscript. MY participated in study design, coordination and drafting the manuscript. All authors read and approved the final manuscript.

Acknowledgements

Data in this manuscript were collected by the Women's Interagency HIV Study (WIHS) Collaborative Study Group with centers (Principal Investigators) at New York City/Bronx Consortium (Kathryn Anastos); Brooklyn, NY (Howard Minkoff); Washington, DC, Metropolitan Consortium (Mary Young); The Connie Wofsy Study Consortium of Northern California (Ruth Greenblatt); Los Angeles County/Southern California Consortium (Alexandra Levine); Chicago Consortium (Mardge Cohen); Data Coordinating Center (Stephen Gange). The WIHS is funded by the National Institute of Allergy and Infectious Diseases (UO1-AI-35004, UO1-AI-31834, UO1-AI-34994, UO1-AI-34989, UO1-AI-34993, and UO1-AI-42590) and by the *Eunice Kennedy Shriver* National Institute of Child Health and Human Development (UO1-HD-32632). The study is co-funded by the National Cancer Institute, the National Institute on Drug Abuse, and the National Institute on Deafness and Other Communication Disorders. Funding is also provided by the National Center for Research Resources (UCSF-CTSI Grant Number UL1 RR024131). This manuscript was also partially supported by K24 AI078884 funded by NIH. The contents of this publication are solely the responsibility of the authors and do not necessarily represent the official views of the National Institutes of Health.

Author details

[1]Department of Medicine, Georgetown University, 2115 Wisconsin Avenue NW, Suite 130, Washington, DC 20007, USA. [2]Division of Infectious Diseases, Weill Cornell Medical College, New York, NY, USA. [3]Department of Epidemiology, Johns Hopkins School of Public Health, Baltimore, MD, USA. [4]Division of Infectious Diseases, Cook County Hospital, Chicago, IL, USA. [5]Department of Obstetrics and Gynecology, Maimonides Medical Center, Brooklyn, NY, USA. [6]Department of Dermatology, University of California at San Francisco, San Francisco, CA, USA. [7]Departments of Pediatrics and Preventive Medicine, University of Southern California, Los Angeles, CA, USA.

References

1. Vanhems P, Voisin L, Gayet-Ageron A, Trepo C, Cotte L, Peyramond D, Chidiac C, Touraine JL, Livrozet JM, Fabry J, Voirin N: **The incidence of herpes zoster is less likely than other opportunistic infections to be reduced by highly active antiretroviral therapy.** *J Acquir Immune Defic Syndr* 2005, **38:**111–113.
2. Levin MJ, Anderson JP, Seage GR 3rd, Williams PL: **Short-term and long-term effects of highly active antiretroviral therapy on the incidence of herpes zoster in HIV-infected children.** *J Acquir Immune Defic Syndr* 2009, **50:**182–191.
3. Glesby MJ, Hoover DR, Tan T, Shi Q, Gao W, French AL, Maurer T, Young M, Dehovitz J, Ru J, Anastos K: **Herpes zoster in women with and at risk for HIV: data from the Women's interagency HIV study.** *J Acquir Immune Defic Syndr* 2004, **37:**1604–1609.
4. Martinez E, Gatell J, Moran Y, Aznar E, Buira E, Guelar A, Mallolas J, Soriano E: **High incidence of herpes zoster in patients with AIDS soon after therapy with protease inhibitors.** *Clin Infect Dis* 1998, **27:**1510–1513.
5. Rodriguez-Rosado R, Soriano V, Dona C, Gonzalez-Lahoz J: **Opportunistic infections shortly after beginning highly active antiretroviral therapy.** *Antivir Ther* 1998, **3:**229–231.
6. Michelet C, Arvieux C, Francois C, Besnier JM, Rogez JP, Breux JP, Souala F, Allavena C, Raffi F, Garre M, Cartier F: **Opportunistic infections occurring during highly active antiretroviral treatment.** *Aids* 1998, **12:**1815–1822.
7. Espinosa E, Pena-Jimenez A, Ormsby CE, Vega-Barrientos R, Reyes-Teran G: **Later onset of herpes zoster-associated immune reconstitution inflammatory syndrome.** *HIV Med* 2009, **10:**454–457.
8. Sharma A, Makrandi S, Modi M, Sharma A, Marfatia Y: **Immune reconstitution inflammatory syndrome.** *Indian J Dermatol Venereol Leprol* 2008, **74:**619–621.
9. Murdoch DM, Venter WD, Feldman C, Van Rie A: **Incidence and risk factors for the immune reconstitution inflammatory syndrome in HIV patients in South Africa: a prospective study.** *Aids* 2008, **22:**601–610.
10. Huruy K, Mulu A, Mengistu G, Shewa-Amare A, Akalu A, Kassu A, Andargie G, Elias D, Torben W: **Immune reconstitution inflammatory syndrome among HIV/AIDS patients during highly active antiretroviral therapy in Addis Ababa, Ethiopia.** *Jpn J Infect Dis* 2008, **61:**205–209.
11. Patel AK, Patel KK, Shah SD, Desai J: **Immune reconstitution syndrome presenting with cerebral varicella zoster vasculitis in HIV-1-infected patient: a case report.** *J Int Assoc Physicians AIDS Care (Chic Ill)* 2006, **5:**157–160.
12. Lehloenya R, Meintjes G: **Dermatologic manifestations of the immune reconstitution inflammatory syndrome.** *Dermatol Clin* 2006, **24:**549–570, vii.
13. Ratnam I, Chiu C, Kandala NB, Easterbrook PJ: **Incidence and risk factors for immune reconstitution inflammatory syndrome in an ethnically diverse HIV type 1-infected cohort.** *Clin Infect Dis* 2006, **42:**418–427.
14. Tangsinmankong N, Kamchaisatian W, Lujan-Zilbermann J, Brown CL, Sleasman JW, Emmanuel PJ: **Varicella zoster as a manifestation of immune restoration disease in HIV-infected children.** *J Allergy Clin Immunol* 2004, **113:**742–746.
15. Domingo P, Torres OH, Ris J, Vazquez G: **Herpes zoster as an immune reconstitution disease after initiation of combination antiretroviral therapy in patients with human immunodeficiency virus type-1 infection.** *Am J Med* 2001, **110:**605–609.
16. Gebo KA, Kalyani R, Moore RD, Polydefkis MJ: **The incidence of, risk factors for, and sequelae of herpes zoster among HIV patients in the highly active antiretroviral therapy era.** *J Acquir Immune Defic Syndr* 2005, **40:**169–174.
17. Ramsay A, Young S, Lightman S: **Failure of antiretroviral therapy to control Varicella zoster retinitis.** *Clin Experiment Ophthalmol* 2001, **29:**433–434.
18. Maurer T, Rodrigues LK, Ameli N, Phanuphak N, Gange SJ, DeHovitz J, French AL, Glesby M, Jordan C, Khalsa A, Hessol NA: **The effect of highly active antiretroviral therapy on dermatologic disease in a longitudinal study of HIV type 1-infected women.** *Clin Infect Dis* 2004, **38:**579–584.
19. Hung CC, Hsiao CF, Wang JL, Chen MY, Hsieh SM, Sheng WH, Chang SC: **Herpes zoster in HIV-1-infected patients in the era of highly active antiretroviral therapy: a prospective observational study.** *Int J STD AIDS* 2005, **16:**673–676.
20. Gona P, Van Dyke RB, Williams PL, Dankner WM, Chernoff MC, Nachman SA, Seage GR 3rd: **Incidence of opportunistic and other infections in HIV-infected children in the HAART era.** *Jama* 2006, **296:**292–300.
21. Wood SM, Shah SS, Steenhoff AP, Rutstein RM: **Primary varicella and herpes zoster among HIV-infected children from 1989 to 2006.** *Pediatrics* 2008, **121:**e150–e156.
22. Martinez PA, Diaz R, Gonzalez D, Oropesa L, Gonzalez R, Perez L, Viera J, Kouri V: **The effect of highly active antiretroviral therapy on outcome of central nervous system herpesviruses infection in Cuban human**

immunodeficiency virus-infected individuals. *J Neurovirol* 2007, **13:**446–451.
23. Barkan SE, Melnick SL, Preston-Martin S, Weber K, Kalish LA, Miotti P, Young M, Greenblatt R, Sacks H, Feldman J: **The women's interagency HIV study. WIHS collaborative study group.** *Epidemiology* 1998, **9:**117–125.
24. Bacon MC, von Wyl V, Alden C, Sharp G, Robison E, Hessol N, Gange S, Barranday Y, Holman S, Weber K, Young MA: **The Women's interagency HIV study: an observational cohort brings clinical sciences to the bench.** *Clin Diagn Lab Immunol* 2005, **12:**1013–1019.
25. DHHS: *Guidelines for the use of antiretroviral agents in HIV-infected adults and adolescents*, DHHS/Henry J. Kaiser family foundation panel on clinical practices for the treatment of HIV infection; 2009. Available at http://aidsinfo.nih.gov. In.
26. Bozzette SA, Hays RD, Berry SH, Kanouse DE, Wu AW: **Derivation and properties of a brief health status assessment instrument for use in HIV disease.** *J Acquir Immune Defic Syndr Hum Retrovirol* 1995, **8:**253–265.
27. Stone SF, Price P, French MA: **Immune restoration disease: a consequence of dysregulated immune responses after HAART.** *Curr HIV Res* 2004, **2:**235–242.
28. Takeoka H, Chong Y, Murata M, Furusyo N, Nabeshima S, Yamaji K, Kishihara Y, Hayashi J: **[Varicella-zoster virus symptoms and polyneuropathy in a patient with human immunodeficiency virus infection not improved until highly active anti-retroviral therapy added to acyclovir therapy].** *Kansenshogaku Zasshi* 2006, **80:**46–50.
29. Wang CC, Yepes LC, Danaher RJ, Berger JR, Mootoor Y, Kryscio RJ, Miller CS: **Low prevalence of varicella zoster virus and herpes simplex virus type 2 in saliva from human immunodeficiency virus-infected persons in the era of highly active antiretroviral therapy.** *Oral Surg Oral Med Oral Pathol Oral Radiol Endod* 2010, **109:**232–237.
30. Carmichael JK: **Treatment of herpes zoster and postherpetic neuralgia.** *Am Fam Physician* 1991, **44:**203–210.
31. Whitley RJ: **The past as prelude to the future: history, status, and future of antiviral drugs.** *Ann Pharmacother* 1996, **30:**967–971.
32. Livengood JM: **The role of stress in the development of herpes zoster and postherpetic neuralgia.** *Curr Rev Pain* 2000, **4:**7–11.
33. Schmader K, George LK, Newton R, Hamilton JD: **The accuracy of self-report of herpes zoster.** *J Clin Epidemiol* 1994, **47:**1271–1276.
34. Wilson TE, Barron Y, Cohen M, Richardson J, Greenblatt R, Sacks HS, Young M: **Adherence to antiretroviral therapy and its association with sexual behavior in a national sample of women with human immunodeficiency virus.** *Clin Infect Dis* 2002, **34:**529–534.

3

NGX-4010, a capsaicin 8% patch, for the treatment of painful HIV-associated distal sensory polyneuropathy

Stephen Brown[1*], David M Simpson[2], Graeme Moyle[3], Bruce J Brew[4], Giovanni Schifitto[5], Nicholas Larbalestier[6], Chloe Orkin[7], Martin Fisher[8], Geertrui F Vanhove[9] and Jeffrey K Tobias[9]

Abstract

Background: HIV-associated distal sensory polyneuropathy (HIV-DSP) is the most frequently reported neurologic complication associated with HIV infection. NGX-4010 is a capsaicin 8% dermal patch with demonstrated efficacy in the treatment of HIV-DSP. Data from two phase III, double-blind studies were integrated to further analyze the efficacy and safety of NGX-4010 and explore the effect of demographic and baseline factors on NGX-4010 treatment in HIV-DSP.

Methods: Data from two similarly designed studies in which patients with HIV-DSP received NGX-4010 or a low-concentration control patch (capsaicin 0.04% w/w) for 30 or 60 minutes were integrated. Efficacy assessments included the mean percent change from baseline in Numeric Pain Rating Scale (NPRS) scores to Weeks 2–12. Safety and tolerability assessments included adverse events (AEs) and pain during and after treatment.

Results: Patients (n = 239) treated with NGX-4010 for 30 minutes demonstrated significantly (p = 0.0026) greater pain relief compared with controls (n = 100); the mean percent change in NPRS scores from baseline to Weeks 2–12 was −27.0% *versus* −15.7%, respectively. Patients who received a 60-minute application of NGX-4010 (n = 243) showed comparable pain reductions (−27.5%) to patients treated for 30 minutes, but this was not statistically superior to controls (n = 115). NGX-4010 was effective regardless of gender, baseline pain score, duration of HIV-DSP, or use of concomitant neuropathic pain medication, although NGX-4010 efficacy was greater in patients not receiving concomitant neuropathic pain medications. NGX-4010 was well tolerated; the most common AEs were application-site pain and erythema, and most AEs were mild to moderate. The transient increase in pain associated with NGX-4010 treatment decreased the day after treatment and returned to baseline by Day 2.

Conclusions: A single 30-minute application of NGX-4010 provides significant pain relief for at least 12 weeks in patients with HIV-DSP and is well tolerated.

Keywords: NGX-4010, Capsaicin 8% patch, HIV-associated distal sensory polyneuropathy, Neuropathic pain

* Correspondence: s.brown@aidsresearch.org
[1]AIDS Research Alliance, Los Angeles, CA, USA

Background

HIV-associated distal sensory polyneuropathy (HIV-DSP) is the most frequently reported neurologic complication associated with HIV infection. It can be caused by the virus itself [1] or by the use of antiretroviral drugs; for example, some nucleoside reverse transcriptase inhibitors have been shown to have a dose-dependent toxic effect in 15–30% of patients [1]. The clinical presentation of HIV-DSP is similar regardless of whether it is caused by HIV itself or is due to the toxicity of antiretroviral drugs.

HIV-DSP presents with predominantly symmetrical signs of distal sensory loss and reduction or loss of ankle reflexes. Symptomatic HIV-DSP reflects the involvement of both small and large sensory nerve fibers and includes distal painful dysesthesias, allodynia, severe burning pain, pins and needles, and numbness [1,2]. These symptoms usually begin in the feet and may progress bilaterally up the legs and to the arms in severe HIV-DSP.

In a recent US study, 881 of 1,539 (57%) individuals infected with HIV showed evidence of HIV-sensory neuropathy, which encompasses HIV-DSP caused by the virus and toxic DSP due to dideoxynucleoside antiretroviral therapy [3]. Of those with DSP, 38% reported neuropathic pain [4]. Very few neuropathic pain treatments, however, have demonstrated efficacy in clinical trials for patients with HIV-associated neuropathy. For example, the tricyclic antidepressant amitriptyline [5], the anticonvulsant pregabalin [6], and topical treatments such as lidocaine [7] and low-dose (0.075%) capsaicin cream [8] have all failed to show significant pain relief when compared with controls. By contrast, three small, randomized, placebo-controlled studies showed that smoking cannabis reduced daily pain compared with smoking identical placebo cigarettes from which the cannabinoids had been removed [9-11]. Other neuropathic pain therapies such as duloxetine and venlafaxine have not been studied in patients with HIV-DSP [12] while the results of a single published study investigating opioid use among patients with HIV suggested those receiving opioids experienced more pain than those patients who did not receive opioids [13]. Furthermore, many of these agents, which are not approved by the Food and Drug Administration or the European Medicines Agency, are associated with unwanted side effects and burdensome treatment regimens [12]. Sedation and dizziness are common adverse events (AEs) associated with gabapentin and pregabalin, whereas nausea can be common with duloxetine [12]. Gabapentin and pregabalin also require slow dose titration, as does amitriptyline [12]. In addition, cumbersome regimens must be followed for treatment with lidocaine patches and low-dose capsaicin creams; the lidocaine patch is licensed to be worn for 12 hours followed by a 12-hour treatment break [12], and capsaicin cream requires application several times a day [8]. A recent systematic review of randomized controlled studies concluded that evidence of efficacy exists only for capsaicin 8%, smoked cannabis, and recombinant-human nerve growth factor (rhNGF) [14]. However, rhNGF did not demonstrate evidence for the expected nerve fiber regeneration [15] and was not developed further for clinical use.

NGX-4010 is a capsaicin 8% (w/w) dermal patch licensed in 2009 in the EU for the treatment of peripheral neuropathic pain in non-diabetic adults either alone or in combination with other medicinal products for pain; and indicated in the US for the management of neuropathic pain associated with post-herpetic neuralgia. NGX-4010 was developed to rapidly deliver a high dose of capsaicin directly to the source of pain with a single application. Capsaicin is a highly selective agonist for the Transient Receptor Potential Vanilloid 1 (TRPV1) receptor, which is a ligand-gated non-selective cation channel that is highly expressed in nociceptors and is critical for pain transmission and modulation [16]. As a component of small nerve fibers, C fibers are involved in HIV-DSP [17] and, as TRPV1 expression is altered on C fibers following nerve injury [18], these fibers may play a role in the neuropathic pain experienced by individuals with HIV-DSP. TRPV1 is therefore a logical target for treating neuropathic pain. Exposure of TRPV1 receptors to high concentrations of capsaicin initially causes depolarization, action potential initiation, and burning pain [19,20]. This is followed by a defunctionalization and reduction in the density of epidermal nerve fibers, resulting in inhibition of pain transmission [19-21]. The effect is reversible, with regrowth of epidermal nerve fibers evident 12 weeks after exposure to capsaicin [21].

Two similarly designed phase III, double-blind, controlled studies have investigated the efficacy of NGX-4010 in patients with HIV-DSP. These studies demonstrated that treatment with NGX-4010 was well tolerated and resulted in a reduction in pain over 12 weeks [22,23] (Table 1). Study C107 investigated the efficacy of NGX-4010 applied for 30, 60, or 90 minutes and demonstrated that the 30-minute NGX-4010 application resulted in a statistically significant reduction in pain; there was no evidence of increased efficacy with longer application durations [22]. Study C119 investigated the efficacy of NGX-4010 applied for 30 or 60 minutes and demonstrated a greater pain reduction in the 30-minute NGX-4010 group *versus* the 30-minute control group. Although this did not attain statistical significance using a prespecified analysis of covariance (ANCOVA) model, it did show a significant difference ($p = 0.035$) when a post hoc non-parametric test was used [23]. In neither study did the 60-minute treatment group show a significant difference as compared with control.

To analyze in more detail the efficacy and safety of NGX-4010 in patients with HIV-DSP, an integrated

Table 1 Summary of randomized, double-blind, controlled trials of NGX-4010 in patients with HIV-DSP

Trial	Number of patients: NGX-4010	Number of patients: Control patch*	Dose	Mean percent change in NPRS "average pain for past 24 hours" during Weeks 2–12 post application compared with baseline (%)	
C107 [22]	225	82	Single 30-, 60-, or 90-minute application of NGX-4010 patch *versus* low-concentration (0.04%) capsaicin control patch	30 minutes	−27.7 (p = 0.0007† *versus* control)
				60 minutes	−15.8 (p = 0.291† *versus* control)
				90 minutes	−24.7 (p = 0.0046† *versus* control)
				Pooled	−22.8 (p = 0.0026† *versus* control)
C119 [23]	332	162	Single 30- or 60-minute application of NGX-4010 patch *versus* low-concentration (0.04%) capsaicin control patch	30 minutes	−26.2 (p = 0.1031‡ *versus* control)
				60 minutes	−32.8 (p = 0.4884‡ *versus* control)
				Pooled	−29.5 (p = 0.0967‡ *versus* control)

NPRS Numeric Pain Rating Score.
*A low-concentration capsaicin patch (0.04% w/w) was used as a control to ensure effective blinding in the randomized studies.
†p-value was computed using gender-stratified ANCOVA to test for a difference between the NGX-4010 group and the total control group, with baseline pain score, pre-topical anesthetic pain score, and percent change in pain score after topical anesthetic treatment as covariates.
‡p-value was computed using a gender-stratified ANCOVA to compare differences between each NGX-4010 group and the respective control group, with baseline pain as the covariate.

analysis of the 30- and 60-minute NGX-4010 applications from the two double-blind, controlled HIV-DSP studies was performed. This integrated analysis also investigated the effects of demographic factors, disease duration and severity, and the use of concomitant neuropathic pain medication, which are often difficult to evaluate in individual studies due to the limited sample size.

Results

Patients

The integrated analysis comprised data from 482 and 215 patients treated with NGX-4010 and a control patch, respectively (Figure 1). Of the patients treated with NGX-4010, 239 and 243 received a 30- and 60-minute application, respectively. Among the control patients, 100 and 115 received a 30- and 60-minute application, respectively. One patient, in the control group, was randomly assigned to receive a 30-minute treatment, but actually received a 60-minute treatment.

Gender, age, race, baseline Numeric Pain Rating Scale (NPRS) score, CD4 cell count, viral load, and the percentage of patients receiving some form of concomitant neuropathic pain treatment at baseline were similar between the two phase III studies and between treatment groups within the two studies (NeurogesX unpublished data) [22,23]. The average duration of HIV-DSP was slightly longer in study C119 (means ranged from 5.7– 6.6 years [23]) compared with study C107 (means ranged from 4.2–5.4 years [22]). Patient demographics and baseline characteristics for the integrated dataset were similar between the NGX-4010 and control groups (Table 2).

The percentage of patients terminating the studies before the end of the 12-week double-blind period was 8% for the combined NGX-4010 group and 8% for the combined control group (Figure 1). Reasons for premature termination were AEs, being lost to follow-up, death, non-compliance, unsatisfactory therapeutic response, and other. Five patients (three in the 60-minute NGX-4010 group, one in the 60-minute control group, and one in the 30-minute control group) withdrew from the study due to AEs. In only two of these patients were the AEs judged to be related to study medication and both consisted of application-site pain. Both patients were in the 60-minute NGX-4010 group. Three patients died during the 12-week observation period; two deaths in the 60-minute NGX-4010 group were due to sepsis and pre-existing arteriosclerosis and one death in the 60-minute control group was due to a presumed drug overdose. No deaths were considered to be related to study drug treatment.

Efficacy

Data for the primary endpoint, the mean change in NPRS score from baseline to Week 2–12, for the integrated 30- and 60-minute treatment groups, along with those of other efficacy endpoints are shown in Table 3.

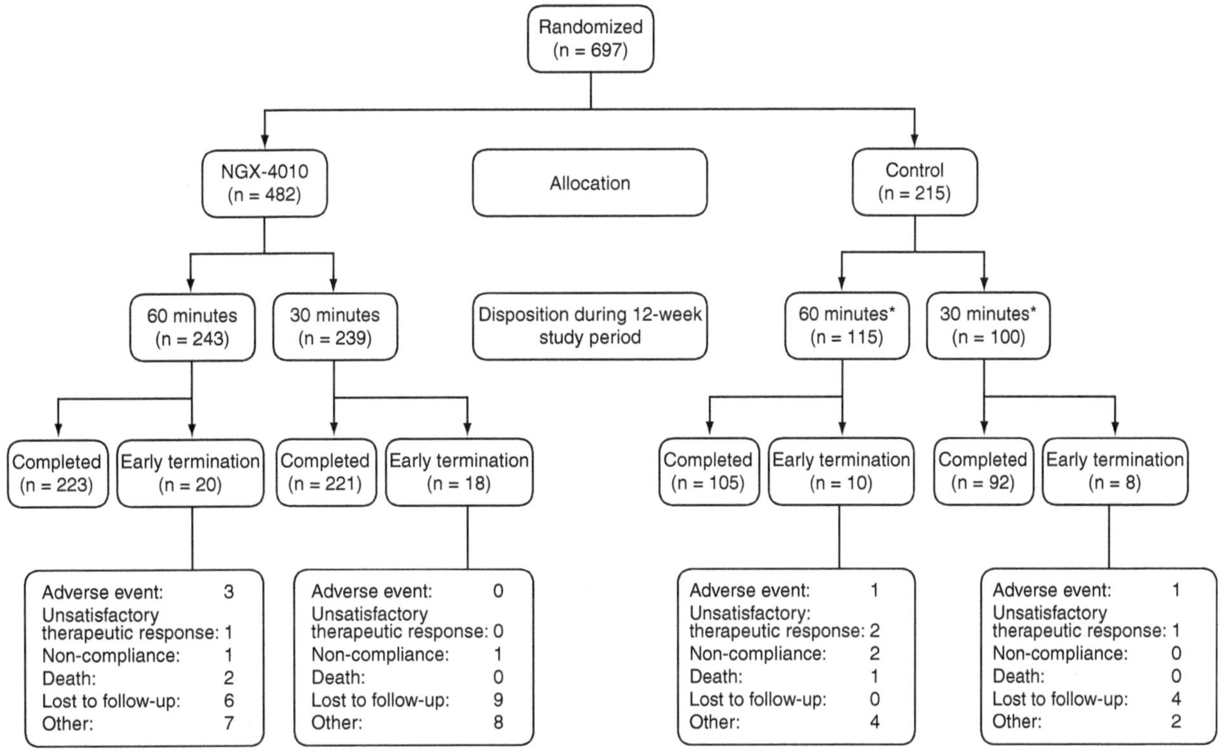

Figure 1 Disposition of all patients from both phase III HIV-DSP studies used in the integrated analysis. *One patient randomly assigned to receive the 30-minute control treatment received the 60-minute control treatment.

These analyses demonstrated that the 30- and 60-minute NGX-4010 doses provided comparable pain reduction (−26.9% and −27.9%, respectively). Only the 30-minute dose was statistically superior to the low-concentration capsaicin control; the 60-minute NGX-4010 group showed a similar pain reduction to the 60-minute control group.

Similarly, a comparable percentage of patients in the 30- and 60-minute groups (40% for each) responded to NGX-4010 treatment (≥30% decrease in NPRS score from baseline to Weeks 2–12), but only the 30-minute NGX-4010 treatment resulted in a significantly greater percentage of responders compared with controls (Table 3). Patients treated with NGX-4010 for 30 minutes had a 2.2-fold higher likelihood of being a responder compared with patients treated with control for 30 minutes. The reduction in pain in response to NGX-4010 treatment was confirmed by the results of the Patient Global Impression of Change (PGIC). A comparable percentage of patients in the 30- and 60-minute groups (65% and 69%, respectively) felt slightly, much, or very much improved, and this was significantly different from control in both treatment groups (Table 3).

A weekly analysis of change in NPRS score from baseline for the 30-minute treatment groups demonstrated a significantly greater pain reduction for patients treated with NGX-4010 compared with control by Week 2, and this was maintained up to Week 12 (Figure 2A). Figure 2B shows daily mean changes in NPRS score from baseline for the 30-minute treatment groups in more detail. On average, NGX-4010 treatment is associated with a transient increase in pain on Day 0 followed by declining pain scores the following day and a return to baseline by Day 2. After Day 2, patients treated with NGX-4010 experienced a progressive reduction in pain which was greater than that of patients in the control group from Day 5 through to Day 84 (Figure 2B).

Patients treated with NGX-4010 showed a greater improvement in NPRS scores compared with those treated with control in all subgroups regardless of gender, baseline pain score, concomitant neuropathic pain medication use, and HIV-DSP duration (Figure 3 and 4). Treatment differences between NGX-4010 and control were similar regardless of gender (Figure 3A) or baseline pain score (Figure 3B). Treatment differences between NGX-4010 and control were larger in patients not using concomitant neuropathic pain medications compared with those using concomitant neuropathic pain medications (−23.7% [95% CI: −38.2, −9.3] *versus* −7.0%, [95% CI: −15.1 to 1.1] respectively; Figure 3C). Notably, treatment differences between NGX-4010 and control were larger in patients with a longer duration of HIV-DSP. This was

Table 2 Demographic and baseline characteristics from the integrated population of the two phase III HIV-DSP studies

	NGX-4010 total (n = 482)	NGX-4010 30 minutes (n = 239)	NGX-4010 60 minutes (n = 243)	Control total (n = 215)	Control 30 minutes (n = 100)	Control 60 minutes (n = 115)
Age, mean (SD), years	49 (8)	50 (9)	49 (8)	50 (8)	49 (8)	50 (9)
Male, n (%)	426 (88)	205 (86)	221 (91)	193 (90)	90 (90)	103 (90)
White, n (%)	315 (65)	156 (65)	159 (65)	144 (67)	68 (68)	76 (66)
Duration of pain, mean (SD), years	5.8 (3.9)	5.6 (3.7)	6.0 (4.1)	5.6 (4.1)	5.9 (3.9)	5.4 (4.4)
Baseline NPRS score, mean (SD)	6.0 (1.6)	6.0 (1.6)	6.0 (1.5)	5.9 (1.5)	6.0 (1.5)	5.8 (1.5)
Receiving concomitant neuropathic pain medication at study entry,* n (%)	339 (70)	180 (75)	159 (65)	143 (67)	72 (72)	71 (62)
Receiving Ntox antiretroviral therapy at baseline,† n (%)	52 (11)	25 (10)	27 (11)	18 (8)	8 (8)	10 (9)
CD4 count, mean x10^6/l (SD)	419 (242)	437 (235)	402 (247)	468 (314)	479 (291)	458 (334)
Viral load, HIV RNA copies/ml, median	400	400	400	400	400	400
(range)	(40–5,510,520)	(40–610,677)	(40–5,510,520)	(40–664,583)	(40–664,583)	(40–460,000)

NPRS Numeric Pain Rating Scale, *SD* standard deviation.
*A patient was defined as receiving concomitant neuropathic pain medication if he or she was taking an anticonvulsant, non-SSRI antidepressant, or opioid on Day −1 and for a total duration of at least 7 consecutive days.
†A patient was defined as receiving antiretroviral therapy if he or she was taking neurotoxic antiretroviral medications for at least 8 weeks prior to the screening date.

largely due to a greater pain reduction in patients with longer HIV-DSP duration receiving NGX-4010 than those with a shorter duration of HIV-DSP receiving NGX-4010 (Figure 3D).

Safety

More patients receiving NGX-4010 than control for the combined 30- and 60-minute groups experienced a treatment-related AE (77% *versus* 52%, respectively). The most common (≥2%) treatment-related AEs were application-site reactions, including pain, and erythema (Table 4), which generally appeared to increase with increasing treatment duration. The majority of AEs were mild to moderate in severity; 21% of NGX-4010-treated patients reported a severe AE compared with 8% of patients in the control group. The most common severe AE was

Table 3 Integrated efficacy data for the 30- and 60-minute treatment groups

	NGX-4010			Control		
	Total (n = 482)	30 minutes (n = 239)	60 minutes (n = 243)	Total (n = 215)	30 minutes (n = 100)	60 minutes (n = 115)
LS mean change (SE) in NPRS score from baseline to Weeks 2–12	−27.4 (1.4)	−26.9 (2.1)	−27.9 (2.0)	−20.0 (2.1)	−15.8 (3.0)	−24.2 (2.9)
95% CI of LS mean	−30.1, −24.7	−30.8, −23.0	−31.7, −24.0	−24.1, −15.9	−21.8, −9.8	−29.8, −18.6
p-value*	0.0034	0.0024	0.2935	—	—	—
Patients with ≥30% reduction in NPRS score from baseline to Weeks 2–12, n (%)	193 (40)	95 (40)	98 (40)	66 (31)	23 (23)	43 (37)
OR	1.65	2.21	1.22	—	—	—
95% CI of OR	1.15, 2.35	1.29, 3.79	0.77, 1.95	—	—	—
p-value†	0.0062	0.0040	0.3949	—	—	—
PGIC at Week 12	n = 438	n = 220	n = 218	n = 196	n = 92	n = 104
Very much/much/slightly improved, n (%)	294 (67)	143 (65)	151 (69)	97 (49)	38 (41)	59 (57)
p-value‡	<0.0001	0.0001	0.0333	—	—	—

CI confidence interval, *LS* least square, *NPRS* Numeric Pain Rating Scale, *OR* odds ratio, *PGIC* Patient Global Impression of Change, *SE* standard error.
*p-value is computed using weighted gender-stratified ANCOVA to test for difference between each NGX-4010 group and the respective control group, with baseline pain, pre-topical anesthetic pain, and percent change in pain during topical anesthetic application as covariates.
†p-value is computed using logistic regression to test for difference between each NGX-4010 group and the respective control group, with gender, baseline pain, pre-topical anesthetic pain, and percent change in pain as covariates.
‡p-values were computed using Fisher's exact test comparing each NGX-4010 group and the respective control group.

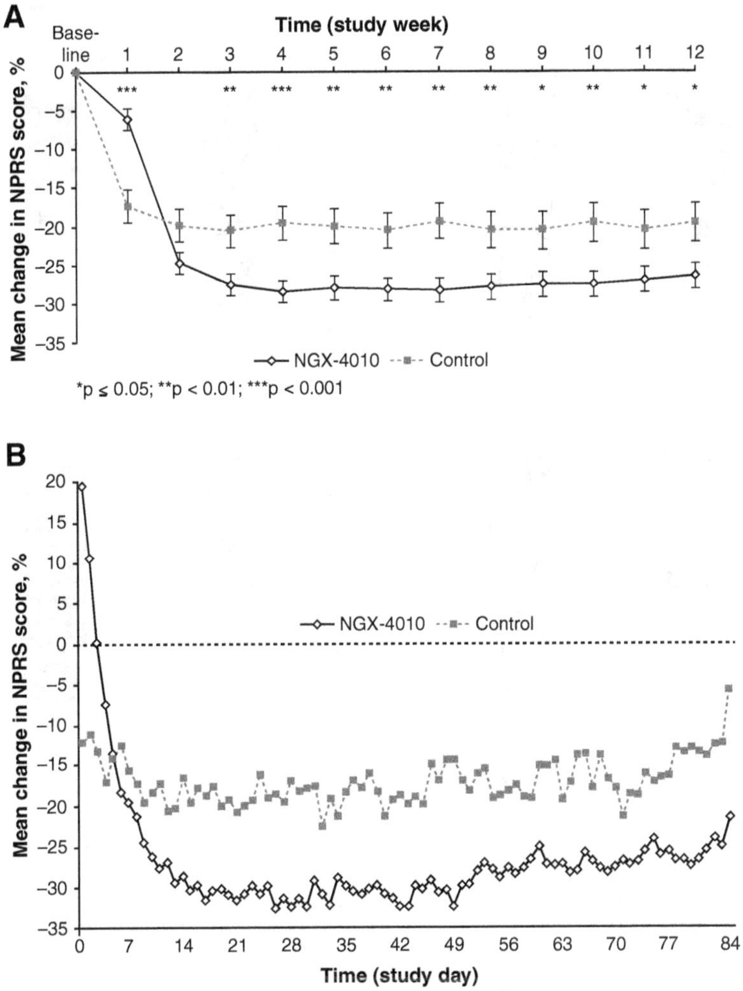

Figure 2 Pain reduction following a single 30-minute application of NGX-4010. (**A**) Weekly analysis of least squares mean change (± standard error) in Numeric Pain Rating Scale (NPRS) score from baseline for the integrated 30-minute treatment group. (**B**) Daily analysis of mean change in NPRS score from baseline for the integrated 30-minute treatment group.

application-site pain and the incidence of severe application-site pain was higher in the 60-minute NGX-4010 group (18%) than in the 30-minute NGX-4010 group (10%).

In the 30-minute treatment groups, 10 (4%) NGX-4010-treated patients and three (3%) control patients reported one or more serious adverse event (SAE). In the 60-minute treatment groups, 19 (8%) NGX-4010-treated patients and eight (7%) control patients reported one or more SAEs. None of the reported SAEs was considered to be related to the study drug.

No clinically important mean changes in hematology, serum chemistry, or vital signs were observed in the NGX-4010 or control groups except for small transient elevations in mean systolic and diastolic blood pressure (<4 mmHg) during and shortly after NGX-4010 application.

Tolerability

NGX-4010 was well tolerated. Nearly all patients in both the 30- and 60-minute NGX-4010 groups completed at least 90% of the intended NGX-4010 application duration (Table 5). Detailed tolerability assessments demonstrated that mean NPRS scores decreased slightly after application of the topical anesthetic and increased after patch application in all treatment groups. In the 60-minute treatment group, mean NPRS scores increased to pre-topical anesthetic levels by 55 minutes post-patch application and remained at that pain level through 1 hour 55 minutes after patch removal; by contrast, the mean NPRS scores for the 30-minute treatment group remained below pretreatment levels through 1 hour 55 minutes after patch removal (data not shown). Application-site pain appeared to be delayed and, at the end of the treatment day, the mean maximum change in "average pain for

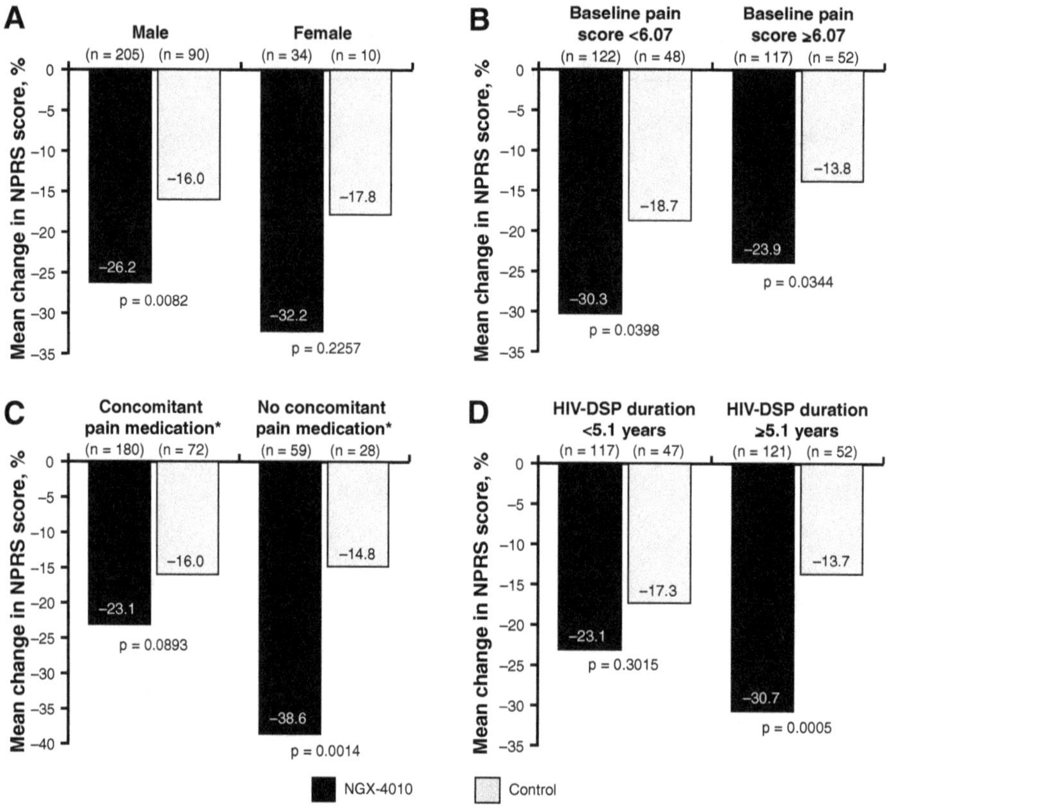

Figure 3 Mean percent change in NPRS score. Change in NPRS score from baseline to Weeks 2–12 for the 30-minute treatment groups. Analysis by subgroup: (**A**) gender; (**B**) baseline pain score; (**C**) concomitant neuropathic pain medication use; and (**D**) duration of HIV-DSP. *A patient was defined as receiving concomitant neuropathic pain medication if he or she was taking an anticonvulsant, non-SSRI antidepressant, or opioid on Day −1 and for a total duration of at least 7 consecutive days.

the past 24 hours" NPRS score from baseline was 2.2 for those treated with NGX-4010 for 60 minutes and 1.5 for those treated with NGX-4010 for 30 minutes. Increases in NPRS score were transient, with pain reductions observed by Day 3 (Figure 2B). The percentage of patients who were administered medication for treatment-related discomfort on the day of treatment or during the 5 days after treatment was higher in the total NGX-4010 group compared with the control group (71% *versus* 31%, $p < 0.0001$). The percentage of patients using medication for treatment-related discomfort was lower in the 30-minute NGX-4010 group compared with the 60-minute treatment group (68% and 74%, respectively).

As expected, on the day of treatment there were significant differences in the distribution of maximum dermal assessment scores between the total NGX-4010 and control groups ($p < 0.0001$). A total of 60% of NGX-4010-treated patients and 44% of control patients had a maximum dermal assessment score of >0. Dermal irritation was commonly mild in the NGX-4010-treatment groups, with dermal assessment scores ≥2 (definite erythema, readily visible, minimal edema, or minimal papular response) being reported in only a few patients (2% and 5%, for the 30- and 60-minute NGX-4010 groups, respectively).

Discussion

The similarity of the demographic and baseline characteristics of the patients from the two multicenter, randomized, double-blind, controlled phase III studies (Table 2), together with comparable study designs, enrollment, and assessment criteria allowed data from the two studies to be combined. The integrated analyses from the two phase III studies demonstrated that a single 30-minute application of NGX-4010 provides significant pain relief — as demonstrated by a decrease in NPRS score — for patients with HIV-DSP for at least 12 weeks. This decrease in the NPRS score of patients receiving a 30-minute NGX-4010 application was supported by the analysis of patient-reported outcomes using the PGIC. The PGIC provides a global assessment of patient improvement that is independent of NPRS score collection. This measurement is recommended in chronic pain studies by the Initiative on Methods, Measurement, and Pain Assessment in Clinical Trials [25] and is more sensitive to treatment effects in

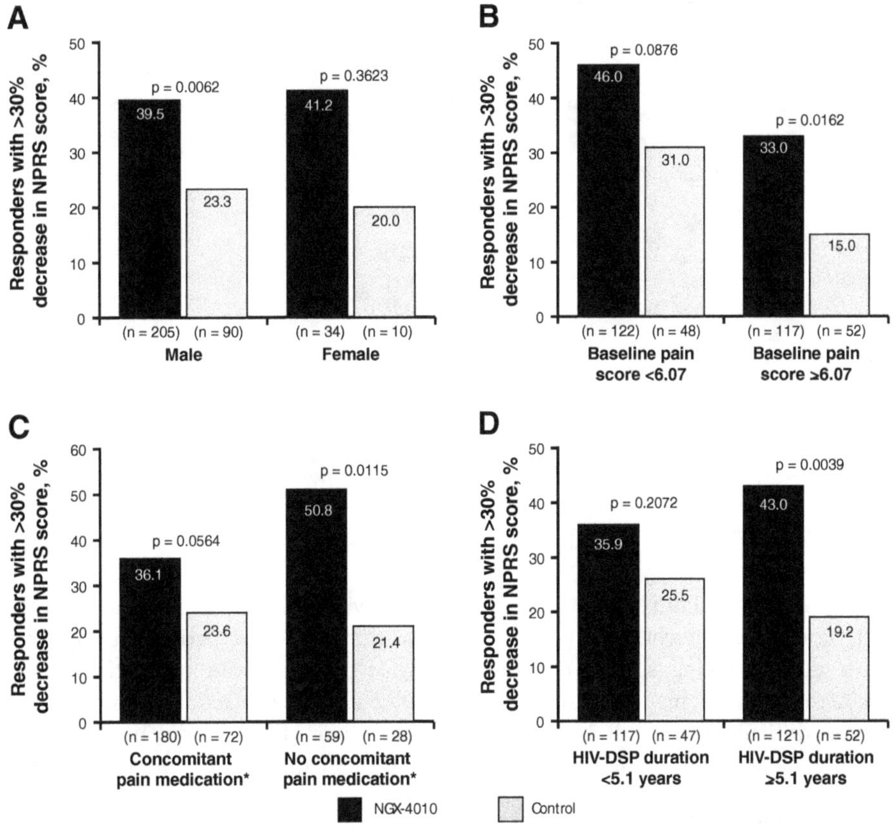

Figure 4 Percentage of patients with ≥30% reduction in NPRS score from baseline to weeks 2–12. Patients in the 30-minute treatment groups; analysis by subgroup: (**A**) gender; (**B**) baseline pain score; (**C**) concomitant neuropathic pain medication use; and (**D**) duration of HIV-DSP. *Concomitant medication was defined as in Figure 3.

neuropathic pain than pain intensity measurements [26]. Using the PGIC, 12 weeks after a single application of NGX-4010, 65% of patients felt slightly, much, or very much improved compared with 41% of control patients.

The reduction in NPRS score following the 60-minute application of NGX-4010 was not significantly different from control. This is likely due to the large effects of the control patch observed in study C119 [23]. Interestingly, there was a significant improvement using the PGIC in the 60-minute treatment compared with the control group.

The data presented here show no evidence of increased efficacy with increased NGX-4010 treatment duration and support the selection of the 30-minute dose for treatment of peripheral neuropathic pain in patients with HIV-associated neuropathy. By contrast, for patients with post-herpetic neuralgia who typically experience neuropathic pain on the torso as opposed to the extremities, treatment duration is 60 minutes [27,28].

A transient increase in pain compared with baseline was seen on Day 0 in patients receiving NGX-4010, due to the treatment procedure. However, treatment-related pain was short-lived, with NPRS scores for patients treated with NGX-4010 for 30 minutes returning to baseline by Day 2. Thereafter, NPRS scores in patients receiving a 30-minute NGX-4010 application continued to decline and NGX-4010-treated patients achieved a greater pain reduction than those in the control group by Day 5 and on each subsequent day through Day 84. Weekly NPRS scores demonstrated significantly greater reductions in pain for NGX-4010-treated patients compared with controls each week from Week 2 to study completion (Week 12).

Subgroup analyses showed greater pain reduction in patients treated with NGX-4010 compared with those treated with control in all subgroups regardless of gender, baseline pain score, concomitant neuropathic pain medication, and HIV-DSP duration. However, NGX-4010 was more effective in patients not using concomitant neuropathic pain medications compared with those using concomitant neuropathic pain medications. This result is not unexpected as it has been shown previously that the additional reduction of neuropathic pain obtained with an add-on drug is generally not as large as the benefit obtained with monotherapy [29,30]. This may be because some of the pathophysiologic mechanisms implicated in the generation and maintenance of neuropathic pain overlap or converge to a common

Table 4 The most common treatment-related AEs*

System organ class preferred term, n(%)	NGX-4010			Control		
	Total (n = 482)	30 minutes (n = 239)	60 minutes (n = 243)	Total (n = 215)	30 minutes (n = 99)	60 minutes (n = 116)
Number of patients reporting ≥1 treatment-related AE	373 (77)	175 (73)	198 (81)	111 (52)	51 (52)	60 (52)
General disorders and administration-site conditions	369 (77)	173 (72)	196 (81)	108 (50)	51 (52)	57 (49)
Application-site dryness	24 (5)	9 (4)	15 (6)	2 (1)	1 (1)	1 (1)
Application-site erythema	177 (37)	80 (33)	97 (40)	58 (27)	24 (24)	34 (29)
Application-site edema	10 (2)	2 (1)	8 (3)	2 (1)	0	2 (2)
Application-site pain	312 (65)	152 (64)	160 (66)	67 (31)	36 (36)	31 (27)
Application-site papules	20 (4)	9 (4)	11 (5)	1 (<1)	0	1 (1)
Application-site paresthesia	10 (2)	7 (3)	3 (1)	3 (1)	1 (1)	2 (2)
Application-site pruritus	38 (8)	18 (8)	20 (8)	4 (2)	1 (1)	3 (3)
Application-site swelling	17 (4)	4 (2)	13 (5)	4 (2)	2 (2)	2 (2)

AE adverse event.
*Includes AEs experienced by ≥2% of patients in any of the total treatment groups.

pathway, resulting in a less than additive effect even for medications that act via different mechanistic pathways. Furthermore, patients already taking several concomitant neuropathic pain medications may be more treatment resistant or more difficult to treat. It is therefore important to note that a significant treatment effect was seen with NGX-4010 compared with control, despite two-thirds of the patients using concomitant neuropathic pain medication at study entry and during the study (Table 2). Gender, baseline pain score, and the duration of HIV-DSP did not influence NGX-4010 efficacy, indicating that pain relief can be achieved with

Table 5 Summary of tolerability on the treatment day

	NGX-4010			Control		
	Total (n = 482)	30 minutes (n = 239)	60 minutes (n = 243)	Total (n = 215)	30 minutes (n = 99)	60 minutes (n = 116)
Change in NPRS score from pre-topical anesthetic time point at the last observation*						
Mean (SD)	1.8 (2.9)	1.5 (3.0)	2.2 (2.8)	−0.2 (2.3)	−0.1 (2.0)	−0.4 (2.5)
p-value†	<0.0001	<0.0001	<0.0001	—	—	—
Patients with at least 90% of the intended patch application duration, n (%)	482 (100)	239 (100)	243 (100)	214 (100)	98 (99)	116 (100)
p-value‡	0.1340	0.2912	0.2872	—	—	—
Patients using medication for treatment-related discomfort on Days 0–5, n (%)	342 (71)	162 (68)	180 (74)	67 (31)	29 (29)	38 (33)
p-value§	<0.0001	<0.0001	<0.0001	—	—	—
Maximum dermal irritation‖ score on Day 0, n (%)						
0	198 (41)	111 (46)	87 (36)	121 (56)	56 (57)	65 (56)
1	135 (28)	66 (28)	69 (28)	69 (32)	33 (33)	36 (31)
2	133 (28)	58 (24)	75 (31)	24 (11)	10 (10)	14 (12)
>2	16 (3)	4 (2)	12 (5)	1 (1)	0 (0)	1 (1)
p-value**	<0.0001	0.001	<0.0001	—	—	—

NPRS Numeric Pain Rating Scale, *SD* standard deviation.
*Includes the evening of the treatment day.
† p-value was computed using a Wilcoxon rank-sum test comparing the means between each NGX-4010 group and the pooled control group.
‡ p-value was computed using a Pearson's chi-square test comparing the percentages of patients between each NGX-4010 group and the pooled control group.
§ p-value was computed using a Fisher's exact test comparing the percentages of patients between each NGX-4010 group and the pooled control group.
‖Dermal irritation assessed by scoring the irritation from 0–7 where 0=no evidence of irritation, 1=minimal erythema, barely perceptible, 2=definite erythema, readily visible, minimal edema or minimal papular response, 3=erythema and papules, 4=definite edema, 5=erythema, edema, and papules, 6=vesicular eruption, and 7=strong reaction spreading beyond test [24].
** p-value was computed using an exact Cochran–Mantel–Haenszel test comparing the distribution of scores between each NGX-4010 group and the pooled control group.

NGX-4010 treatment even in those patients with high pain levels or long disease duration.

Although NGX-4010 application does cause some treatment-related pain, it is generally mild or moderate and transient. The vast majority of patients were able to tolerate >90% of the intended NGX-4010 application. Most common treatment-related AEs were application-site reactions; systemic effects were limited to small, transient elevations in mean systolic and diastolic blood pressure shortly after NGX-4010 application due to treatment-associated increases in pain.

Conclusions

With the current lack of effective treatment for pain associated with HIV-DSP, a therapy such as NGX-4010, which can deliver rapid and prolonged pain relief for at least 3 months after a single 30-minute application, may be of great benefit to patients with HIV-DSP. In addition to its efficacy, there are few systemic AEs associated with NGX-4010 [31], unlike other available therapies, and repeated applications of NGX-4010 do not result in an increased incidence of application-site AEs, dermal irritation, intolerability, or impaired neurologic function [32]. Efficacy has been demonstrated when NGX-4010 is used alone as well as in combination with other systemic medications for neuropathic pain. Treatment with NGX-4010 neither increases the pill burden nor the potential for systemic drug–drug interactions, two important considerations for patients with HIV-DSP, who may already be taking several medications. Data from these two phase III clinical trials have led to the approval of NGX-4010 for the treatment of HIV-DSP in the EU and have resulted in NGX-4010 being given a level A efficacy rating in the European Federation of Neurological Sciences guidelines for HIV neuropathy [33].

Methods

Enrollment

Details of each of the studies included in this analysis have been reported previously [22,23]. Both studies were approved by institutional review boards/independent ethics committees and conducted in accordance with the ethical principles of the Declaration of Helsinki, Good Clinical Practice guidelines, and applicable regulatory requirements.

Both studies recruited patients who were ≥18 years of age with a diagnosis of HIV-DSP for ≥2 months and an average baseline NPRS score [34] of 3–9. Patients taking other pain medications such as anticonvulsants, non-selective serotonin reuptake inhibitor (non-SSRI) antidepressants (e.g., tricyclic antidepressants, serotonin–norepinephrine reuptake inhibitors), opioids, non-steroidal anti-inflammatory drugs, salicylates, or acetaminophen had to be on stable doses for ≥21 days before patch application and remain on stable doses throughout the study period. Exclusion criteria in both studies included the prior use of NGX-4010 and use of a topical medication on the painful area within 21 days before the NGX-4010 application day.

Treatment

Patients were randomly assigned to receive treatment with an NGX-4010 (QUTENZA™/Qutenza®) patch (capsaicin 640 μg/cm^2, 8% w/w; NeurogesX, Inc., San Mateo, CA, USA) or a low-concentration control patch (capsaicin 3.2 μg/cm^2, 0.04% w/w). The control patch produced local erythema and a burning sensation to provide effective blinding in the studies.

Patients were pre-treated with a topical local anesthetic cream (L.M.X.4 lidocaine 4%; Ferndale Laboratories, Inc., Ferndale, MI, USA) for 60 minutes before patch application. Both the NGX-4010 and control patches were applied for 30, 60, or 90 minutes in study C107 [22] and for 30 or 60 minutes in study C119 [23]. After patch removal, the treatment area was cleansed with a proprietary cleansing gel (NeurogesX, Inc.) formulated to remove residual capsaicin. A rapid-onset, opioid-based oral pain medication (e.g., oxycodone hydrochloride oral solution, 1 mg/ml) could be administered at the onset of treatment-associated discomfort and as needed while in the clinic. Following patch removal, local cooling could be used. Patients could also take a short-term regimen of an opioid-based oral pain medication (e.g., hydrocodone bitartrate/acetaminophen 5 mg/500 mg) for treatment-related discomfort for up to 5 or 7 days post treatment, depending on the study.

Assessments

The studies included either a ≥5 day [22] or ≥14 day [23] baseline screening period. Assessments were also carried out on the day of treatment (Day 0), at the termination visit (Week 12), and, depending on the study, at interim visits at Weeks 1 and 4 or 4 and 8 during the 12-week blinded observation period. The primary efficacy endpoint was the mean percent change from baseline in NPRS scores for "average pain for the past 24 hours" from Weeks 2–12. Patients recorded their "average pain for the past 24 hours" every evening at 9:00 pm in paper pain diaries from the baseline screening period until the evening before the termination visit.

Other efficacy measurements included the percentage of patients with ≥30% mean decrease in NPRS score from baseline during Weeks 2–12 and the percentage of those feeling improved according to the PGIC at Week 12. In this assessment patients reported how they felt after treatment compared with before treatment on a 7-point scale with −3 indicating "very much worse" to +3 indicating "very much improved" and 0 indicating "no change".

Safety and tolerability assessments included AEs, vital signs, clinical laboratory tests, physical examination, dermal assessment (0- to 7-point severity score) [24], "pain now" NPRS scores during and after patch application, early patch removal, and use of medication for treatment-related discomfort during Days 0 to 5.

Efficacy analyses

Data from patients receiving NGX-4010 and control patches for 30 or 60 minutes were integrated from both phase III HIV-DSP studies. The 90-minute NGX-4010 dose was not included in these analyses as it was not evaluated in study C119 [23]. Intent-to-treat efficacy analyses consisted of all patients who received any study treatment and had at least 3 days of available NPRS scores during the baseline period. The primary efficacy endpoint was the percent change in NPRS scores from baseline during Weeks 2–12. Changes in NPRS scores from baseline to Weeks 2–12 were compared between treatment groups using a pre-specified gender-stratified ANCOVA model with baseline pain score, pre-topical anesthetic pain score, and percent change in pain score after topical anesthetic treatment as covariates. To avoid the potentially confounding effect of opioid medications allowed during Days 0–5, Week 1 NPRS scores were not included in the primary endpoint analysis. In addition, least square means of the difference between treatment groups and the 95% confidence interval (CI) were calculated.

Missing post-treatment NPRS scores were imputed using a modified last observation carried forward approach. If the NPRS score was missing on post-treatment Days 0–8 or on Day 8 and one or more consecutive days, then the baseline score was imputed for those days. If the NPRS score was missing for any day after Day 8, then the missing score was imputed by the last available non-imputed score recorded before that day. If all post-treatment NPRS scores were missing (including Day 0), all scores were imputed using the baseline score. NPRS baseline scores were calculated using all available screening scores that were not biased by pain medication changes [22] or using all available screening scores between Day −14 and Day −1 [23]. For the weekly and the daily NPRS scores, missing scores were not imputed.

The percentage of responders (classified as those achieving ≥30% reduction in NPRS score from baseline) was compared between groups using logistic regression analyses, with baseline pain score, gender, pre-topical anesthetic pain score, and percent change in pain score after topical anesthetic treatment as covariates. In addition, odds ratios and the 95% CI of observing responses in the NGX-4010 group compared with the control group were estimated. The percentage of patients reporting improvements according to the PGIC was compared between treatment groups using Fisher's exact test. For both the primary endpoint and responder analysis, the treatment effect was assessed by gender, baseline pain score (median NPRS score of < and ≥6.07), HIV-DSP duration (median of < and ≥5.2 years), and concomitant neuropathic pain medication use at study entry (defined as receiving an anticonvulsant, non-SSRI antidepressant or opioid on Day −1 and for at least 7 consecutive days) in patients treated for 30 minutes.

Safety and tolerability analyses

AEs were coded using the Medical Dictionary for Regulatory Activities version 9.0. Medication use for treatment-related discomfort (from Days 0–5) and the percentage of patients completing the intended patch duration were compared using Fisher's exact test. The percentages of patients reporting each level of dermal response were compared using the Cochran–Mantel–Haenszel test. The maximum changes in "pain now" NPRS score from the pre-topical anesthetic time point during and after patch application were summarized and compared using the Wilcoxon rank sum test.

Patients were analyzed as randomized for the efficacy analyses and as treated for the safety analyses.

Abbreviations

AE: Adverse event; ANCOVA: Analysis of covariance; CI: Confidence interval; HIV-DSP: HIV-associated neuropathy; LS: Least square; NPRS: Numerical Pain Rating Scale; OR: Odds ratio; PGIC: Patient Global Impression of Change; rhNGF: Recombinant-human nerve growth factor; SD: Standard deviation; SE: Standard error; TRPV1: Transient Receptor Potential Vanilloid 1.

Competing interests

DMS has received consultancy fees and/or honorarium or speaker fees from NeurogesX, Astellas Pharma Europe Ltd., Eli Lilly and Pfizer. DMS's institute has received grants from NeurogesX, Astra Zeneca and Pfizer. MF has received speaker fees and funding to attend a conference from Astellas. SB's institute, AIDS Research Alliance, received grants to conduct the research. GS received funds as site investigator. JKT and GFV are former employees of NeurogesX and still own stock in NeurogesX.

Authors' contributions

SB, DMS, GM, BJB, GS, NL, CO, and MF conducted the study, interpreted the data, and edited the manuscript. GFV and JKT designed the study, analyzed and interpreted the data, and prepared the manuscript. All authors read and approved the final manuscript.

Acknowledgements

Funding for these studies was provided by NeurogesX, Inc. Editorial assistance was provided by Adelphi Communications, supported by Astellas Pharma Europe Ltd.

Author details

[1]AIDS Research Alliance, Los Angeles, CA, USA. [2]Mount Sinai School of Medicine, New York, NY, USA. [3]Chelsea and Westminster Hospital, London, United Kingdom. [4]St Vincent's Hospital, Darlinghurst, Australia. [5]University of Rochester, Rochester, NY, USA. [6]St Thomas' Hospital, London, United Kingdom. [7]Andrews Out Patients Unit, London, United Kingdom. [8]HIV/GUM Research, Elton John Centre, Brighton, United Kingdom. [9]NeurogesX, Inc, San Mateo, CA, USA.

References

1. Ferrari S, Vento S, Monaco S, Cavallaro T, Cainelli F, Rizzuto N, Temesgen Z: **Human immunodeficiency virus-associated peripheral neuropathies.** *Mayo Clin Proc* 2006, **81**:213–219.
2. Gonzalez-Duarte A, Robinson-Papp J, Simpson DM: **Diagnosis and management of HIV-associated neuropathy.** *Neurol Clin* 2008, **26**:821–832.
3. McArthur JC, Brew BJ, Nath A: **Neurological complications of HIV infection.** *Lancet Neurol* 2005, **4**:543–555.
4. Ellis RJ, Rosario D, Clifford DB, McArthur JC, Simpson D, Alexander T, Gelman BB, Vaida F, Collier A, Marra CM, Ances B, Atkinson JH, Dworkin RH, Morgello S, Grant I: **Continued high prevalence and adverse clinical impact of human immunodeficiency virus-associated sensory neuropathy in the era of combination antiretroviral therapy: the CHARTER study.** *Arch Neurol* 2010, **67**:552–558.
5. Kieburtz K, Simpson D, Yiannoutsos C, Max MB, Hall CD, Ellis RJ, Marra CM, McKendall R, Singer E, Dal Pan GJ, Clifford DB, Tucker T, Cohen B: **A randomized trial of amitriptyline and mexiletine for painful neuropathy in HIV infection. AIDS clinical trial group 242 protocol team.** *Neurology* 1998, **51**:1682–1688.
6. Simpson DM, Schifitto G, Clifford DB, Murphy TK, Durso-De Cruz E, Glue P, Whalen E, Emir B, Scott GN, Freeman R: **Pregabalin for painful HIV neuropathy: a randomized, double-blind, placebo-controlled trial.** *Neurology* 2010, **74**:413–420.
7. Estanislao L, Carter K, McArthur J, Olney R, Simpson D: **A randomized controlled trial of 5% lidocaine gel for HIV-associated distal symmetric polyneuropathy.** *J Acquir Immune Defic Syndr* 2004, **37**:1584–1586.
8. Paice JA, Ferrans CE, Lashley FR, Shott S, Vizgirda V, Pitrak D: **Topical capsaicin in the management of HIV-associated peripheral neuropathy.** *J Pain Symptom Manage* 2000, **19**:45–52.
9. Abrams DI, Jay CA, Shade SB, Vizoso H, Reda H, Press S, Kelly ME, Rowbotham MC, Petersen KL: **Cannabis in painful HIV-associated sensory neuropathy: a randomized placebo-controlled trial.** *Neurology* 2007, **68**:515–521.
10. Ellis RJ, Toperoff W, Vaida F, van den BG, Gonzales J, Gouaux B, Bentley H, Atkinson JH: **Smoked medicinal cannabis for neuropathic pain in HIV: a randomized, crossover clinical trial.** *Neuropsychopharmacology* 2009, **34**:672–680.
11. Ware MA, Wang T, Shapiro S, Robinson A, Ducruet T, Huynh T, Gamsa A, Bennett GJ, Collet JP: **Smoked cannabis for chronic neuropathic pain: a randomized controlled trial.** *CMAJ* 2010, **182**:E694–E701.
12. O'Connor AB, Dworkin RH: **Treatment of neuropathic pain: an overview of recent guidelines.** *Am J Med* 2009, **122**(10 Suppl):S22–S32.
13. Koeppe J, Armon C, Lyda K, Nielsen C, Johnson S: **Ongoing pain despite aggressive opioid pain management among persons with HIV.** *Clin J Pain* 2010, **26**:190–198.
14. Phillips TJ, Cherry CL, Cox S, Marshall SJ, Rice AS: **Pharmacological treatment of painful HIV-associated sensory neuropathy: a systematic review and meta-analysis of randomised controlled trials.** *PLoS One* 2010, **5**:e14433.
15. Schifitto G, Yiannoutsos C, Simpson DM, Adornato BT, Singer EJ, Hollander H, Marra CM, Rubin M, Cohen BA, Tucker T, Koralnik IJ, Katzenstein D, Haidich B, Smith ME, Shriver S, Millar L, Clifford DB, McArthur JC: **Long-term treatment with recombinant nerve growth factor for HIV-associated sensory neuropathy.** *Neurology* 2001, **57**:1313–1316.
16. Caterina MJ, Julius D: **The vanilloid receptor: a molecular gateway to the pain pathway.** *Annu Rev Neurosci* 2001, **24**:487–517.
17. Polydefkis M, Yiannoutsos CT, Cohen BA, Hollander H, Schifitto G, Clifford DB, Simpson DM, Katzenstein D, Shriver S, Hauer P, Brown A, Haidich AB, Moo L, McArthur JC: **Reduced intraepidermal nerve fiber density in HIV-associated sensory neuropathy.** *Neurology* 2002, **58**:115–119.
18. Ma W, Zhang Y, Bantel C, Eisenach JC: **Medium and large injured dorsal root ganglion cells increase TRPV-1, accompanied by increased alpha2C-adrenoceptor co-expression and functional inhibition by clonidine.** *Pain* 2005, **113**:386–394.
19. Bley KR: **TRPV1 agonist approaches for pain management.** In *Vanilloid Receptor TRPV1 in Drug Discovery*. Edited by Gomtsyan A, Faltynek CR. Hoboken, NJ, USA: John Wiley & Sons, Inc; 2010:325–347.
20. Szallasi A, Blumberg PM: **Vanilloid (capsaicin) receptors and mechanisms.** *Pharmacol Rev* 1999, **51**:159–212.
21. Kennedy WR, Vanhove GF, Lu SP, Tobias J, Bley KR, Walk D, Wendelschafer-Crabb G, Simone DA, Selim MM: **A randomized, controlled, open-label study of the long-term effects of NGX-4010, a high-concentration capsaicin patch, on epidermal nerve fiber density and sensory function in healthy volunteers.** *J Pain* 2010, **11**:579–587.
22. Simpson DM, Brown S, Tobias J: **Controlled trial of high-concentration capsaicin patch for treatment of painful HIV neuropathy.** *Neurology* 2008, **70**:2305–2313.
23. Clifford DB, Simpson DM, Brown S, Moyle G, Brew BJ, Conway B, Tobias JK, Vanhove GF: **A randomized, double-blind, controlled study of NGX-4010, a capsaicin 8% dermal patch, for the treatment of painful HIV-associated distal sensory polyneuropathy.** *J Acquir Immune Defic Syndr* 2012, **59**:126–133.
24. US Food and Drug Administration Center for Drug Evaluation and Research: *Guidance for industry: Skin irritation and sensitization testing of generic transdermal drug products.* Washington, DC, USA: US Department of Health and Human Services; 1999. www.fda.gov/ohrms/dockets/98fr/990236Gd.pdf#search=%22HillTop%20Research%2C%20Inc.%20dermal%20irritation%22.
25. Dworkin RH, Turk DC, Farrar JT, Haythornthwaite JA, Jensen MP, Katz NP, Kerns RD, Stucki G, Allen RR, Bellamy N, Carr DB, Chandler J, Cowan P, Dionne R, Galer BS, Hertz S, Jadad AR, Kramer LD, Manning DC, Martin S, McCormick CG, McDermott MP, McGrath P, Quessy S, Rappaport BA, Robbins W, Robinson JP, Rothman M, Royal MA, Simon L, Stauffer JW, Stein W, Tollett J, Wernicke J, Witter J: **Core outcome measures for chronic pain clinical trials: IMMPACT recommendations.** *Pain* 2005, **113**:9–19.
26. Haanpää M, Attal N, Backonja M, Baron R, Bennett M, Bouhassira D, Cruccu G, Hansson P, Haythornthwaite JA, Iannetti GD, Jensen TS, Kauppila T, Nurmikko TJ, Rice AS, Rowbotham M, Serra J, Sommer C, Smith BH, Treede RD: **NeuPSIG guidelines on neuropathic pain assessment.** *Pain* 2011, **152**:14–27.
27. Backonja M, Wallace MS, Blonsky ER, Cutler BJ, Malan P Jr, Rauck R, Tobias J: **NGX-4010, a high-concentration capsaicin patch, for the treatment of postherpetic neuralgia: a randomised, double-blind study.** *Lancet Neurol* 2008, **7**:1106–1112.
28. Webster LR, Malan TP, Tuchman MM, Mollen MD, Tobias JK, Vanhove GF: **A multicenter, randomized, double-blind, controlled dose finding study of NGX-4010, a high-concentration capsaicin patch, for the treatment of postherpetic neuralgia.** *J Pain* 2010, **11**:972–982.
29. Gilron I, Bailey JM, Tu D, Holden RR, Weaver DF, Houlden RL: **Morphine, gabapentin, or their combination for neuropathic pain.** *N Engl J Med* 2005, **352**:1324–1334.
30. Gilron I, Bailey JM, Tu D, Holden RR, Jackson AC, Houlden RL: **Nortriptyline and gabapentin, alone and in combination for neuropathic pain: a double-blind, randomised controlled crossover trial.** *Lancet* 2009, **374**:1252–1261.
31. Vanhove GF, Wallace M, Irving G, Backonja M, Webster LR, Tobias JK: **Integrated safety analyses of NGX-4010, an 8% capsaicin patch, in patients with peripheral neuropathic pain.** In *13th World Congress on Pain; August 29-September 2, 2010*. Montréal, Québec, Canada; 2010. Abstract [PH 101].
32. Simpson DM, Gazda S, Brown S, Webster LR, Lu SP, Tobias JK, Vanhove GF: **Long-term safety of NGX-4010, a high-concentration capsaicin patch, in patients with peripheral neuropathic pain.** *J Pain Symptom Manage* 2010, **39**:1053–1064.
33. Attal N, Cruccu G, Baron R, Haanpaa M, Hansson P, Jensen TS, Nurmikko T: **EFNS guidelines on the pharmacological treatment of neuropathic pain: 2010 revision.** *Eur J Neurol* 2010, **17**:1113–1188.
34. Farrar JT, Young JP Jr, LaMoreaux L, Werth JL, Poole RM: **Clinical importance of changes in chronic pain intensity measured on an 11-point numerical pain rating scale.** *Pain* 2001, **94**:149–158.

4

Risk factors of chronic hepatitis in antiretroviral-treated HIV infection, without hepatitis B or C viral infection

Thep Chalermchai[1,2], Narin Hiransuthikul[1*], Pisit Tangkijvanich[3], Suteeraporn Pinyakorn[4], Anchalee Avihingsanon[4,5] and Jintanat Ananworanich[2,4,5]

Abstract

Background: Increasing rates of non-AIDS defining illnesses, and in particular liver diseases, have been found after the initiation of highly active antiretroviral therapy. However, there is little evidence concerning the risk factors for and clinical characteristics of liver disease in antiretroviral (ARV)-treated HIV infection, in the absence of hepatitis B or C viral co-infection.

Methods: A nested case–control study of HIV infected volunteers, matched by starting date of anti-retroviral treatment, was conducted in a Thai cohort studied from Nov 2002 - July 2012. Cases were defined as those subjects with an elevated alanine aminotransferase (ALT ≥ 40 IU/L) at two consecutive visits six months apart, while controls were defined as individuals who never demonstrated two consecutive elevated ALT results and had a normal ALT result (< 40 IU/L) at their last visit. Both groups had normal ALT levels prior to ARV initiation. Clinical demographics and risk factors for chronic hepatitis including HIV-related illness, ARV treatment and metabolic diseases were collected and analyzed. Conditional logistic regression was used to determine risk factors for chronic hepatitis in HIV infection.

Results: A total of 124 matched pairs with HIV infection were followed over 3,195 person-years. The mean age (±SD) was 33.0 ± 7.3 years, with 41.1% of subjects being male. The incidence of chronic hepatitis was 5.4 per 100 person-years. The median time from initiation of ARV to chronic hepatitis was 1.3 years (IQR, 0.5-3.5). From univariate analysis; male sex, plasma HIV-1 RNA level > 5 $\log_{10}$ copies/ml, metabolic syndrome at baseline visit, high BMI > 23 kg/m^2, abnormal HDL cholesterol at time of ALT elevation and treatment experience with NNRTI plus boosted PI were selected (p value < 0.2) to the final model of multivariate analysis. Male sex had 3.1 times greater risk of chronic hepatitis than the females by multivariate analysis (adjusted OR, 95% CI: 3.1, 1.5-6.3, p =0.002). High BMI ≥ 23 kg/m^2 was also associated with 2.4 times greater risk of chronic hepatitis (adjusted OR, 95% CI: 2.4, 1.2-4.8, p = 0.01).

Conclusions: Chronic hepatitis in ARV-treated HIV-infected patients is common and may lead to a major health care problem. Male sex and high BMI ≥ 23 kg/m^2 carry higher risks for developing chronic hepatitis in this study. Therefore, these patients should be closely monitored for long-term hepatotoxicity.

Keywords: Chronic hepatitis, HIV infection, Risk factors

* Correspondence: nhiransu@gmail.com
[1]Department of Preventive and Social Medicine, Faculty of Medicine, Chulalongkorn University, Bangkok, Thailand

Background

Human immunodeficiency virus (HIV) infection continues to be a major global health problem. An estimated 33.4 million people are currently living with HIV worldwide [1]. The era of highly active antiretroviral therapy (HAART) for the treatment of HIV-infected individuals has led to a dramatic reduction in AIDS-defining illnesses and mortality [2]. However, an inverse trend has also been observed with increasing rates of non-AIDS defining illnesses including liver diseases manifesting themselves in the context of longer life expectancy [3,4]. Little is known about the risk factors for and clinical characteristics of liver disease in Asian HIV infection. Manifestations of liver disease in HIV infection include mild, asymptomatic rises in liver transaminase levels, chronic steatohepatitis, liver cirrhosis and more severe forms resulting in hepatic failure. In general, chronic liver disease in HIV mono-infected patients usually present with no or only mild symptoms and rising serum transaminase levels [5]. Research into the HIV-infected subgroup with mildly elevated transaminase levels is so far minimal. Previous studies suggested that the majority of mild, asymptomatic chronic hepatitis in HIV infection were undiagnosed [5]. Failure or delay in the diagnosis and treatment of liver disease in HIV infection may result in long-term liver morbidities such as chronic steatohepatitis, liver cirrhosis or hepatocellular carcinoma and, importantly, may also increase the rate of liver-related mortality [6].

The etiologies of liver disease seen in HIV infection include hepatitis B or C virus co-infection, medication-induced hepatitis from antiretroviral (ARV) or non-ARV drugs (such as anti-tuberculous and anti-lipemic agents), metabolic syndrome, excessive alcohol consumption and HIV infection itself [3].

ARV medications that commonly result in rising transaminase in HIV infection include stavudine (d4T), nevirapine (NVP) and high dose ritonavir (RTV) [7-9]. Other reported risk factors were being men who has sex with men (MSM), and having a history of arterial hypertension or a body mass index (BMI) greater than 25 kg/m^2 [9-11].

Chronic hepatitis in HIV infection has also been associated with poor HIV-specific treatment outcomes, such as current CD4+ T-lymphocyte counts < 200 cells/mm^3 and detectable HIV-1 RNA levels [11].

Previous studies of chronic hepatitis in HIV infection were mostly cross-sectional. Most of the studies were conducted in developed countries. There is a lack of clinical evidence in developing countries especially in patients treated with ARV. Results from this study will support healthcare personnel in understanding and selecting appropriate treatment for a resource-limited setting.

This study aims to determine clinical demographic and the risk factors of chronic hepatitis in ARV-treated, HIV-infected Thai patients without hepatitis B or C co-infection who were followed longitudinally for up to 10 years.

Materials and methods

We conducted a nested case–control study utilizing data from a long term observational study (Clinical trial.gov, NCT 00411983) for HIV-infected individuals who had previously participated in clinical studies and continued into a long term cohort after the completion of the specific study. The study participants were scheduled for follow-up at The HIV Netherlands Australia Thailand Research Collaboration or HIV-NAT clinic in Bangkok, Thailand on a semi-annual basis to monitor their long-term outcomes for AIDS-defining and non-AIDS defining illnesses as well as adverse events from ARV treatment. Medical history, physical examination and history of ARV treatment were recorded. Subjects underwent blood draw for complete blood count (CBC), serum alanine aminotransferase level (ALT) and serum creatinine level. CD4+ T lymphocyte counts and HIV-1 RNA levels were also measured at each study visit.

Our study focused on liver complications in HIV without hepatitis B or C co-infection. The inclusion criteria were HIV-infected individuals, older than 18 years of age, negative hepatitis B surface antigen (HBs Ag) or HBV DNA and negative HCV antibody (anti-HCV) or HCV RNA. Exclusion criteria were patients who did not have a recorded viral hepatitis serology result, had an abnormal ALT level at their baseline visit or prior to ARV treatment (ALT ≥40 IU/L), unavailable baseline ALT level or had less than 12 months of follow up. Written, informed consent was obtained from all enrollees. This specific study was approved by the Ethics Committee of the Faculty of Medicine, Chulalongkorn University, Bangkok, Thailand.

For this case–control study, the cases, or chronic hepatitis was defined as those with elevated ALT ≥ 40 IU/L at 2 consecutive visits 6 months apart after the initiation of ARV [7,8]. The controls was defined as those patients who never had two consecutive ALT ≥ 40 IU/L and still had normal ALT at the last visit. Both groups had normal ALT at pre-ARV initiation (baseline).

The case and control were matched 1:1 for duration from ARV initiation (± 6 months).

All clinical data and laboratory testing for comparison were selected by utilizing data at baseline and at the time chronic hepatitis occurred in the cases and the data at the same period (± 6 months) for the matched controls.

All analytic data for this study were censored on July 1, 2012.

The duration of the study was calculated from the time of initiation of ARV to the last follow-up visit.

The onset of chronic hepatitis was calculated from the time of ARV initiation to the diagnosis of chronic hepatitis.

Definitions

HIV infection was defined by a positive result for HIV-specific antibodies by enzyme-linked immunosorbent assay (ELISA) and/or HIV-1 RNA by the Roche Amplicor HIV-1 Monitor Test v1.5.

Hepatitis B virus infection was defined by a positive result for HBsAg using the ARCHITECT HBsAg qualitative assay (ABBOTT Max-Planck-Ring 2, Germany) and/or detectable HBV DNA by polymerase chain reaction (PCR).

Hepatitis C virus infection was defined by a positive result for HCV-specific antibodies using the ARCHITECT Anti-HCV assay or detectable HCV RNA by PCR.

Severity grading of chronic hepatitis was classified according to the following ranges of ALT level: grade 1, 1.0 – 2.5 times the upper limit of normal (1.0-2.5 × ULN); grade 2, 2.6–5.0 × ULN; grade 3, 5.1–10 × ULN; grade 4, >10 × ULN. Severe hepatitis was defined by at least grade 3 ALT elevation [12].

Severity of HIV infection was classified by Centers for Disease Control and Prevention (CDC) 1993 guidelines [13].

Body mass index (BMI) was calculated as weight in kilograms divided by height in meters squared. BMI categories specific for Asian individuals were assigned as follows: BMI <18.5 (underweight), BMI = 18.5 – 22.9 (normal), BMI = 23–24.9 (overweight) and BMI ≥25.0 (obese) [14].

Dyslipidemia was defined as serum triglyceride level ≥ 150 mg/dL, HDL-cholesterol ≤ 40 mg/dL for males, ≤ 50 mg/dL for females, LDL-cholesterol ≥ 130 mg/dL and total cholesterol ≥200 mg/dL [15,16].

Elevated blood pressure was defined as a systolic blood pressure > 130 mmHg or diastolic blood pressure > 85 mmHg, or known history of hypertension [16].

Impaired fasting plasma glucose was defined as a fasting plasma glucose ≥ 100 mg/dL or known history of diabetes mellitus [16].

Metabolic syndrome was defined as having at least 3 of 5 criteria serum triglyceride level ≥150 mg/dL, serum HDL-cholesterol ≤40 mg/dL for male or ≤50 mg/dL for females, elevated blood pressure, impaired fasting plasma glucose and BMI ≥ 23 kg/m2 or waist circumference ≥ 90 cm. for male or ≥ 80 cm. for females [14].

Clinically-diagnosed lipodystrophy was defined as those with lipoatrophy or lipohypertrophy, truncal obesity or facial lipodystrophy [17].

The main risk factors that were evaluated included clinical characteristics [age, gender, sexual risk behavior, HIV-related illness and disease severity, baseline CD4^{+} T lymphocyte counts, plasma HIV-1 RNA level and metabolic diseases] and clinical parameters and laboratory assessments at an event visit [previous history of ARV treatment, concomitant medications, clinical and laboratory findings of HIV-related illnesses and metabolic diseases].

Statistical and data analysis

Clinical characteristics were described as frequency and percentage for categological data. Continuous data were

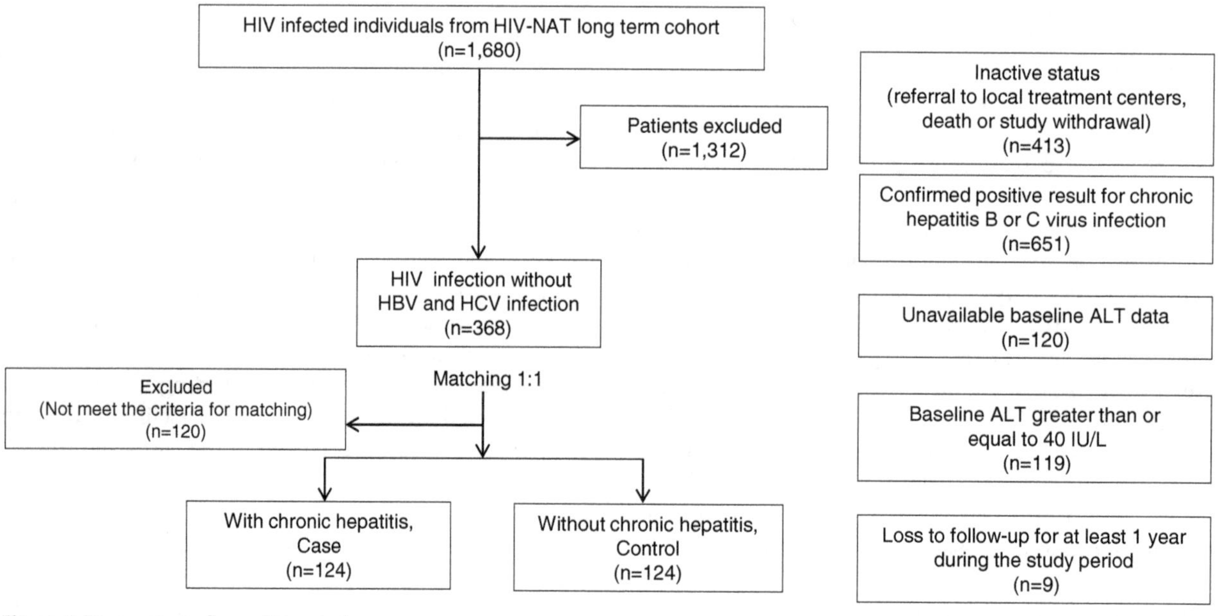

Figure 1 Demonstrate flow of the study.

reported as mean ($\bar{x}$) and standard deviation (SD) if normally distributed or as median and inter-quartile range (IQR) if not normally distributed [18]. For inferential data analysis, the McNemar's test was used for categorical data. For continuous data, the paired student's t-test was used if the data had normal distribution, while the Wilcoxon signed-rank test was used if they showed non-normal distribution. Factors with p value less than 0.2 from univariate analysis were selected to the model of multivariate analysis. Conditional stepwise, logistic regression was used to evaluate the risk factors of chronic hepatitis. Odds ratio (OR) and adjusted OR with 95% confidence intervals (CI) were reported to demonstrate an association between significant factors with chronic hepatitis. Statistical significance was defined as a p value less than 0.05. We used STATA/LC version 11.2 for Windows.

Results

A total of 1,680 HIV-infected individuals participated in the long term HIV-NAT cohort during the period of November 2002 to July 2012. We excluded individuals from the present study owing to inactive status (referral to local treatment centers, death or study withdrawal) at the time of data analysis (n = 413), a confirmed positive result for chronic hepatitis B or C virus infection (n = 651), unavailable baseline ALT data (n = 120), baseline ALT ≥ 40 IU/L (n = 119) and loss to follow-up for at least 1 year (n = 9) (Figure 1).

Characteristics of chronic hepatitis in cases

There were 124 study cases. An incidence rate of chronic hepatitis was 5.4 per 100 person-years (Table 1). The mean ALT level at the time of diagnosis of chronic hepatitis was 73 ± 107 IU/L [median ALT level was 52 IU/L, (IQR, 46–65)]. There were 98.4% of these individuals who were initially found to have mild ALT (grade 1 or 2) elevation, while 1.6% (n = 2) were found to have severe hepatitis. The mean (±SD) AST level was slightly higher than the normal value (58 ± 49 IU/L). The median duration from the time of an initiation of ARV to the diagnosis of chronic hepatitis was 1.3 years (IQR, 0.5-3.5). The following symptoms were reported at time of ALT elevation; however, their relatedness to ALT elevation cannot be confirmed: nausea and/or vomiting (24.2%), fatigue (11.3%), anorexia (7.3%), flatulence (4.0%) and others (4.8%). All were grades 1 or 2. No abnormal severe symptoms, liver failure or hepatic encephalopathy was reported.

Table 1 Characteristics of chronic hepatitis in cases of HIV patients with chronic non HBV/HCV hepatitis*

Clinical parameters	Case (n =124)
Incidence rate , per 100 person-years	5.4
Median (IQR), duration from starting ARV to hepatitis, years	1.3(0.5–3.5)
Mean ALT level at time of ALT elevation, IU/L (±SD)	73 ± 107
Mean AST level at time of ALT elevation, IU/L (±SD)	58 ± 49
Mean alkaline phosphatase level at time of ALT elevation, IU/L (±SD)	97 ± 54
Severity grading of chronic hepatitis **, n (%)	
o Mild (grade 1 or 2)	122 (98.4)
o Severe, at least grade 3	2 (1.6)
Symptoms at time of ALT elevation, n (%)	
o Any	64(51.6)
o Nausea/ vomiting	30(24.2)
o Fatigue	14(11.3)
o Anorexia	9(7.3)
o Flatulence	5(4.0)
o Weight loss	4(3.2)
o Jaundice	1(0.8)
o Liver tenderness	1(0.8)

Abbreviation: HIV Human immunodeficiency virus, *HBV* Hepatitis B virus, *HCV* Hepatitis C virus, *ALT* Alanine aminotransferase, *AST* Aspartate aminotransferase, *SD* Standard deviation.
* Chronic hepatitis was defined as those with elevated ALT ≥40 IU/L at 2 consecutive visits 6 months apart.
**Severity grading of chronic hepatitis was classified by using ALT level: grade 1, 1.0 – 2.5 times the upper limit of normal (1.0-2.5 × ULN); grade 2, 2.6–5.0 × ULN; grade 3, 5.1–10 × ULN; grade 4, >10 × ULN [12]. Severe hepatitis was defined as having at least grade 3 ALT level.

Baseline demographics

From a total of 124 HIV-infected, matched pairs by the date of starting ARV treatment were selected. Male gender was more commonly found in the cases than the controls. The mean ages in the cases and the controls were similar. The proportion of men who have sex with men (MSM) were slightly higher in the cases than the controls with borderline significance (p = 0.08) (Table 2).

Advanced, HIV-related illnesses were found in 11.3% and 5.6% of the case and control groups respectively. There was no significant difference in the proportions of CD4+ cell count less than 200 cells/mm3 and HIV-1 RNA level greater than 5 log $_{10}$ copies/ml between the two groups.

The proportion of individuals with BMI greater than 23 kg/m^2 was slightly higher in the cases than the controls but did not reach statistical significant difference (p = 0.09). There were only 12 patients who met the criteria for metabolic syndrome because of missing data for lipid profiles and waist circumference. There was no significant difference of metabolic syndrome between groups.

There was no difference in the prevalence of elevated blood pressure and hypertension, impaired fasting plasma glucose and lipid profiles between the groups.

Table 2 Clinical characteristics of HIV patients with or without chronic non HBV/HCV hepatitis at baseline visit**

Clinical parameters	Case (n = 124)	Control (n = 124)	p value
Male sex (n,%)	65(52.4)	37(29.8)	0.001*
Mean age (years), ± SD	32.7 ± 7.4	33.3 ± 7.2	0.56
o ≤ 25 (n,%)	16(12.9)	12(9.7)	0.85
o 25–34.9 (n,%)	68(54.8)	70(56.4)	
o 35–44.9 (n,%)	31(25.0)	34(27.4)	
o ≥ 45 (n,%)	9(7.3)	8(6.5)	
BMI ≥ 23 kg/m^2 (n,%)	39(31.4)	27(21.8)	0.09
Elevated blood pressure/ hypertension (n,%)	18(14.5)	18(14.5)	1.00
Metabolic syndrome (n,%)	9(7.3)	3(2.4)	0.08
Sexual risk behavior (n,%)			0.08
o Heterosexual	83(66.9)	98(79.0)	
o MSM	37(29.9)	23(18.6)	
o Others	4(3.2)	3(2.4)	
CDC classification (n,%)			0.21
o Category A or B	110(88.7)	117(94.4)	
o Category C	14(11.3)	7(5.6)	
Laboratory measurement (n,%)			
o CD4+ cell count ≤ 200 cells/mm3	53(42.7)	50(40.3)	0.66
o Nadir CD4+ cell count ≤ 200 cells/mm3	67(54)	67(54)	1.00
o HIV-1 RNA level ≥ 5 log 10 copies/ml	41(33.1)	31(25)	0.13
o Impaired fasting plasma glucose ≥ 100 mg/dL	21(16.9)	16(12.9)	0.87
o Total cholesterol ≥ 200 mg/dL	25(22.7)	27(24.1)	0.87
o Triglycerides ≥ 150 mg/dL	25(22.7)	26(23.2)	0.88
o HDL cholesterol ≤ 40 mg/dL (male) or ≤ 50 mg/dL (female)	55(51.4)	57(52.3)	0.70
o LDL cholesterol ≥ 130 mg/dL	2(1.8)	1(0.9)	0.57
Median, duration of study (years) (IQR)	9.6(6.7–11.9)	9.6(6.7–11.9)	0.97

Abbreviation: HIV Human immunodeficiency virus, *HBV* Hepatitis B virus, *HCV* Hepatitis C virus, *SD* Standard deviation, *BMI* Body mass index, *MSM* Men who have sex with men, *CDC* The centers for disease control and prevention, *HDL Cholesterol* High density lipoprotein cholesterol, *LDL Cholesterol* Low density lipoprotein cholesterol and *IQR* Interquartile range.
*Significant value with p value less than 0.05.
**Chronic hepatitis was defined as those with elevated ALT ≥ 40 IU/L at 2 consecutive visits 6 months apart.

Clinical characteristics at the time of chronic hepatitis (at event visit)

The proportion of individuals with BMI greater than 23 kg/m^2 was significantly higher in the cases (44.4%) than the controls (20.9%, p = 0.001) (Table 3).

There was no difference in the proportion with individuals of CD4+ cell count less than 200 cells/mm3, plasma HIV-1 RNA level greater than 400 copies/ml, elevated blood pressure and hypertension, impaired fasting plasma glucose and metabolic syndrome between the groups. The cases tended to have lower HDL than the controls (p = 0.09).

Anti-retroviral regimens

All patients were treated with ARV (Table 4). The combination of dual nucleoside reverse transcriptase inhibitors (NRTI) with PI (protease inhibitor) (48.4%) or non-nucleoside reverse transcriptase inhibitors (NNRTI) (37.1%) were the most common first regimens. For triple NRTI, the most common regimen was zidovudine (ZDV) combined with lamivudine (3TC) plus didanosine (ddI) (33%). For dual NRTI plus NNRTI, the most common regimens were efavirenz (EFV) combined with tenofovir (TDF) plus 3TC (35.7%) and NVP combined with 3TC and d4T (17.3%). For dual NRTI plus boosted PI, the most common regimens were saquinavir/ritonavir combined with 3TC plus TDF (24.4%) and lopinavir/ritonavir combined with 3TC plus TDF (12.2%). For NNRTI plus boosted PI, the most common regimen was indinavir/ritonavir combined with EFV (44.4%).

Eleven patients developed early acute adverse events from ARV treatment such as severe hepatitis, drug

Table 3 Clinical characteristics of HIV patients with or without chronic non HBV/HCV hepatitis at time of ALT elevation**

Clinical parameters	Case (n = 124)	Control (n = 124)	p value
BMI ≥ 23 kg/m 2 (n,%)	55(44.4)	26(20.9)	0.001*
Elevated blood pressure/ hypertension (n, %)	24(19.3)	18(14.5)	0.32
Metabolic syndrome (n, %)	3(4.3)	3(3.0)	0.66
Clinically-diagnosed lipodystrophy	14(11.3)	10(8.1)	0.32
Laboratory measurement (n, %)			
o CD4+ cell count ≤ 200 cells/mm3	15(12.1)	10(8.1)	0.30
o HIV-1 RNA level ≥ 400 copies/ml	11(8.8)	16(9.6)	0.21
o Impaired fasting plasma glucose ≥ 100 mg/dL	15(14.1)	10(9.6)	0.21
o Total cholesterol ≥ 200 mg/dL	56(50.4)	48(42.8)	0.49
o Triglycerides ≥ 150 mg/dL	40(36.0)	31(27.7)	0.29
o HDL cholesterol ≤ 40 mg/dL (male) or ≤ 50 mg/dL (female)	36(34.3)	22(21.6)	0.09
o LDL cholesterol ≥ 130 mg/dL	36(34.3)	25(24.5)	0.32

Abbreviation: HIV Human immunodeficiency virus, *HBV* Hepatitis B virus, *HCV* Hepatitis C virus, *BMI* Body mass index, *HDL* High density lipoprotein and *LDL* Low density lipoprotein.
*Significant value with p value less than 0.05.
**Chronic hepatitis was defined as those with elevated ALT ≥ 40 IU/L at 2 consecutive visits 6 months apart.

hypersensitivity reaction and severe fatigue. ARV was discontinued and the hepatitis completely resolved. The new regimens for these patients were used as the first ARV regimen for our analysis.

Concomitant medication

The concomitant medications were similar between the 2 groups (Table 5).

Risk factor variables for chronic hepatitis

From the univariate analysis; male sex, plasma HIV-1 RNA level > 5 log $_{10}$ copies/ml and metabolic syndrome

Table 4 Antiretroviral use* of HIV patients with or without chronic non HBV/HCV hepatitis**

Clinical parameters	Case (n = 124)	Control (n = 124)	p value
Median, duration of ARV exposure (years) (IQR)	2.2(0.9-5.2)	1.6(0.9-4.4)	0.18
Antiretroviral regimens (n, %)			
o Triple NRTIs	18(14.5)	-	NA
o Dual NRTIs plus NNRTI	46(37.1)	52(41.9)	0.37
o Dual NRTIs plus boosted PIs	58(46.8)	65(54.4)	0.29
o NNRTIs plus boosted PIs	2(1.6)	7(5.7)	0.12

Abbreviation: NRTIs Nucleoside reverse transcriptase inhibitors, *NNRTI* Non-nucleoside reverse transcriptase inhibitor, *PIs* Protease inhibitors, *ARV* Antiretroviral, *IQR* Interquartile range, *NA* Non applicable.
* Ever exposed to antiretroviral medication.
**Chronic hepatitis was defined as those with elevated ALT ≥ 40 IU/L at 2 consecutive visits 6 months apart.

at baseline visit, high BMI ≥ 23 kg/m^2 and abnormal HDL cholesterol at time of ALT elevation and treatment experience with NNRTI plus boosted PI were selected to the final model of multivariate analysis (Table 6).

From the multivariate analysis, male sex (AOR, 95% CI; 3.1, 1.5-6.3, p =0.002) and high BMI ≥ 23 kg/m^2 (AOR, 95% CI; 2.4, 1.2-4.8, p = 0.01) were the independent risk factors for chronic hepatitis.

Discussion

Our study examined clinical characteristics and the risk factors of chronic hepatitis by evaluating ALT level as a surrogate marker. We reported a case–control study of 124 matched pairs, ARV-treated HIV-infected individuals without HBV or HCV infection with a follow-up time of 3,195 person-years. Our incidence rate of hepatitis was slightly higher (5.4 cases per 100 person-years) than previously reported in Kovari et al. (3.9 cases per 100 person-years) [9].

The ALT elevation in our study was mostly mild (grade 1–2, 98.4%). There was no report of serious liver disease or hepatic encephalopathy, however, its long-term deleterious consequence is not well defined. The majority of previous studies mainly reported patients with severe elevation of ALT (≥ 5 times, UNL) who also tended to have symptomatic disease [19]. In general, chronic liver disease in HIV usually presents with no or mild symptoms with rising serum transaminase levels. Because such individuals are mostly asymptomatic, delayed diagnosis is common [5,20]. Delayed diagnosis and treatment may lead to long term consequences from

Table 5 Concomitant medication use* of HIV patients with or without chronic non HBV/HCV hepatitis**

Concomitant medications	Case (n = 124)	Control (n = 124)	p value
o Isoniazid	17(13.7)	22(17.7)	0.36
o Pyrazinamide	7(5.6)	6(4.8)	0.78
o Gemfibrosil	7(5.6)	7(5.6)	1.0
o Fenofibrate	11(8.8)	8(6.5)	0.47
o Simvastatin	7(5.6)	5(4.0)	0.53
o Cotrimoxazole	50(40.3)	50(40.3)	1.0
o Dapsone	4(3.2)	3(2.4)	0.71
o Fluconazole	19(15.3)	14(11.3)	0.30
o Analgesic	14(11.3)	17(13.7)	0.33

Footnote:
* Ever exposed to any concomitant medications.
** Chronic hepatitis was defined as those with elevated ALT ≥ 40 IU/L at 2 consecutive visits 6 months apart.

chronic hepatitis such as liver fibrosis, resulting in cirrhosis and importantly liver cancer [21,22].

We found that the median time from ARV initiation to chronic hepatitis was 1.3 years (IQR, 0.5-3.5) which was similar to previous report of 1.2 year [9]. As our definition required two consecutive abnormal ALT 6-month apart, this suggests that early detection of chronic hepatitis will require monitoring of symptoms and liver enzymes within the first year of ARV initiation.

Our study confirmed that males had 3.1 times (95% CI, 1.5-6.3) greater risk of chronic hepatitis than females. This finding supports the report by Guaraldi G et al. that non-alcoholic fatty liver disease (NAFLD) was associated with male sex and elevated ALT level [23]. Previous study in HIV-negative US adolescents also supported an association between NAFLD and male sex [24].

Our study concurred that high BMI greater than 23 kg / m^2 was associated with 2.4 times (95% CI, 1.2-4.8) greater risk of chronic hepatitis. Previous studies showed that high BMI (>25 kg / m^2) and overt obesity were associated with chronic hepatitis [5,9,11]. However, this study did not show an effect of other metabolic components, likely due to missing information on lipid profiles and waist circumference to diagnose the metabolic syndrome. The metabolic syndrome and high BMI can directly cause insulin resistance and impaired fatty acid oxidation in hepatocytes and subsequently lead to hepatic cellular injury [25,26].

Our findings confirmed the study from the Swiss HIV cohort that HIV-related parameters such as baseline CD4+ cell count and HIV-1 RNA level are not associated with chronic hepatitis. Our finding disagrees with the study of Sterling et al. which reported that detectable HIV-1 RNA level was associated with chronic, rising ALT enzymes. However, that study was a cross-sectional study. Plasma HIV-1 RNA and ALT level were tested only one visit during the study period [11].

We did not find exposure to ARV or concomitant medication to demonstrate an association with chronic hepatitis in contrast to previous reports [7,10]. The Swiss cohort reported that chronic elevated ALT levels were associated with stavudine use of at least 2 years duration but this study examined only a history of any ARV exposure, regardless of the duration of that exposure [9].

The strengths of this study include the availability of prospective longitudinal data collection of ALT that has been shown to accurately reflect liver steatosis. The determination of chronic hepatitis by using ALT level as a surrogate laboratory test increases the generalizability of the data to other resource-limited settings. This test is inexpensive, widely available and easy to perform. However, liver injury may exist in the absence of transaminases elevation. Limitations of this study include a lack of histological and clinical imaging data to confirm liver

Table 6 Univariate and multivariate analysis to evaluate each variable and medication for the risk of chronic non HBV/HCV hepatitis***

Clinical parameters and ARV	Univariate OR (95% CI)	p value*	Multivariate AOR (95% CI)	p value**
Male sex	3.0(1.6–5.5)	<0.001	3.1(1.5–6.3)	0.002*
BMI ≥ 23 kg/m2 at time of ALT elevation	3.1(1.7–5.6)	<0.001	2.4(1.2–4.8)	0.01*
Metabolic syndrome at baseline visit	4.0(0.8–18.8)	0.08		
Plasma HIV-1 RNA level ≥ 5 log 10 copies/ml at baseline visit	1.6(0.9–3.0)	0.13		
HDL cholesterol ≤ 40 mg/dL (male) or ≤ 50 mg/dL (female) at time of ALT elevation	1.8(0.9–3.7)	0.09		
Exposure to NNRTIs + boosted PIs regimens	0.3(0.1–1.4)	0.12		

Abbreviation: OR Odds ratio, *AOR* Adjusted odds ratio, *BMI* Body mass index, *HDL* High density lipoprotein, *NNRTI* Non-nucleoside reverse transcriptase inhibitor, *PIs* Protease inhibitors,
*P value less than 0.20 from univariate analysis to the model for multivariable analysis **Significant value with p value less than 0.05.
*** Chronic hepatitis was defined as those with elevated ALT ≥ 40 IU/L at 2 consecutive visits 6 months apart.

injury as well as missing data on alcohol use and parameters to diagnose metabolic syndrome. In addition, lipodystrophy may be under diagnosed or under reported. This study did not exclude other causes of chronic hepatitis including metabolic diseases such as hemochromatosis, Wilson's disease and autoimmune hepatitis and infectious causes including cytomegalovirus or Epstein-Barr virus, chronic hepatitis E virus. Finally, this study also did not examine an association between duration of ARV treatment and chronic hepatitis because it had already matched for the date of ARV initiation.

Conclusion

In conclusion, chronic hepatitis in ARV-treated HIV infected patients is common and may lead to a major health care problem. Male sex and high BMI ≥ 23 kg/m^2 carry higher risks for developing chronic hepatitis in this study. Therefore, these patients should be closely monitored for long-term hepatotoxicity.

Abbreviations

AOR: Adjusted odds ratio; BMI: Body mass index; CDC: Centers for disease control and prevention; HBV: Hepatitis B virus; HCV: Hepatitis C virus; HDL cholesterol: High density lipoprotein cholesterol; HIV: Human immunodeficiency virus; IQR: Interquartile range; LDL cholesterol: Low density lipoprotein cholesterol; MSM: Men who have sex with men; NNRTI: Non-nucleoside reverse transcriptase inhibitor; NRTI: Nucleoside reverse transcriptase inhibitors; OR: Odds ratio; PI: Protease inhibitors; SD: Standard deviation; ULN: Upper limit of normal.

Competing interests

The authors declare that they have no competing interests.

Authors' contributions

NH, PT, AA, JA, TC and SP designed and conducted the study, interpreted the data, and prepared and edited the manuscript. All authors read and approved the final manuscript.

Acknowledgements

We thank our study participants, the 90th Anniversary of Chulalongkorn University Fund and the HIV-NAT intramural fund, Supalak Klungkang M.Sc. and Duangjai Chatvong BBA for helping with data collection and James LK Fletcher MD. for English editing of this manuscript.

Author details

[1]Department of Preventive and Social Medicine, Faculty of Medicine, Chulalongkorn University, Bangkok, Thailand. [2]SEARCH, The Thai Red Cross AIDS Research Center, Bangkok, Thailand. [3]Department of Biochemistry, Faculty of Medicine, Chulalongkorn University, Bangkok, Thailand. [4]HIV-NAT, The Thai Red Cross AIDS Research Center, Bangkok, Thailand. [5]Department of Medicine, Faculty of Medicine, Chulalongkorn University, Bangkok, Thailand.

References

1. De Cock KM, Jaffe HW, Curran JW: **The evolving epidemiology of HIV/AIDS.** *AIDS* 2012, **26**(10):1205–13.
2. Palella FJ Jr, Delaney KM, Moorman AC, Loveless MO, Fuhrer J, Satten GA, *et al*: **Declining morbidity and mortality among patients with advanced human immunodeficiency virus infection. HIV Outpatient Study Investigators.** *N Engl J Med* 1998, **338**(13):853–60.
3. Joshi D, O'Grady J, Dieterich D, Gazzard B, Agarwal K: **Increasing burden of liver disease in patients with HIV infection.** *Lancet* 2011, **377**(9772):1198–209.
4. Weber R, Sabin CA, Friis-Moller N, Reiss P, El-Sadr WM, Kirk O, *et al*: **Liver-related deaths in persons infected with the human immunodeficiency virus: the D:A:D study.** *Arch Intern Med* 2006, **166**(15):1632–41.
5. Crum-Cianflone N, Collins G, Medina S, Asher D, Campin R, Bavaro M, *et al*: **Prevalence and factors associated with liver test abnormalities among human immunodeficiency virus-infected persons.** *Clin Gastroenterol Hepatol* 2010, **8**(2):183–91.
6. Marine-Barjoan E, Saint-Paul MC, Pradier C, Chaillou S, Anty R, Michiels JF, *et al*: **Impact of antiretroviral treatment on progression of hepatic fibrosis in HIV/hepatitis C virus co-infected patients.** *AIDS* 2004, **18**(16):2163–70.
7. Sulkowski MS, Thomas DL, Chaisson RE, Moore RD: **Elevated liver enzymes following initiation of antiretroviral therapy.** *JAMA* 2000, **283**(19):2526–7.
8. Servoss JC, Kitch DW, Andersen JW, Reisler RB, Chung RT, Robbins GK: **Predictors of antiretroviral-related hepatotoxicity in the adult AIDS Clinical Trial Group (1989–1999).** *J Acquir Immune Defic Syndr* 2006, **43**(3):320–3.
9. Kovari H, Ledergerber B, Battegay M, Rauch A, Hirschel B, Foguena AK, *et al*: **Incidence and risk factors for chronic elevation of alanine aminotransferase levels in HIV-infected persons without hepatitis b or c virus co-infection.** *Clin Infect Dis* 2010, **50**(4):502–11.
10. Maida I, Nunez M, Rios MJ, Martin-Carbonero L, Sotgiu G, Toro C, *et al*: **Severe liver disease associated with prolonged exposure to antiretroviral drugs.** *J Acquir Immune Defic Syndr* 2006, **42**(2):177–82.
11. Sterling RK, Chiu S, Snider K, Nixon D: **The prevalence and risk factors for abnormal liver enzymes in HIV-positive patients without hepatitis B or C coinfections.** *Dig Dis Sci* 2008, **53**(5):1375–82.
12. AIDS Clinical Trials Group: *Table for grading severity of adult adverse experiences.* Rockville, MD: Division of AIDS, National Institute of Allergy and Infectious Diseases; 1992.
13. From the Centers for Disease Control and Prevention: **1993 revised classification system for HIV infection and expanded surveillance case definition for AIDS among adolescents and adults.** *JAMA* 1993, **269**(6):729–30.
14. Choo V: **WHO reassesses appropriate body-mass index for Asian populations.** *Lancet* 2002, **360**(9328):235.
15. Alberti KG, Zimmet P, Shaw J: **The metabolic syndrome--a new worldwide definition.** *Lancet* 2005, **366**(9491):1059–62.
16. Grundy SM: **Approach to lipoprotein management in 2001 National Cholesterol Guidelines.** *Am J Cardiol* 2002, **90**(8A):11i–21i.
17. Baril JG, Junod P, Leblanc R, Dion H, Therrien R, Laplante F, *et al*: **HIV-associated lipodystrophy syndrome: a review of clinical aspects.** *Can J Infect Dis Med Microbiol* 2005, **16**(4):233–43.
18. Fleiss JL, Levin B, Paik MC: *Statistical methods for rates and proportions 3.* United States of America: John Wiley & Sons Inc; 2003.
19. Sulkowski MS, Thomas DL, Chaisson RE, Moore RD: **Hepatotoxicity associated with antiretroviral therapy in adults infected with human immunodeficiency virus and the role of hepatitis C or B virus infection.** *JAMA* 2000, **283**(1):74–80.
20. Ingiliz P, Valantin MA, Duvivier C, Medja F, Dominguez S, Charlotte F, *et al*: **Liver damage underlying unexplained transaminase elevation in human immunodeficiency virus-1 mono-infected patients on antiretroviral therapy.** *Hepatology* 2009, **49**(2):436–42.
21. Crum-Cianflone N, Dilay A, Collins G, Asher D, Campin R, *et al*: **Nonalcoholic fatty liver disease among HIV-infected persons.** *J Acquir Immune Defic Syndr* 2009, **50**:464–473.
22. Becker S: **Liver toxicity in epidemiological cohorts.** *Clin Infect Dis* 2004, **38**(Suppl 2):S49–55.
23. Guaraldi G, Squillace N, Stentarelli C, Orlando G, D'Amico R, Ligabue G, *et al*: **Nonalcoholic fatty liver disease in HIV-infected patients referred to a metabolic clinic: prevalence, characteristics, and predictors.** *Clin Infect Dis* 2008, **47**(2):250–7.
24. Graham RC, Burke A, Stettler N: **Ethnic and sex differences in the association between metabolic syndrome and suspected nonalcoholic fatty liver disease in a nationally representative sample of US adolescents.** *J Pediatr Gastroenterol Nutr* 2009, **49**:442–449.
25. Sanyal AJ, Campbell-Sargent C, Mirshahi F, Rizzo WB, Contos MJ, Sterling RK, Luketic VA, Shiffman ML, Clore JN: **Nonalcoholic steatohepatitis:**

5

Serious Non-AIDS events: Immunopathogenesis and interventional strategies

Denise C Hsu[1*], Irini Sereti[2] and Jintanat Ananworanich[3]

Abstract

Despite the major advances in the management of HIV infection, HIV-infected patients still have greater morbidity and mortality than the general population. Serious non-AIDS events (SNAEs), including non-AIDS malignancies, cardiovascular events, renal and hepatic disease, bone disorders and neurocognitive impairment, have become the major causes of morbidity and mortality in the antiretroviral therapy (ART) era. SNAEs occur at the rate of 1 to 2 per 100 person-years of follow-up. The pathogenesis of SNAEs is multifactorial and includes the direct effect of HIV and associated immunodeficiency, underlying co-infections and co-morbidities, immune activation with associated inflammation and coagulopathy as well as ART toxicities. A number of novel strategies such as ART intensification, treatment of co-infection, the use of anti-inflammatory drugs and agents that reduce microbial translocation are currently being examined for their potential effects in reducing immune activation and SNAEs. However, currently, initiation of ART before advanced immunodeficiency, smoking cessation, optimisation of cardiovascular risk factors and treatment of HCV infection are most strongly linked with reduced risk of SNAEs or mortality. Clinicians should therefore focus their attention on addressing these issues prior to the availability of further data.

Keywords: Serious non-AIDS events, Immune activation, HIV infection

Introduction

Since the first description of AIDS in 1981, there have been tremendous advances in understanding the biology of the virus, the host's immune response and the clinical management of HIV infection. The introduction of combination antiretroviral therapy (ART) in 1996 has revolutionized HIV treatment, increasing the average life expectancy after HIV diagnosis from 10.5 to 22.5 years from 1996 to 2005 [1]. The estimated life expectancy for a 30 year old male infected with a drug-sensitive virus in 2010 and starting ART at about 6 years post infection can be as high as 75 years in some predictive models [2].

Despite the success of ART, life expectancy in HIV-infected patients is still lower than uninfected persons [2-4] and mortality in HIV-infected patients can be up to 15 times higher when compared with the general population, matched for sex and age [3]. In the pre-ART era, AIDS was the primary cause of death in HIV-infected patients [5-7]. With the use of ART, mortality due to serious non-AIDS events (SNAEs) has become more prominent especially in resource-rich settings [6,8-13] and in patients with higher CD4 T cell counts [7,14].

* Correspondence: d.hsu@amr.org.au

[1]The Kirby Institute for Infection and Immunity in Society, University of New South Wales, Sydney, Australia

Definition of serious non-AIDS events

Non-AIDS events (NAEs) are clinical events that do not meet the definition of AIDS-defining events based on the 1993 US Centers for Disease Control and Prevention (CDC) AIDS indicator conditions [15]. They encompass multiple diseases involving different organ systems, including cardiovascular, liver and renal disease, non-AIDS-defining malignancies, diabetes, neuropsychiatric disorders and bone-related abnormalities [16].

SNAEs are NAEs that result in death, are life-threatening, cause prolonged hospitalization and persistent incapacity or are associated with significant morbidity [12,14,17]. Most studies include cardiovascular, liver and end stage renal disease, as well as non-AIDS-defining cancers [11,14,18,19]. Other studies include an even broader range of conditions such as non-AIDS-related infections and psychiatric events [7,12,16,17,20].

Incidence of SNAEs

The incidence of SNAEs in ART-treated patients is around 1 to 2 per 100 person-years of follow-up (PYFU) [11,14,17-19,21], (Table 1), but can be up to 60 per 100 PYFU in a cohort of treatment-experienced patients with multidrug resistant virus [12]. The relative contribution of non-AIDS malignancy, cardiovascular, liver and end stage renal disease to SNAEs vary across studies due to inconsistencies in the definition of SNAEs and differences in the rates of underlying co-morbidities e.g. Hepatitis B virus (HBV) and Hepatitis C virus (HCV) co-infection. However, non-AIDS malignancy, cardiovascular disease (CVD) and liver disease combined seem to account for >80% of SNAEs according to several published studies [9,11,14,17,18]. The incidence of non-AIDS malignancy and cardiovascular disease is about 2-fold higher in HIV-infected patients in the ART era when compared to the general population [22-26].

SNAEs are associated with worse outcome than AIDS events in the ART era. Compared with ART-treated patients without events, the risk of death is increased by 7 to 11-fold in those with SNAEs and by 4 to 5-fold in those with AIDS events [11,14]. Amongst SNAEs, liver-related events are associated with the highest mortality [11,14], followed by renal events, malignancies and cardiovascular events, with estimated 12-month mortality of 39.7, 32.7, 29.5 and 6.1% respectively [11].

SNAEs pathogenesis

Prior to the Strategies for Management of Antiretroviral Therapy (SMART) Study, ART toxicities were thought to be a major contributor to SNAEs. In the SMART Study, over 5000 HIV-infected patients with CD4 T cell count >350 cells/μL were randomized to either episodic ART (when CD4 T cell count fell below 250 cells/μL) or continuous ART. Patients on episodic ART had 1.8-fold increase in mortality and 1.7-fold increase in SNAEs (defined as major cardiovascular, renal or hepatic disease) when compared to those on continuous ART [27], thereby highlighting the role of HIV viraemia and immunodeficiency in the pathogenesis of SNAEs [28].

The pathogenesis of SNAEs is in fact multifactorial and complex (Figure 1). The direct effect of HIV and associated immunodeficiency, underlying co-morbidities and co-infections, immune activation with associated inflammation and coagulopathy as well as ART toxicities can all contribute.

The direct effect of HIV

Uncontrolled HIV replication causes immune activation and progressive decline in CD4 T cell count [29]. In addition, HIV can also contribute directly to organ dysfunction and SNAEs. HIV can infect human hepatic stellate cells and induce collagen expression and pro-inflammatory cytokines secretion *in vitro* [30,31]. HIV can also mediate dysregulation of glomerular podocytes in HIV-transgenic mouse models [32], as well as apoptosis of human renal tubular cell lines [33]. Therefore, direct effect of HIV may contribute to decline in renal function and increase risk of chronic kidney disease [34]. HIV may contribute directly to non-AIDS malignancy [35], as it can be oncogenic by activating proto-oncogenes [36] or by blocking tumour suppressor genes [37] in cell lines. Increased rates of microsatellite instability in tumours of HIV-infected patients have also been found [38].

Immunodeficiency

Lower nadir or pre-ART CD4 T cell count is associated with increased risk of SNAEs [11,14,16,39]. In addition, the degree of CD4 T cell recovery after ART initiation also influences the incidence of SNAEs [14,18,21,39]. A 100 cells/μL lower latest CD4 T cell count in ART-treated patients is associated with a 30% increase in the risk of SNAEs, even after adjusting for smoking status, diabetes mellitus, hyperlipidaemia, HCV and HBV co-infection and alcohol abuse [18]. Lower latest CD4 T cell count in ART-treated patients is also associated with an increase in mortality [40,41].

Suboptimal restoration of CD4 T cells may be secondary to a number of factors including decreased thymic function [42,43] and impaired homeostatic responses and survival of T cells [44]. HIV replication and immune activation stimulate the secretion of transforming growth factor (TGF-β), mainly by regulatory T cells, with macrophages also contributing. TGF-β triggers collagen production by fibroblasts [45-47]. The resultant structural damage and fibrosis of the lymphoid tissues restricts T cell access to interleukin-7 (IL-7) on the fibroblastic reticular cell (FRC) network [45] thus limiting naïve CD4 T cell survival [48,49]. Furthermore, ongoing immune activation leads to rapid CD4 T cell turnover, overwhelming the already impaired renewal mechanisms [44], resulting in suboptimal CD4 recovery [50,51].

Co-infections

Due to common routes of transmission, HIV-infected patients also have increased risk of exposure to other infections that can cause organ dysfunction.

About 6-14% of HIV-infected patients have HBV and about 25-30% have HCV infection, with the rates varying depending on endemicity of HBV in the population and the prevalence of injecting drug use [52]. HBV and/or HCV co-infection greatly increases the risk of SNAEs despite ART [9,11,14,18,39,53]. Co-infection with HCV is associated with increased risk of renal disease (1.5-fold) [54,55], cardiovascular disease (1.5-fold) [56], cirrhosis (19-fold) and hepatocellular carcinoma (5-fold) [57]

Table 1 Summary of studies describing the incidence of SNAEs in various patient populations

Study	Study population	N	Median follow-up (yrs)	Male (%)	Median age (yrs)	Median nadir CD4 count (cells/μL)	Median baseline CD4 count (cells/μL)	HBV + (%)	HCV + (%)	Rate of SNAEs per 100 PYFU	Ref
EuroSIDA	A prospective observational cohort of HIV-infected patients in Europe, Israel and Argentina followed from 2001-09.	12844		73	39	178	403	6	24	1.8	[14]
SMART (S) ESPRIT(E)	S: HIV-infected patients with CD4 count >350 cells/μL were randomized to either CD4 count guided episodic use of ART or to continuous use of ART. E: HIV-infected patients with CD4 count >300 cells/μL were randomized to interleukin-2 plus ART or to ART alone.	S: 5472 E: 4111	S: 2.4 E: 6.8	S: 73 E: 81	S: 43 E: 40	S: 250 E: 197	S: 597 E: 457	S: 2	S: 15	1	[11,27,127]
	An observational cohort of HIV-infected patients with CD4 count >500 cells/μL in Spain from 1996-2011.	547	10	80	43	348	630	5	28	1.4	[17]
CoRIS	A prospective multicenter observational cohort of HIV-infected patients in Spain followed from 2004-2010.	5185	2.1	79	36		342	4	12	2.9	[16]
	A retrospective study of HIV-infected patients receiving ART in Botswana (B) and Nashville, USA (US); from 2002 (B) and 2003 (US)-2007.	B: 650 US: 1129	B: 3 US: 1.5	B: 31 US: 74	B: 33 US: 40		B: 199 US: 243			B: 1 US: 1.2	[19]
LATINA	A retrospective study of HIV-infected patients in Latin America from 1997-2007.	6007	2.5	70						0.9	[18]
APROCO/ COPILOTE	A prospective observational cohort of HIV-infected patients in France followed from 1997-2006.	1231	7.3	77	36		279	5	23	10.5	[20]
OPTIMA	HIV-infected patients with resistance to at least 2 different multidrug regimens were randomized to (a) re-treatment with either standard (≤4) or intensive (≥5) antiretroviral drugs and (b) either treatment starting immediately or after a 12-week monitored ART interruption.	368	4	98	48		107	11	22	61.0	[12]
ATHENA	An observational cohort of ART naive HIV-infected patients starting ART in the Netherlands, 1996-2010.	6440	3.9	75	39		200	7	6	1.2	[21]

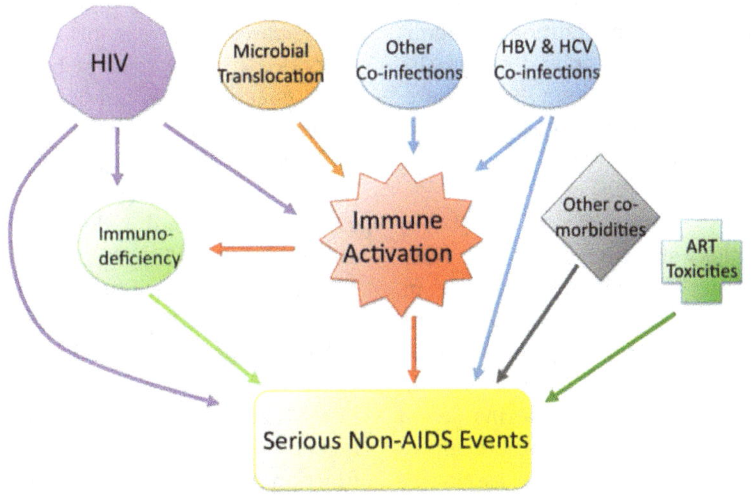

Figure 1 Pathogenesis of serious non-AIDS events. HIV infection causes progressive decline in CD4 T cells through direct cytopathic effects and immune mediated killing of infected cells, as well as indirectly via immune activation. Other drivers of immune activation include co-infections and microbial translocation. HIV can contribute to organ dysfunction through detrimental effects on hepatic stellate cells and renal tubular cells. HIV may also be oncogenic. Co-infection with HBV and HCV is especially important in liver related events. In addition, patients' underlying co-morbidities e.g. smoking, cardiovascular risk factors, and ART related toxicities also contribute to SNAEs.

when compared with HIV mono-infected patients in the ART era.

HIV-infected patients also have increased risk of exposure to Human papillomavirus (HPV) [58], that is implicated in the pathogenesis of cervical and anal cancer [59,60].

Other co-morbidities

HIV-infected patients also have higher prevalence of traditional cardiovascular risk factors such as smoking [61-63], elevated total cholesterol/HDL ratio [61-64] and substance abuse [65]. Some studies also found higher rates of hypertension and diabetes [64,66], but these findings have not been confirmed by others [62,63,67].

Smoking is a major cause of increased mortality in ART-treated patients, accounting for a loss of >12 life years, and is associated with >4-fold increase in all-cause mortality, >5-fold increase in non-AIDS mortality, >4-fold increase in cardiovascular-related mortality and >3-fold increase in cancer-related mortality [68].

Though uncontrolled HIV replication, immunodeficiency, co-infection and co-morbid conditions are important contributors to the pathogenesis of SNAEs, these factors only partially account for the increased risk of SNAEs in HIV-infected patients. HIV elite controllers have increased coronary plaques and carotid intima media thickness when compared to uninfected controls even after adjustment for traditional cardiovascular risk factors [69,70], demonstrating that factors other than uncontrolled viral replication, immunodeficiency, traditional risk factors, and ART toxicities contribute to increased cardiovascular risks in HIV-infected patients.

Immune activation

Inflammation is central to the process of atherosclerosis [71,72], tumour progression [73,74] and liver fibrosis [75,76] in the general population. High levels of biomarkers associated with inflammation (C-reactive protein, CRP, and IL-6) and coagulopathy (D-dimer and fibrinogen) are associated with increased risk of cardiovascular disease [77-80], increased cancer risks [81-83] and mortality [80,84-86] in the general population.

In HIV-infected patients, CRP, IL-6 and D-dimer levels [61] as well as markers of T cell activation [50,87] remain higher than uninfected controls despite suppressive ART. Furthermore, higher CRP, IL-6 and D-dimer [88-90], soluble CD14 (sCD14, a marker of LPS-induced monocyte activation) [91] and lymphocyte activation markers [92] are associated with higher mortality.

In ART-treated patients, CRP, IL-6 and D-dimer levels are also associated with increased risk of CVD, independent of other CVD risk factors [93,94]. These markers are also associated with increased risks of both infection-related and infection unrelated cancers even after adjusting for demographics and CD4 T cell count [95]. Recently, higher levels of tumour necrosis factor (TNF) were also found to be significantly associated with increased risk of SNAEs [96]. Therefore these data suggest that immune activation plays a very important role in SNAEs pathogenesis.

Intermittent viraemia

The drivers of immune activation are diverse. Intermittent HIV viraemia can occur in 20-30% of ART-treated patients [97,98]. The presence of viraemia whilst on

ART is associated with higher IL-6, D-dimer and sCD14 levels [62] and SNAEs [11,39]. In addition, viraemia below the limit of detection of conventional assays also correlates with persistent T cell activation [99]. Therefore, residual viraemia may partially be responsible for persistent immune activation despite ART.

Co-infections

The presence of co-infections also contributes to continual stimulation and activation of the immune system. Asymptomatic CMV infection has been associated with CD8 T cell activation in ART-treated patients [100]. CMV specific CD4 T cells can cause a systemic inflammatory response that is sustained even during latent infection [101] and is associated with atherogenesis [102,103]. Hepatitis C co-infection is also associated with increased CD8 T cell activation when compared with HIV mono-infected patients despite ART [104,105].

Microbial translocation

Microbial translocation due to impaired mucosal barrier integrity may be another cause of immune activation in HIV infection. Rhesus macaques with chronic SIV infection have disruptions of the epithelial barrier of the colon and increased lipopolysaccharide (LPS) staining. The levels of LPS staining in the colon also correlated with the levels of LPS in the draining lymph nodes and remote peripheral lymph nodes [106]. African green monkeys are natural hosts of SIV. In chronic SIV infection, they display little immune activation, maintain mucosal barrier integrity and do not progress to AIDS [107]. However, the injection of LPS into SIV-infected African green monkeys was associated with increases in T cell activation, sCD14 and SIV viraemia [108]. In HIV-infected patients, plasma LPS also correlated with plasma interferon (IFN)-α and T cell activation levels [109]. These data suggest that impaired mucosal barrier integrity and microbial translocation may induce immune activation.

Markers of microbial translocation e.g. LPS, sCD14 [110] and bacterial 16 s rDNA [111] do not always normalise with ART. LPS can induce tissue factor expression on monocytes [112]. Tissue factor is the initiator of the coagulation cascade [113] and its expression on monocytes is correlated with D-dimer levels [112]; suggesting that microbial translocation may contribute to atherogenesis and increased CVD [112].

Antiretroviral therapy

Finally, adverse effects of ART may also contribute to SNAEs. A detail review of ART-related toxicities is beyond the scope of this review. Protease inhibitors as a class, as well as indinavir, lopinavir and abacavir may be associated with increased risk of CVD [25,114,115].

Some studies found that the rate of liver-related deaths is increased per year of ART [116,117]. The cohort described by Weber et al have high rates of HBV and HCV infection, 17% and 66%, respectively [116]. Though patients with HBV or HCV infection have about 5-fold greater risk of hepatotoxicity after ART initiation [118-120], ART is essential as it slows fibrosis progression [121] and reduces liver-related mortality by about 10-fold [122]. In patients without chronic viral hepatitis, ART toxicity rarely causes liver-related mortality, at a rate of 0.04 per 1000 person years [123].

ART has been associated with improved renal function and a slower rate of eGFR decline in HIV-infected patients [124,125]. Though tenofovir use is associated with higher risk of acute renal injury and greater loss of renal function than other ART regimen, the overall risk of serious renal event is not high, in 0.5% of patients [126].

Interventions to reduce SNAEs

Strategies to reduce SNAEs include preventing and reversing immunodeficiency, the modification of traditional risk factors, treatment of co-infections and addressing drivers of immune activation. A wide variety of agents are currently being examined for their potential effects in reducing immune activation and SNAEs (Table 2). However, the majority of studies that have been performed are small, are heterogeneous in terms of ART status and show conflicting findings. The majority of studies used markers of immune activation, in particular CD8 T cell activation as outcome measures. Some recent studies have also included sCD14 and D-dimer. However, randomized placebo-controlled trials that use clinical outcome measures are rare [127].

Preventing and reversing immunodeficiency

ART initiation prior to advanced immunodeficiency

Data from randomized controlled trials suggest that deferral of ART initiation until CD4 T cell count <250 cells/μL was associated with increased SNAEs, AIDS-related events and mortality [128-130]. Observational studies suggest that ART initiation at CD4 T cell count >350 cells/μL is associated with lower risk of SNAEs [14], AIDS-defining illness or death when compared to deferring ART [131-134]. The benefit of ART initiation at CD4 T cell count >350 cells/μL when compared to deferring until CD4 T cell count ~350 cells/μL is insignificant in some studies when the analysis is restricted to mortality alone [131,134]. Results from the START study (NCT00867048), a multicenter international trial designed to assess the risks and benefits of initiating ART at CD4 T cell count at >500 or <350 cells/μL will likely shed further light on this issue. Nonetheless, given that the majority of HIV-infected patients start ART with CD4 T cell count <250 cells/μL [135,136], earlier HIV diagnosis and initiation

Table 2 Potential strategies to reduce SNAEs

Potential strategies to reduce SNAEs	Interventions investigated or under evaluation	References
Preventing immunodeficiency	Initiate ART prior to advanced immunodeficiency	[14,128-134]
Increasing CD4 T cell recovery		
Cytokine therapy	Subcutaneous IL-2	[127]
	Subcutaneous IL-7	[137,138]
Modulating lymphoid tissue fibrosis	Pirfenidone	Human data pending
	Angiotensin receptor antagonist	Human data pending
	ACE inhibitor	Human data pending
Managing co-morbidities	Smoking cessation	[68,145]
	Optimise blood pressure, lipids and diabetic control	[146,147]
	ART switch	[152-160]
Reducing chronic antigen stimulation		
Residual viraemia	Raltegravir intensification	[161-170]
	Maraviroc intensification	[171-174]
HBV and HCV co-infection	Hepatitis B and C treatment	[105,175,176]
CMV co-infection	Valganciclovir	[178]
HSV co-infection	Valacyclovir	[179]
Reducing inflammation	Statins	[182-187]
	COX-2 inhibitors	[195,196]
	Aspirin	[199]
	Hydroxychloroquine & Chloroquine	[191-193]
	Leflunomide	[200]
	Prednisone	[201-204]
Reducing microbial translocation		
Balancing microbiota	Prebiotic, probiotic and synbiotic	[210-213]
Reducing bacterial/endotoxin load	Rifaximin	Human data pending
	Bovine colostrum	[167]
	Sevelamer	Human data pending
Improving mucosal integrity	Lubiprostone	Human data pending
Reducing inflammation in the gut	Mesalamine	Human data pending

of ART before advanced immunodeficiency will likely reduce SNAEs.

Improving CD4 T cell recovery

A number of studies have investigated the use of cytokines critical for T cell homeostasis e.g. IL-2 and IL-7 to enhance CD4 T cell recovery. Though subcutaneous IL-2 administration in concert with ART resulted in sustained increase in CD4 T cell count, this did not translate into clinical benefit [127]. Subcutaneous IL-7 administration also leads to increase in CD4 T cells in phase I and II studies [137,138] but clinical outcomes have not yet been assessed. The restoration of TH17 cells and improvement in TH17/T regulatory cell ratio may be especially important given their roles in mucosal immunity [139,140].

Modulating the effects of lymphoid tissue fibrosis

Lymphoid tissue fibrosis is associated with poor CD4 T cell restoration after ART initiation [49]. TGF-β is key in the process of lymphoid tissue fibrosis. Pirfenidone can reduce TGF-β production and has anti-fibrotic effects [45,141]. Pirfenidone administered to rhesus macaques prior to SIV infection was associated with reduced lymph node fibrosis and preservation of lymph node CD4 T cells [142]. TNF blockade with adalimumab was also associated with attenuated TGF-β expression, reduced lymph node fibrosis and preserved lymph node architecture in a recent rhesus macaque study [47]. The effect of pirfenidione or adalimumab on lymph node fibrosis in HIV infection has not been studied to date.

The renin-angiotensin pathway is involved in cardiac, renal and liver fibrosis. Binding of angiotensin II to the angiotensin 1 receptor on cardiac fibroblast, hepatic stellate cells or mesangial cells leads to proliferation as well as collagen and TGF-β synthesis [143,144]. Trials on the effect of angiotensin converting enzyme (ACE) inhibitor e.g. lisinopril (ClinicalTrials.gov identifier: NCT01535235), angiotensin II receptor antagonists e.g. losartan (NCT01852942, NCT01529749) and telmisartan (NCT01928927) in modulating lymphoid tissue fibrosis are currently underway.

Optimizing cardiovascular risk factors

In the D.A.D study, patients who stopped smoking had about 30% reduction in the risk of CVD [145]. Surprisingly, a reduction in mortality was not seen. This may be because patients ceased smoking after the diagnosis of a serious illness and succumb before the benefit of smoking cessation on mortality can be seen [145]. In the Danish HIV cohort, previous smokers had a >1.5-fold reduction in mortality when compared with current smokers. In addition, though previous smokers have higher rates of AIDS-related deaths when compared with never smokers, the incidence of non-AIDS-related death was not different between previous and never smokers [68]. These data suggest that smoking cessation alone would result in significant benefits and should be encouraged.

Modification of other cardiovascular risk factors e.g. treatment of hypertension, dyslipidaemia and optimal glycaemic control in diabetic patients is critical. Suggested target levels have been published [146,147]. Each 10 mmHg reduction in systolic blood pressure and each 38 mg/dL reduction in total cholesterol is associated with a 5 and 20% reduction in risk of CVD, respectively [148]. However, in patients with known hypertension, diabetes or dyslipidaemia meeting indication for treatment, over 40% were not on treatment [149]. Given that a significant proportion of SNAEs are cardiovascular events, more aggressive detection and management of cardiovascular risk factors will likely reduce SNAEs.

ART modification is a potential strategy to reduce cardiovascular risk [150]. A recent review of switch studies have been published [151]. Switching from stavudine to tenofovir was associated with a reduction in total cholesterol and triglycerides and an increase in limb fat [152]. Switching from protease inhibitors to efavirenz or nevirapine was associated with reduction in total cholesterol [153]. However, this switch is not possible in patients with non-nucleoside reverse transcriptase inhibitor resistance. Switching from lopinavir/ritonavir to atazanavir (both boosted with ritonavir 100 mg or unboosted) was associated with reduction of total cholesterol and triglycerides, though greater reductions were seen with unboosted atazanavir [154-156]. Switching to atazanavir was also associated with a reduction in cardiovascular risk score [157]. Though switching from lopinavir/ritonavir to raltegravir was associated with improvement in lipid profile [158,159], no change in endothelial function was detected [160]. The importance of having fully active backbone antiretrovirals was highlighted in the SWITCHMRK study where patients switched to raltegravir had higher rates of virologic failure [158].

Suppressing chronic antigen stimulation

Reducing residual viraemia

Intensification studies have been performed to assess the impact of adding antiretroviral agents to a suppressive ART regimen (as measured by conventional assays). None of the raltegravir intensification studies were able to demonstrate reduction in ultra-sensitive plasma HIV-RNA levels [161-167]. In addition, the majority of studies also found no reduction in markers of T cell [161-164,167] or monocyte activation [167]. However, some studies have noted a reduction in D-dimer levels [168], T cell activation [165,166,169] as well as an early transient increase in 2-LTR circles post raltegravir intensification [168,170], suggesting that residual viraemia was occurring prior to raltegravir intensification and was contributing to immune activation in some patients.

Maraviroc intensification studies have also been performed and yielded conflicting data. Some found reduction in T cell activation [171-173] whilst others found increase in CD4 and CD8 T cell activation both in the peripheral blood and in the rectal mucosa after maraviroc intensification [174]. Hunt et al postulated that the binding of maraviroc to CCR5 prevents the interaction between CCR5 and its natural ligands. Excess CCR5 ligands may then bind to other chemokine receptor such as CCR3 and CCR4 on T cells, leading to T cell activation [174]. Therefore, the beneficial effect of adding antiretroviral agents to an already suppressive ART regimen is uncertain based on currently available data.

Treating other co-infections

HCV treatment and suppression of HCV viraemia is associated with reductions in CD4 and CD8 T cell activation [105]. Sustained virologic response is associated with reduced liver-related complications as well as both liver-related and non liver-related mortality in co-infected patients [175,176]. Unfortunately, HCV treatment may be limited by contraindications, adverse events, high costs, and drug interactions. Next generation agents with higher efficacy and better side effect profiles may revolutionise the management of HIV/HCV co-infected patients [177].

Treatment of other persistent viral infection has also been investigated. Eight weeks of valganciclovir in ART-treated, CMV seropositive patients led to a significant reduction of CMV viraemia as well as a reduction in CD8

T cell activation [178]. In a study targeting HSV co-infection using 12 weeks of valacyclovir in ART-treated, HSV-1 and HSV-2 seropositive patients, no change in T cell activation, CRP or IL-6 levels was demonstrated [179].

Anti-inflammatory agents

Statins are 3-hydroxy-3-methyl-glutaryl-coenzyme A reductase inhibitors. Not only do statins reduce serum cholesterol [180], they may also have anti-inflammatory properties [181]. Statin use is associated with reduced monocyte activation (unpublished data McComsey et al), decline in CRP levels [182] as well as reduced T cell activation [183] in ART-treated and in untreated, HIV-infected patients [184]. A retrospective observational study of ART-treated patients showed that statin use is associated with a 3-fold reduction in mortality [185]. Though not statistically significant, a trend for reduction in SNAEs [186] and mortality [187] has also been seen in other retrospective observational studies.

Hydroxychloroquine (HCQ) and its analogue chloroquine (CQ) have immunomodulatory, anti-inflammatory and anti-HIV properties [188-190]. In patients with uncontrolled viral replication, the use of CQ was associated with reduced CD8 T cell activation [191] whereas the same effect was not seen with HCQ [192]. However a non-randomized study of HCQ in 20 ART-treated patients showed decline in plasma LPS, IL-6 and reduced T cell and monocyte activation [193]. Thus findings are inconclusive.

COX-2 inhibitors inhibit cyclooxygenase type 2, reducing Prostaglandin E2 production, thereby reducing activation of T cells through the cyclic adenosine monophosphate (cAMP) pathway [194]. Studies on COX-2 inhibitors have been small and reduction in T cell activation tended to occur in viraemic patients [195,196]. However, it is important to bear in mind that COX-2 inhibitors are associated with increased cardiovascular risk, via a direct pharmacologic consequence of inhibition of COX-2 [197]. Therefore assessing the utility of COX-2 inhibitors without using clinical outcome measures may be insufficient.

Aspirin is a cornerstone in the secondary prevention of vascular disease [198]. In a pilot study, aspirin use was associated with reduced platelet activation, a decrease in sCD14 in monocytes and reductions in CD38 and HLA-DR on CD4 and CD8 T cells. However, there was no change in IL-6, D-dimer and CRP [199]. An aspirin study with larger number of participants is in development with the AIDS Clinical Trials Group.

Leflunomide is an immunomodulatory agent that is used in the treatment of rheumatoid arthritis. The administration of leflunomide in untreated, HIV-infected patients for 28 days was associated with a decrease in CD8 T cell activation [200].

The use of prednisone in patients with untreated chronic HIV infection was associated with less CD4 T cell depletion, a decline in CD4 T cell activation and stable HIV viral load [201,202]. Prednisone at 0.5 mg/kg/day in ART-treated patients was also associated with a reduction in CD8 T cell activation and TNF levels as well as a transient decrease in IL-6 [203]. However, in another study using prednisone at 40 mg/day, no reduction in CD4 or CD8 T cell activation, plasma IL-6 or TNF levels was found [204]. Furthermore, long-term prednisone use, especially at doses >7.5 mg/day is associated with significant adverse effects such as osteoporosis, impaired glucose tolerance, dyslipidaemia, weight gain, cataract formation and increased risk of infections [205]. Even short courses have been associated with an increased risk of osteonecrosis in HIV-infected patients [206].

Targeting microbial translocation

Given that HIV infection has been associated with depressed levels of beneficial gut microbiota and elevated levels of pathogenic microbiota [207], a range of prebiotics (selectively fermented ingredients that changes the growth and/or activity of certain gut microflora, resulting in health benefits [208]), probiotics (live microorganisms that when consumed, confer a health benefit [209]) and synbiotics (combinations of pre and probiotics) are under investigation.

A prebiotic oligosaccharide mixture has been associated with improvement in microbiota composition and reduction in sCD14 in untreated HIV-infected patients [210]. A retrospective cohort study on both ART-treated and untreated HIV-infected patients found that probiotic yogurt consumption was associated with a greater increase in CD4 T cell count even after adjustment for ART [211]. A double-blind randomized placebo-controlled trial in 20 untreated HIV-infected patients found reductions in plasma bacterial DNA and IL-6 levels in patients receiving synbiotics [212]. However, a synbiotic agent in ART-treated women found no change in microbial translocation nor immune activation status despite improvement in the levels of probiotic species [213]. Therefore, more randomized controlled clinical trial data are needed to clarify the effects of pre and probiotics in reducing immune activation.

Bovine colostrum contains oligosaccharides, growth factors, immunoglobulins and antimicrobial peptides and has some activity in alleviating HIV-associated diarrhoea in single arm studies [214-216]. However a randomized controlled trial on the addition of bovine colostrum to suppressive ART found no change in CD4 T cell count, markers of microbial translocation nor T cell activation [167].

A number of new agents that target microbial translocation are under evaluation. Rifaximin is a minimally absorbed oral rifamycin antibiotic that has activity against both gram-positive and gram-negative enteric bacteria [217]. It is effective in the treatment of hepatic encephalopathy, by reducing ammonia-producing enteric bacteria [218,219]. There are currently 3 clinical trials of rifaximin in HIV-infected patients (ClinicalTrials.gov identifier: NCT01654939, NCT01866826 and NCT01466595). Lubiprostone is a chloride channel activator that is used in the treatment of constipation [220]. It has been found to enhance recovery of mucosal barrier function in ischaemic porcine colon [221]. A pilot study of lubiprostone in ART treated, virologically suppressed patients with CD4 T cell count <350 cells/μL (NCT01839734) is currently recruiting. Sevelamer is a phosphate binder that is used in patients with end-stage renal failure [222]. It can also bind to endotoxins and reduce CRP, IL-6 and sCD14 in patients on haemodialysis [223,224]. The trial in untreated, HIV-infected patients (NCT01543958) was completed in June 2013 and results are pending. Mesalamine (5-aminosalicylic acid) is an anti-inflammatory agent used in the management of inflammatory bowel disease [225]. A trial using mesalamine in ART treated, virologically suppressed patients with CD4 T cell count <350 cells/μL (NCT01090102) is currently enrolling.

Conclusions

Despite the use of ART, HIV-infected patients still have higher mortality and morbidity when compared to the general population. SNAEs occur at the rate of about 1-2 per 100 PYFU and are the predominant causes of morbidity and mortality in HIV-infected patients in the ART era. Many factors contribute to the pathogenesis of SNAEs including the direct effect of HIV and associated immunodeficiency, underlying co-morbidities, immune activation and ART toxicities. Though multiple interventions have been investigated or are ongoing, most of the studies are small, of short duration and clinical outcome measures have not been ascertained. The cost required to investigate the effectiveness of an intervention to reduce SNAEs may be prohibitively high as it will require thousands of participants with possibly several years of follow up.

Currently, the interventions with evidence to suggest an association with reduced risk of SNAEs or mortality are starting ART before advanced immunodeficiency, smoking cessation, optimisation of cardiovascular risk factors and treatment of HCV infection. Clinicians should focus their attention on addressing these issues prior to the availability of further data.

Abbreviations

ACE: Angiotensin converting enzyme; ART: Antiretroviral therapy; cAMP: Cyclic adenosine monophosphate; CDC: Centers for disease control and prevention; CQ: Chloroquine; CRP: C-reactive protein; CVD: Cardiovascular disease; EBV: Epstein-Barr virus; FRC: Fibroblastic reticular cell; HBV: Hepatitis B virus; HCV: Hepatitis C virus; HCQ: Hydroxychloroquine; HPV: Human papillomavirus; IL-7: Interleukin-7; IFN: Interferon; LPS: Lipopolysaccharide; NAEs: Non-AIDS events; PYFU: Person-years of follow-up; sCD14: Soluble CD14; SIR: Standardized incidence ratio; SMART: Strategies for management of antiretroviral therapy; SNAEs: Serious non-AIDS events; START: Strategic timing of antiretroviral treatment; TGF: Transforming growth factor; TNF: Tumour necrosis factor.

Competing interests

The authors declare that they have no competing interests.

Authors' contributions

DH, JA, IS contributed to the writing of the manuscript. All authors read and approved the final manuscript.

Author details

[1]The Kirby Institute for Infection and Immunity in Society, University of New South Wales, Sydney, Australia. [2]HIV Pathogenesis Unit, Laboratory of Immunoregulation, NIAID/NIH, Bethesda, MD, USA. [3]HIV Netherlands Australia Thailand Research Collaboration and SEARCH, Thai Red Cross AIDS Research Centre, Bangkok, Thailand.

References

1. Harrison KM, Song R, Zhang X: **Life expectancy after HIV diagnosis based on national HIV surveillance data from 25 states, United States.** *J Acquir Immune Defic Syndr* 2010, **53**:124–130.
2. Nakagawa F, Lodwick RK, Smith CJ, Smith R, Cambiano V, Lundgren JD, Delpech V, Phillips AN: **Projected life expectancy of people with HIV according to timing of diagnosis.** *AIDS* 2012, **26**:335–343.
3. Lohse N, Hansen AB, Pedersen G, Kronborg G, Gerstoft J, Sorensen HT, Vaeth M, Obel N: **Survival of persons with and without HIV infection in Denmark, 1995-2005.** *Ann Intern Med* 2007, **146**:87–95.
4. **Life expectancy of individuals on combination antiretroviral therapy in high-income countries: a collaborative analysis of 14 cohort studies.** *Lancet* 2008, **372**:293–299.
5. Krentz HB, Kliewer G, Gill MJ: **Changing mortality rates and causes of death for HIV-infected individuals living in Southern Alberta, Canada from 1984 to 2003.** *HIV Med* 2005, **6**:99–106.
6. Palella FJ Jr, Baker RK, Moorman AC, Chmiel JS, Wood KC, Brooks JT, Holmberg SD: **Mortality in the highly active antiretroviral therapy era: changing causes of death and disease in the HIV outpatient study.** *J Acquir Immune Defic Syndr* 2006, **43**:27–34.
7. Lau B, Gange SJ, Moore RD: **Risk of non-AIDS-related mortality may exceed risk of AIDS-related mortality among individuals enrolling into care with CD4+ counts greater than 200 cells/mm3.** *J Acquir Immune Defic Syndr* 2007, **44**:179–187.
8. Reisler RB, Han C, Burman WJ, Tedaldi EM, Neaton JD: **Grade 4 events are as important as AIDS events in the era of HAART.** *J Acquir Immune Defic Syndr* 2003, **34**:379–386.
9. **Causes of death in HIV-1-infected patients treated with antiretroviral therapy, 1996-2006: collaborative analysis of 13 HIV cohort studies.** *Clin Infect Dis* 2010, **50**:1387–1396.
10. Lewden C, May T, Rosenthal E, Burty C, Bonnet F, Costagliola D, Jougla E, Semaille C, Morlat P, Salmon D, *et al*: **Changes in causes of death among adults infected by HIV between 2000 and 2005: the "Mortalite 2000 and 2005" surveys (ANRS EN19 and Mortavic).** *J Acquir Immune Defic Syndr* 2005, **2008**(48):590–598.
11. Neuhaus J, Angus B, Kowalska JD, La Rosa A, Sampson J, Wentworth D, Mocroft A: **Risk of all-cause mortality associated with nonfatal AIDS and serious non-AIDS events among adults infected with HIV.** *AIDS* 2010, **24**:697–706.
12. Anis AH, Nosyk B, Sun H, Guh DP, Bansback N, Li X, Barnett PG, Joyce V, Swanson KM, Kyriakides TC, *et al*: **Quality of life of patients with advanced HIV/AIDS: measuring the impact of both AIDS-defining events and non-AIDS serious adverse events.** *J Acquir Immune Defic Syndr* 2009, **51**:631–639.
13. Kowalska JD, Reekie J, Mocroft A, Reiss P, Ledergerber B, Gatell J, d'Arminio Monforte A, Phillips A, Lundgren JD, Kirk O: **Long-term exposure to**

combination antiretroviral therapy and risk of death from specific causes: no evidence for any previously unidentified increased risk due to antiretroviral therapy. *AIDS* 2012, **26**:315–323.

14. Mocroft A, Reiss P, Gasiorowski J, Ledergerber B, Kowalska J, Chiesi A, Gatell J, Rakhmanova A, Johnson M, Kirk O, Lundgren J: **Serious fatal and nonfatal non-AIDS-defining illnesses in Europe.** *J Acquir Immune Defic Syndr* 2010, **55**:262–270.
15. CDC: **1993 revised classification system for HIV infection and expanded surveillance case definition for AIDS among adolescents and adults.** *MMWR Recomm Rep* 1992, **41**:1–19.
16. Masia M, Padilla S, Alvarez D, Lopez JC, Santos I, Soriano V, Hernandez-Quero J, Santos J, Tural C, del Amo J, Gutierrez F: **Risk, predictors, and mortality associated with non-AIDS events in newly diagnosed HIV-infected patients: role of antiretroviral therapy.** *AIDS* 2013, **27**:181–189.
17. Lucero C, Torres B, Leon A, Calvo M, Leal L, Perez I, Plana M, Arnedo M, Mallolas J, Gatell JM, Garcia F: **Rate and Predictors of Non-AIDS Events in a Cohort of HIV-Infected Patients with a CD4 T Cell Count Above 500 Cells/mm(3.).** *AIDS Res Hum Retroviruses* 2013, **29**:1161–1167.
18. Belloso WH, Orellana LC, Grinsztejn B, Madero JS, La Rosa A, Veloso VG, Sanchez J, Ismerio Moreira R, Crabtree-Ramirez B, Garcia Messina O, *et al*: **Analysis of serious non-AIDS events among HIV-infected adults at Latin American sites.** *HIV Med* 2010, **11**:554–564.
19. Wester CW, Koethe JR, Shepherd BE, Stinnette SE, Rebeiro PF, Kipp AM, Hong H, Bussmann H, Gaolathe T, McGowan CC, *et al*: **Non-AIDS-defining events among HIV-1-infected adults receiving combination antiretroviral therapy in resource-replete versus resource-limited urban setting.** *AIDS* 2011, **25**:1471–1479.
20. Ferry T, Raffi F, Collin-Filleul F, Dupon M, Dellamonica P, Waldner A, Strady C, Chene G, Leport C, Moing VL: **Uncontrolled viral replication as a risk factor for non-AIDS severe clinical events in HIV-infected patients on long-term antiretroviral therapy: APROCO/COPILOTE (ANRS CO8) cohort study.** *J Acquir Immune Defic Syndr* 2009, **51**:407–415.
21. Zhang S, van Sighem A, Kesselring A, Gras L, Smit C, Prins JM, Kauffmann R, Richter C, de Wolf F, Reiss P: **Episodes of HIV viremia and the risk of non-AIDS diseases in patients on suppressive antiretroviral therapy.** *J Acquir Immune Defic Syndr* 2012, **60**:265–272.
22. Powles T, Robinson D, Stebbing J, Shamash J, Nelson M, Gazzard B, Mandelia S, Moller H, Bower M: **Highly active antiretroviral therapy and the incidence of non-AIDS-defining cancers in people with HIV infection.** *J Clin Oncol* 2009, **27**:884–890.
23. Bedimo RJ, McGinnis KA, Dunlap M, Rodriguez-Barradas MC, Justice AC: **Incidence of non-AIDS-defining malignancies in HIV-infected versus noninfected patients in the HAART era: impact of immunosuppression.** *J Acquir Immune Defic Syndr* 2009, **52**:203–208.
24. Shiels MS, Cole SR, Kirk GD, Poole C: **A meta-analysis of the incidence of non-AIDS cancers in HIV-infected individuals.** *J Acquir Immune Defic Syndr* 2009, **52**:611–622.
25. Islam FM, Wu J, Jansson J, Wilson DP: **Relative risk of cardiovascular disease among people living with HIV: a systematic review and meta-analysis.** *HIV Med* 2012, **13**:453–468.
26. Martinez E, Milinkovic A, Buira E, de Lazzari E, Leon A, Larrousse M, Lonca M, Laguno M, Blanco JL, Mallolas J, *et al*: **Incidence and causes of death in HIV-infected persons receiving highly active antiretroviral therapy compared with estimates for the general population of similar age and from the same geographical area.** *HIV Med* 2007, **8**:251–258.
27. El-Sadr WM, Lundgren J, Neaton JD, Gordin F, Abrams D, Arduino RC, Babiker A, Burman W, Clumeck N, Cohen CJ, *et al*: **CD4+ count-guided interruption of antiretroviral treatment.** *N Engl J Med* 2006, **355**:2283–2296.
28. Strategies for Management of Antiretroviral Therapy Study Group, Lundgren JD, Babiker A, El-Sadr W, Emery S, Grund B, Neaton JD, Neuhaus J, Phillips AN: **Inferior clinical outcome of the CD4+ cell count-guided antiretroviral treatment interruption strategy in the SMART study: role of CD4+ Cell counts and HIV RNA levels during follow-up.** *J Infect Dis* 2008, **197**:1145–1155.
29. Lawn SD, Butera ST, Folks TM: **Contribution of immune activation to the pathogenesis and transmission of human immunodeficiency virus type 1 infection.** *Clin Microbiol Rev* 2001, **14**:753–777.
30. Tuyama AC, Hong F, Saiman Y, Wang C, Ozkok D, Mosoian A, Chen P, Chen BK, Klotman ME, Bansal MB: **Human immunodeficiency virus (HIV)-1 infects human hepatic stellate cells and promotes collagen I and monocyte chemoattractant protein-1 expression: implications for the pathogenesis of HIV/hepatitis C virus-induced liver fibrosis.** *Hepatology* 2010, **52**:612–622.
31. Hong F, Saiman Y, Si C, Mosoian A, Bansal MB: **X4 Human immunodeficiency virus type 1 gp120 promotes human hepatic stellate cell activation and collagen I expression through interactions with CXCR4.** *PLoS One* 2012, **7**:e33659.
32. Zuo Y, Matsusaka T, Zhong J, Ma J, Ma LJ, Hanna Z, Jolicoeur P, Fogo AB, Ichikawa I: **HIV-1 genes vpr and nef synergistically damage podocytes, leading to glomerulosclerosis.** *J Am Soc Nephrol* 2006, **17**:2832–2843.
33. Kapasi AA, Fan S, Singhal PC: **p300 modulates HIV-1 gp120-induced apoptosis in human proximal tubular cells: associated with alteration of TGF-beta and Smad signaling.** *Nephron Exp Nephrol* 2006, **102**:e30–e38.
34. Wyatt CM, Meliambro K, Klotman PE: **Recent progress in HIV-associated nephropathy.** *Annual review of medicine* 2012, **63**:147–159.
35. Deeken JF, Tjen ALA, Rudek MA, Okuliar C, Young M, Little RF, Dezube BJ: **The rising challenge of non-AIDS-defining cancers in HIV-infected patients.** *Clin Infect Dis* 2012, **55**:1228–1235.
36. Wright S, Lu X, Peterlin BM: **Human immunodeficiency virus type 1 tat directs transcription through attenuation sites within the mouse c-myc gene.** *J Mol Biol* 1994, **243**:568–573.
37. Harrod R, Nacsa J, Van Lint C, Hansen J, Karpova T, McNally J, Franchini G: **Human immunodeficiency virus type-1 Tat/co-activator acetyltransferase interactions inhibit p53Lys-320 acetylation and p53-responsive transcription.** *J Biol Chem* 2003, **278**:12310–12318.
38. Bedi GC, Westra WH, Farzadegan H, Pitha PM, Sidransky D: **Microsatellite instability in primary neoplasms from HIV + patients.** *Nat Med* 1995, **1**:65–68.
39. Baker JV, Peng G, Rapkin J, Abrams DI, Silverberg MJ, MacArthur RD, Cavert WP, Henry WK, Neaton JD: **CD4+ count and risk of non-AIDS diseases following initial treatment for HIV infection.** *AIDS* 2008, **22**:841–848.
40. Marin B, Thiebaut R, Bucher HC, Rondeau V, Costagliola D, Dorrucci M, Hamouda O, Prins M, Walker S, Porter K, *et al*: **Non-AIDS-defining deaths and immunodeficiency in the era of combination antiretroviral therapy.** *AIDS* 2009, **23**:1743–1753.
41. Smith C, Sabin CA, Lundgren JD, Thiebaut R, Weber R, Law M, Monforte A, Kirk O, Friis-Moller N, Phillips A, *et al*: **Factors associated with specific causes of death amongst HIV-positive individuals in the D:A:D Study.** *AIDS* 2010, **24**:1537–1548.
42. Haynes BF, Markert ML, Sempowski GD, Patel DD, Hale LP: **The role of the thymus in immune reconstitution in aging, bone marrow transplantation, and HIV-1 infection.** *Annu Rev Immunol* 2000, **18**:529–560.
43. Douek DC, McFarland RD, Keiser PH, Gage EA, Massey JM, Haynes BF, Polis MA, Haase AT, Feinberg MB, Sullivan JL, *et al*: **Changes in thymic function with age and during the treatment of HIV infection.** *Nature* 1998, **396**:690–695.
44. Zeng M, Haase AT, Schacker TW: **Lymphoid tissue structure and HIV-1 infection: life or death for T cells.** *Trends Immunol* 2012, **33**:306–314.
45. Zeng M, Smith AJ, Wietgrefe SW, Southern PJ, Schacker TW, Reilly CS, Estes JD, Burton GF, Silvestri G, Lifson JD, *et al*: **Cumulative mechanisms of lymphoid tissue fibrosis and T cell depletion in HIV-1 and SIV infections.** *J Clin Invest* 2011, **121**:998–1008.
46. Estes JD, Wietgrefe S, Schacker T, Southern P, Beilman G, Reilly C, Milush JM, Lifson JD, Sodora DL, Carlis JV, Haase AT: **Simian immunodeficiency virus-induced lymphatic tissue fibrosis is mediated by transforming growth factor beta 1-positive regulatory T cells and begins in early infection.** *J Infect Dis* 2007, **195**:551–561.
47. Tabb B, Morcock DR, Trubey CM, Quinones OA, Hao XP, Smedley J, Macallister R, Piatak M Jr, Harris LD, Paiardini M, *et al*: **Reduced inflammation and lymphoid tissue immunopathology in rhesus macaques receiving anti-tumor necrosis factor treatment during primary simian immunodeficiency virus infection.** *J Infect Dis* 2013, **207**:880–892.
48. Schacker TW, Brenchley JM, Beilman GJ, Reilly C, Pambuccian SE, Taylor J, Skarda D, Larson M, Douek DC, Haase AT: **Lymphatic tissue fibrosis is associated with reduced numbers of naive CD4+ T cells in human immunodeficiency virus type 1 infection.** *Clin Vaccine Immunol* 2006, **13**:556–560.
49. Zeng M, Southern PJ, Reilly CS, Beilman GJ, Chipman JG, Schacker TW, Haase AT: **Lymphoid tissue damage in HIV-1 infection depletes naive T**

cells and limits T cell reconstitution after antiretroviral therapy. *PLoS Pathog* 2012, **8:**e1002437.

50. Hunt PW, Martin JN, Sinclair E, Bredt B, Hagos E, Lampiris H, Deeks SG: **T cell activation is associated with lower CD4+ T cell gains in human immunodeficiency virus-infected patients with sustained viral suppression during antiretroviral therapy.** *J Infect Dis* 2003, **187:**1534–1543.
51. Lederman MM, Calabrese L, Funderburg NT, Clagett B, Medvik K, Bonilla H, Gripshover B, Salata RA, Taege A, Lisgaris M, *et al*: **Immunologic failure despite suppressive antiretroviral therapy is related to activation and turnover of memory CD4 cells.** *J Infect Dis* 2011, **204:**1217–1226.
52. Alter MJ: **Epidemiology of viral hepatitis and HIV co-infection.** *J Hepatol* 2006, **44:**S6–S9.
53. Thio CL, Seaberg EC, Skolasky R Jr, Phair J, Visscher B, Munoz A, Thomas DL: **HIV-1, hepatitis B virus, and risk of liver-related mortality in the Multicenter Cohort Study (MACS).** *Lancet* 2002, **360:**1921–1926.
54. Fischer MJ, Wyatt CM, Gordon K, Gibert CL, Brown ST, Rimland D, Rodriguez-Barradas MC, Justice AC, Parikh CR: **Hepatitis C and the risk of kidney disease and mortality in veterans with HIV.** *J Acquir Immune Defic Syndr* 2010, **53:**222–226.
55. Wyatt CM, Malvestutto C, Coca SG, Klotman PE, Parikh CR: **The impact of hepatitis C virus coinfection on HIV-related kidney disease: a systematic review and meta-analysis.** *AIDS* 2008, **22:**1799–1807.
56. Freiberg MS, Chang CC, Skanderson M, McGinnis K, Kuller LH, Kraemer KL, Rimland D, Goetz MB, Butt AA, Rodriguez Barradas MC, *et al*: **The risk of incident coronary heart disease among veterans with and without HIV and hepatitis C.** *Circ Cardiovasc Qual Outcomes* 2011, **4:**425–432.
57. Giordano TP, Kramer JR, Souchek J, Richardson P, El-Serag HB: **Cirrhosis and hepatocellular carcinoma in HIV-infected veterans with and without the hepatitis C virus: a cohort study, 1992-2001.** *Arch Intern Med* 2004, **164:**2349–2354.
58. Mooij SH, van der Klis FR, van der Sande MA, Schepp RM, Speksnijder AG, Bogaards JA, de Melker HE, de Vries HJ, Snijders PJ, van der Loeff MF: **Seroepidemiology of High-Risk HPV in HIV-Negative and HIV-Infected MSM: The H2M Study.** *Cancer Epidemiol Biomarkers Prev* 2013, **22:**1698–1708.
59. Palmer JG, Scholefield JH, Coates PJ, Shepherd NA, Jass JR, Crawford LV, Northover JM: **Anal cancer and human papillomaviruses.** *Dis Colon Rectum* 1989, **32:**1016–1022.
60. Munoz N, Castellsague X, de Gonzalez AB, Gissmann L: **Chapter 1: HPV in the etiology of human cancer.** *Vaccine* 2006, **24**(Suppl 3):S3/1-10.
61. Neuhaus J, Jacobs DR Jr, Baker JV, Calmy A, Duprez D, La Rosa A, Kuller LH, Pett SL, Ristola M, Ross MJ, *et al*: **Markers of inflammation, coagulation, and renal function are elevated in adults with HIV infection.** *J Infect Dis* 2010, **201:**1788–1795.
62. Armah KA, McGinnis K, Baker J, Gibert C, Butt AA, Bryant KJ, Goetz M, Tracy R, Oursler KK, Rimland D, *et al*: **HIV status, burden of comorbid disease, and biomarkers of inflammation, altered coagulation, and monocyte activation.** *Clin Infect Dis* 2012, **55:**126–136.
63. Saves M, Chene G, Ducimetiere P, Leport C, Le Moal G, Amouyel P, Arveiler D, Ruidavets JB, Reynes J, Bingham A, Raffi F: **Risk factors for coronary heart disease in patients treated for human immunodeficiency virus infection compared with the general population.** *Clin Infect Dis* 2003, **37:**292–298.
64. Triant VA, Lee H, Hadigan C, Grinspoon SK: **Increased acute myocardial infarction rates and cardiovascular risk factors among patients with human immunodeficiency virus disease.** *J Clin Endocrinol Metab* 2007, **92:**2506–2512.
65. Goulet JL, Fultz SL, Rimland D, Butt A, Gibert C, Rodriguez-Barradas M, Bryant K, Justice AC: **Aging and infectious diseases: do patterns of comorbidity vary by HIV status, age, and HIV severity?** *Clin Infect Dis* 2007, **45:**1593–1601.
66. Cockerham L, Scherzer R, Zolopa A, Rimland D, Lewis CE, Bacchetti P, Grunfeld C, Shlipak M, Tien PC: **Association of HIV infection, demographic and cardiovascular risk factors with all-cause mortality in the recent HAART era.** *J Acquir Immune Defic Syndr* 2010, **53:**102–106.
67. Bergersen BM, Sandvik L, Dunlop O, Birkeland K, Bruun JN: **Prevalence of hypertension in HIV-positive patients on highly active retroviral therapy (HAART) compared with HAART-naive and HIV-negative controls: results from a Norwegian study of 721 patients.** *Eur J Clin Microbiol Infect Dis* 2003, **22:**731–736.
68. Helleberg M, Afzal S, Kronborg G, Larsen CS, Pedersen G, Pedersen C, Gerstoft J, Nordestgaard BG, Obel N: **Mortality attributable to smoking among HIV-1-infected individuals: a nationwide, population-based cohort study.** *Clin Infect Dis* 2013, **56:**727–734.
69. Pereyra F, Lo J, Triant VA, Wei J, Buzon MJ, Fitch KV, Hwang J, Campbell JH, Burdo TH, Williams KC, *et al*: **Increased coronary atherosclerosis and immune activation in HIV-1 elite controllers.** *AIDS* 2012, **26:**2409–2412.
70. Hsue PY, Hunt PW, Schnell A, Kalapus SC, Hoh R, Ganz P, Martin JN, Deeks SG: **Role of viral replication, antiretroviral therapy, and immunodeficiency in HIV-associated atherosclerosis.** *AIDS* 2009, **23:**1059–1067.
71. Libby P, Ridker PM, Maseri A: **Inflammation and atherosclerosis.** *Circulation* 2002, **105:**1135–1143.
72. Ross R: **Atherosclerosis–an inflammatory disease.** *N Engl J Med* 1999, **340:**115–126.
73. Coussens LM, Werb Z: **Inflammation and cancer.** *Nature* 2002, **420:**860–867.
74. Grivennikov SI, Greten FR, Karin M: **Immunity, inflammation, and cancer.** *Cell* 2010, **140:**883–899.
75. Bataller R, Brenner DA: **Liver fibrosis.** *J Clin Invest* 2005, **115:**209–218.
76. Hernandez-Gea V, Friedman SL: **Pathogenesis of liver fibrosis.** *Annu Rev Pathol* 2011, **6:**425–456.
77. Kaptoge S, Di Angelantonio E, Lowe G, Pepys MB, Thompson SG, Collins R, Danesh J: **C-reactive protein concentration and risk of coronary heart disease, stroke, and mortality: an individual participant meta-analysis.** *Lancet* 2010, **375:**132–140.
78. Danesh J, Kaptoge S, Mann AG, Sarwar N, Wood A, Angleman SB, Wensley F, Higgins JP, Lennon L, Eiriksdottir G, *et al*: **Long-term interleukin-6 levels and subsequent risk of coronary heart disease: two new prospective studies and a systematic review.** *PLoS Med* 2008, **5:**e78.
79. Danesh J, Whincup P, Walker M, Lennon L, Thomson A, Appleby P, Rumley A, Lowe GD: **Fibrin D-dimer and coronary heart disease: prospective study and meta-analysis.** *Circulation* 2001, **103:**2323–2327.
80. Danesh J, Lewington S, Thompson SG, Lowe GD, Collins R, Kostis JB, Wilson AC, Folsom AR, Wu K, Benderly M, *et al*: **Plasma fibrinogen level and the risk of major cardiovascular diseases and nonvascular mortality: an individual participant meta-analysis.** *JAMA* 2005, **294:**1799–1809.
81. Il'yasova D, Colbert LH, Harris TB, Newman AB, Bauer DC, Satterfield S, Kritchevsky SB: **Circulating levels of inflammatory markers and cancer risk in the health aging and body composition cohort.** *Cancer Epidemiol Biomarkers Prev* 2005, **14:**2413–2418.
82. Siemes C, Visser LE, Coebergh JW, Splinter TA, Witteman JC, Uitterlinden AG, Hofman A, Pols HA, Stricker BH: **C-reactive protein levels, variation in the C-reactive protein gene, and cancer risk: the Rotterdam Study.** *J Clin Oncol* 2006, **24:**5216–5222.
83. Heikkila K, Harris R, Lowe G, Rumley A, Yarnell J, Gallacher J, Ben-Shlomo Y, Ebrahim S, Lawlor DA: **Associations of circulating C-reactive protein and interleukin-6 with cancer risk: findings from two prospective cohorts and a meta-analysis.** *Cancer Causes Control* 2009, **20:**15–26.
84. Harris TB, Ferrucci L, Tracy RP, Corti MC, Wacholder S, Ettinger WH Jr, Heimovitz H, Cohen HJ, Wallace R: **Associations of elevated interleukin-6 and C-reactive protein levels with mortality in the elderly.** *Am J Med* 1999, **106:**506–512.
85. Cohen HJ, Harris T, Pieper CF: **Coagulation and activation of inflammatory pathways in the development of functional decline and mortality in the elderly.** *Am J Med* 2003, **114:**180–187.
86. Shorr AF, Thomas SJ, Alkins SA, Fitzpatrick TM, Ling GS: **D-dimer correlates with proinflammatory cytokine levels and outcomes in critically ill patients.** *Chest* 2002, **121:**1262–1268.
87. Valdez H, Connick E, Smith KY, Lederman MM, Bosch RJ, Kim RS, St Clair M, Kuritzkes DR, Kessler H, Fox L, *et al*: **Limited immune restoration after 3 years' suppression of HIV-1 replication in patients with moderately advanced disease.** *AIDS* 2002, **16:**1859–1866.
88. Kuller LH, Tracy R, Belloso W, De Wit S, Drummond F, Lane HC, Ledergerber B, Lundgren J, Neuhaus J, Nixon D, *et al*: **Inflammatory and coagulation biomarkers and mortality in patients with HIV infection.** *PLoS Med* 2008, **5:**e203.
89. Tien PC, Choi AI, Zolopa AR, Benson C, Tracy R, Scherzer R, Bacchetti P, Shlipak M, Grunfeld C: **Inflammation and mortality in HIV-infected adults: analysis of the FRAM study cohort.** *J Acquir Immune Defic Syndr* 2010, **55:**316–322.

90. Andrade BB, Hullsiek KH, Boulware DR, Rupert A, French MA, Ruxrungtham K, Montes ML, Price H, Barreiro P, Audsley J, *et al*: **Biomarkers of inflammation and coagulation are associated with mortality and hepatitis flares in persons coinfected with HIV and hepatitis viruses.** *J Infect Dis* 2013, **207:**1379–1388.
91. Sandler NG, Wand H, Roque A, Law M, Nason MC, Nixon DE, Pedersen C, Ruxrungtham K, Lewin SR, Emery S, *et al*: **Plasma levels of soluble CD14 independently predict mortality in HIV infection.** *J Infect Dis* 2011, **203:**780–790.
92. Hunt PW, Cao HL, Muzoora C, Ssewanyana I, Bennett J, Emenyonu N, Kembabazi A, Neilands TB, Bangsberg DR, Deeks SG, Martin JN: **Impact of CD8+ T-cell activation on CD4+ T-cell recovery and mortality in HIV-infected Ugandans initiating antiretroviral therapy.** *AIDS* 2011, **25:**2123–2131.
93. Duprez DA, Neuhaus J, Kuller LH, Tracy R, Belloso W, De Wit S, Drummond F, Lane HC, Ledergerber B, Lundgren J, *et al*: **Inflammation, coagulation and cardiovascular disease in HIV-infected individuals.** *PLoS One* 2012, **7:**e44454.
94. Ford ES, Greenwald JH, Richterman AG, Rupert A, Dutcher L, Badralmaa Y, Natarajan V, Rehm C, Hadigan C, Sereti I: **Traditional risk factors and D-dimer predict incident cardiovascular disease events in chronic HIV infection.** *AIDS* 2010, **24:**1509–1517.
95. Borges AH, Silverberg MJ, Wentworth D, Grulich AE, Fatkenheuer G, Mitsuyasu R, Tambussi G, Sabin CA, Neaton JD, Lundgren JD: **Predicting risk of cancer during HIV infection: the role of inflammatory and coagulation biomarkers.** *AIDS* 2013, **27:**1433–1441.
96. McComsey GA, Kitch D, Sax PE, Tierney C, Jahed NC, Melbourne K, Ha B, Brown TT, Bloom A, Fedarko N, Daar ES: **Associations of Inflammatory Markers with AIDS and non-AIDS Clinical Events after Initiation of Antiretroviral Therapy: AIDS Clinical Trials Group A5224s, a substudy of ACTG A5202.** *J Acquir Immune Defic Syndr* 2013:. Epub.
97. Havlir DV, Bassett R, Levitan D, Gilbert P, Tebas P, Collier AC, Hirsch MS, Ignacio C, Condra J, Gunthard HF, *et al*: **Prevalence and predictive value of intermittent viremia with combination hiv therapy.** *JAMA* 2001, **286:**171–179.
98. Grennan JT, Loutfy MR, Su D, Harrigan PR, Cooper C, Klein M, Machouf N, Montaner JS, Rourke S, Tsoukas C, *et al*: **Magnitude of virologic blips is associated with a higher risk for virologic rebound in HIV-infected individuals: a recurrent events analysis.** *J Infect Dis* 2012, **205:**1230–1238.
99. Mavigner M, Delobel P, Cazabat M, Dubois M, L'Faqihi-Olive FE, Raymond S, Pasquier C, Marchou B, Massip P, Izopet J: **HIV-1 residual viremia correlates with persistent T-cell activation in poor immunological responders to combination antiretroviral therapy.** *PLoS One* 2009, **4:**e7658.
100. Wittkop L, Bitard J, Lazaro E, Neau D, Bonnet F, Mercie P, Dupon M, Hessamfar M, Ventura M, Malvy D, *et al*: **Effect of cytomegalovirus-induced immune response, self antigen-induced immune response, and microbial translocation on chronic immune activation in successfully treated HIV type 1-infected patients: the ANRS CO3 Aquitaine Cohort.** *J Infect Dis* 2013, **207:**622–627.
101. van de Berg PJ, Heutinck KM, Raabe R, Minnee RC, Young SL, van Donselaar-van der Pant KA, Bemelman FJ, van Lier RA, ten Berge IJ: **Human cytomegalovirus induces systemic immune activation characterized by a type 1 cytokine signature.** *J Infect Dis* 2010, **202:**690–699.
102. Hsue PY, Hunt PW, Sinclair E, Bredt B, Franklin A, Killian M, Hoh R, Martin JN, McCune JM, Waters DD, Deeks SG: **Increased carotid intima-media thickness in HIV patients is associated with increased cytomegalovirus-specific T-cell responses.** *AIDS* 2006, **20:**2275–2283.
103. Sacre K, Hunt PW, Hsue PY, Maidji E, Martin JN, Deeks SG, Autran B, McCune JM: **A role for cytomegalovirus-specific CD4+CX3CR1+ T cells and cytomegalovirus-induced T-cell immunopathology in HIV-associated atherosclerosis.** *AIDS* 2012, **26:**805–814.
104. Kovacs A, Al-Harthi L, Christensen S, Mack W, Cohen M, Landay A: **CD8+ T cell activation in women coinfected with human immunodeficiency virus type 1 and hepatitis C virus.** *J Infect Dis* 2008, **197:**1402–1407.
105. Gonzalez VD, Falconer K, Blom KG, Reichard O, Morn B, Laursen AL, Weis N, Alaeus A, Sandberg JK: **High levels of chronic immune activation in the T-cell compartments of patients coinfected with hepatitis C virus and human immunodeficiency virus type 1 and on highly active antiretroviral therapy are reverted by alpha interferon and ribavirin treatment.** *J Virol* 2009, **83:**11407–11411.
106. Estes JD, Harris LD, Klatt NR, Tabb B, Pittaluga S, Paiardini M, Barclay GR, Smedley J, Pung R, Oliveira KM, *et al*: **Damaged intestinal epithelial integrity linked to microbial translocation in pathogenic simian immunodeficiency virus infections.** *PLoS Pathog* 2010, **6:**e1001052.
107. Pandrea IV, Gautam R, Ribeiro RM, Brenchley JM, Butler IF, Pattison M, Rasmussen T, Marx PA, Silvestri G, Lackner AA, *et al*: **Acute loss of intestinal CD4+ T cells is not predictive of simian immunodeficiency virus virulence.** *J Immunol* 2007, **179:**3035–3046.
108. Pandrea I, Gaufin T, Brenchley JM, Gautam R, Monjure C, Gautam A, Coleman C, Lackner AA, Ribeiro RM, Douek DC, Apetrei C: **Cutting edge: experimentally induced immune activation in natural hosts of simian immunodeficiency virus induces significant increases in viral replication and CD4+ T cell depletion.** *J Immunol* 2008, **181:**6687–6691.
109. Brenchley JM, Price DA, Schacker TW, Asher TE, Silvestri G, Rao S, Kazzaz Z, Bornstein E, Lambotte O, Altmann D, *et al*: **Microbial translocation is a cause of systemic immune activation in chronic HIV infection.** *Nat Med* 2006, **12:**1365–1371.
110. Cassol E, Malfeld S, Mahasha P, van der Merwe S, Cassol S, Seebregts C, Alfano M, Poli G, Rossouw T: **Persistent microbial translocation and immune activation in HIV-1-infected South Africans receiving combination antiretroviral therapy.** *J Infect Dis* 2010, **202:**723–733.
111. Jiang W, Lederman MM, Hunt P, Sieg SF, Haley K, Rodriguez B, Landay A, Martin J, Sinclair E, Asher AI, *et al*: **Plasma levels of bacterial DNA correlate with immune activation and the magnitude of immune restoration in persons with antiretroviral-treated HIV infection.** *J Infect Dis* 2009, **199:**1177–1185.
112. Funderburg NT, Mayne E, Sieg SF, Asaad R, Jiang W, Kalinowska M, Luciano AA, Stevens W, Rodriguez B, Brenchley JM, *et al*: **Increased tissue factor expression on circulating monocytes in chronic HIV infection: relationship to in vivo coagulation and immune activation.** *Blood* 2010, **115:**161–167.
113. Martin DM, Boys CW, Ruf W: **Tissue factor: molecular recognition and cofactor function.** *FASEB J* 1995, **9:**852–859.
114. Bavinger C, Bendavid E, Niehaus K, Olshen RA, Olkin I, Sundaram V, Wein N, Holodniy M, Hou N, Owens DK, Desai M: **Risk of cardiovascular disease from antiretroviral therapy for HIV: a systematic review.** *PLoS One* 2013, **8:**e59551.
115. Mocroft A, Phillips AN, Gatell J, Horban A, Ledergerber B, Zilmer K, Jevtovic D, Maltez F, Podlekareva D, Lundgren JD: **CD4 cell count and viral load-specific rates of AIDS, non-AIDS and deaths according to current antiretroviral use.** *AIDS* 2013, **27:**907–918.
116. Weber R, Sabin CA, Friis-Moller N, Reiss P, El-Sadr WM, Kirk O, Dabis F, Law MG, Pradier C, De Wit S, *et al*: **Liver-related deaths in persons infected with the human immunodeficiency virus: the D:A:D study.** *Arch Intern Med* 2006, **166:**1632–1641.
117. Mocroft A, Soriano V, Rockstroh J, Reiss P, Kirk O, de Wit S, Gatell J, Clotet B, Phillips AN, Lundgren JD: **Is there evidence for an increase in the death rate from liver-related disease in patients with HIV?** *AIDS* 2005, **19:**2117–2125.
118. Aceti A, Pasquazzi C, Zechini B, De Bac C: **Hepatotoxicity development during antiretroviral therapy containing protease inhibitors in patients with HIV: the role of hepatitis B and C virus infection.** *J Acquir Immune Defic Syndr* 2002, **29:**41–48.
119. Wit FW, Weverling GJ, Weel J, Jurriaans S, Lange JM: **Incidence of and risk factors for severe hepatotoxicity associated with antiretroviral combination therapy.** *J Infect Dis* 2002, **186:**23–31.
120. Sulkowski MS, Thomas DL, Chaisson RE, Moore RD: **Hepatotoxicity associated with antiretroviral therapy in adults infected with human immunodeficiency virus and the role of hepatitis C or B virus infection.** *JAMA* 2000, **283:**74–80.
121. Brau N, Salvatore M, Rios-Bedoya CF, Fernandez-Carbia A, Paronetto F, Rodriguez-Orengo JF, Rodriguez-Torres M: **Slower fibrosis progression in HIV/HCV-coinfected patients with successful HIV suppression using antiretroviral therapy.** *J Hepatol* 2006, **44:**47–55.
122. Qurishi N, Kreuzberg C, Luchters G, Effenberger W, Kupfer B, Sauerbruch T, Rockstroh JK, Spengler U: **Effect of antiretroviral therapy on liver-related mortality in patients with HIV and hepatitis C virus coinfection.** *Lancet* 2003, **362:**1708–1713.
123. Kovari H, Sabin CA, Ledergerber B, Ryom L, Worm SW, Smith C, Phillips A, Reiss P, Fontas E, Petoumenos K, *et al*: **Antiretroviral drug-related liver mortality among HIV-positive persons in the absence of hepatitis B or C**

virus coinfection: the data collection on adverse events of anti-HIV drugs study. *Clin Infect Dis* 2013, **56**:870–879.

124. Kalayjian RC, Lau B, Mechekano RN, Crane HM, Rodriguez B, Salata RA, Krishnasami Z, Willig JH, Martin JN, Moore RD, *et al*: **Risk factors for chronic kidney disease in a large cohort of HIV-1 infected individuals initiating antiretroviral therapy in routine care.** *AIDS* 2012, **26**:1907–1915.
125. Choi AI, Shlipak MG, Hunt PW, Martin JN, Deeks SG: **HIV-infected persons continue to lose kidney function despite successful antiretroviral therapy.** *AIDS* 2009, **23**:2143–2149.
126. Cooper RD, Wiebe N, Smith N, Keiser P, Naicker S, Tonelli M: **Systematic review and meta-analysis: renal safety of tenofovir disoproxil fumarate in HIV-infected patients.** *Clin Infect Dis* 2010, **51**:496–505.
127. Abrams D, Levy Y, Losso MH, Babiker A, Collins G, Cooper DA, Darbyshire J, Emery S, Fox L, Gordin F, *et al*: **Interleukin-2 therapy in patients with HIV infection.** *N Engl J Med* 2009, **361**:1548–1559.
128. Emery S, Neuhaus JA, Phillips AN, Babiker A, Cohen CJ, Gatell JM, Girard PM, Grund B, Law M, Losso MH, *et al*: **Major clinical outcomes in antiretroviral therapy (ART)-naive participants and in those not receiving ART at baseline in the SMART study.** *J Infect Dis* 2008, **197**:1133–1144.
129. Cohen MS, Chen YQ, McCauley M, Gamble T, Hosseinipour MC, Kumarasamy N, Hakim JG, Kumwenda J, Grinsztejn B, Pilotto JH, *et al*: **Prevention of HIV-1 infection with early antiretroviral therapy.** *N Engl J Med* 2011, **365**:493–505.
130. Severe P, Juste MA, Ambroise A, Eliacin L, Marchand C, Apollon S, Edwards A, Bang H, Nicotera J, Godfrey C, *et al*: **Early versus standard antiretroviral therapy for HIV-infected adults in Haiti.** *N Engl J Med* 2010, **363**:257–265.
131. Sterne JA, May M, Costagliola D, de Wolf F, Phillips AN, Harris R, Funk MJ, Geskus RB, Gill J, Dabis F, *et al*: **Timing of initiation of antiretroviral therapy in AIDS-free HIV-1-infected patients: a collaborative analysis of 18 HIV cohort studies.** *Lancet* 2009, **373**:1352–1363.
132. Kitahata MM, Gange SJ, Abraham AG, Merriman B, Saag MS, Justice AC, Hogg RS, Deeks SG, Eron JJ, Brooks JT, *et al*: **Effect of early versus deferred antiretroviral therapy for HIV on survival.** *N Engl J Med* 2009, **360**:1815–1826.
133. Lee L: **Timing of HAART initiation and clinical outcomes in human immunodeficiency virus type 1 seroconverters.** *Arch Intern Med* 2011, **171**:1560–1569.
134. Cain LE, Logan R, Robins JM, Sterne JA, Sabin C, Bansi L, Justice A, Goulet J, van Sighem A, de Wolf F, *et al*: **When to initiate combined antiretroviral therapy to reduce mortality and AIDS-defining illness in HIV-infected persons in developed countries: an observational study.** *Ann Intern Med* 2011, **154**:509–515.
135. Keiser O, Anastos K, Schechter M, Balestre E, Myer L, Boulle A, Bangsberg D, Toure H, Braitstein P, Sprinz E, *et al*: **Antiretroviral therapy in resource-limited settings 1996 to 2006: patient characteristics, treatment regimens and monitoring in sub-Saharan Africa, Asia and Latin America.** *Trop Med Int Health* 2008, **13**:870–879.
136. Egger M: **Immunodeficiency at the start of combination antiretroviral therapy in low-, middle-and high-income countries.** *J Acquir Immune Defic Syndr* 2013. In press.
137. Sereti I, Dunham RM, Spritzler J, Aga E, Proschan MA, Medvik K, Battaglia CA, Landay AL, Pahwa S, Fischl MA, *et al*: **IL-7 administration drives T cell-cycle entry and expansion in HIV-1 infection.** *Blood* 2009, **113**:6304–6314.
138. Levy Y, Lacabaratz C, Weiss L, Viard JP, Goujard C, Lelievre JD, Boue F, Molina JM, Rouzioux C, Avettand-Fenoel V, *et al*: **Enhanced T cell recovery in HIV-1-infected adults through IL-7 treatment.** *J Clin Invest* 2009, **119**:997–1007.
139. Hunt PW: **Th17, gut, and HIV: therapeutic implications.** *Curr Opin HIV and AIDS* 2010, **5**:189–193.
140. Kanwar B, Favre D, McCune JM: **Th17 and regulatory T cells: implications for AIDS pathogenesis.** *Curr Opin HIV and AIDS* 2010, **5**:151–157.
141. Macias-Barragan J, Sandoval-Rodriguez A, Navarro-Partida J, Armendariz-Borunda J: **The multifaceted role of pirfenidone and its novel targets.** *Fibrogenesis Tissue Repair* 2010, **3**:16.
142. Plaeger SF, Collins BS, Musib R, Deeks SG, Read S, Embry A: **Immune activation in the pathogenesis of treated chronic HIV disease: a workshop summary.** *AIDS Res Hum Retroviruses* 2012, **28**:469–477.
143. Kim S, Iwao H: **Molecular and cellular mechanisms of angiotensin II-mediated cardiovascular and renal diseases.** *Pharmacol Rev* 2000, **52**:11–34.
144. Abbas G, Silveira MG, Lindor KD: **Hepatic fibrosis and the renin-angiotensin system.** *Am J Ther* 2011, **18**:e202–e208.
145. Petoumenos K, Worm S, Reiss P, de Wit S, d'Arminio Monforte A, Sabin C, Friis-Moller N, Weber R, Mercie P, Pradier C, *et al*: **Rates of cardiovascular disease following smoking cessation in patients with HIV infection: results from the D:A:D study(*).** *HIV Med* 2011, **12**:412–421.
146. **EACS Guidelines.** http://www.eacsociety.org/Portals/0/Guidelines_Online_131014.pdf.
147. Dube MP, Stein JH, Aberg JA, Fichtenbaum CJ, Gerber JG, Tashima KT, Henry WK, Currier JS, Sprecher D, Glesby MJ: **Guidelines for the evaluation and management of dyslipidemia in human immunodeficiency virus (HIV)-infected adults receiving antiretroviral therapy: recommendations of the HIV Medical Association of the Infectious Disease Society of America and the Adult AIDS Clinical Trials Group.** *Clin Infect Dis* 2003, **37**:613–627.
148. Friis-Moller N, Thiebaut R, Reiss P, Weber R, Monforte AD, De Wit S, El-Sadr W, Fontas E, Worm S, Kirk O, *et al*: **Predicting the risk of cardiovascular disease in HIV-infected patients: the data collection on adverse effects of anti-HIV drugs study.** *Eur J Cardiovasc Prev Rehabil* 2010, **17**:491–501.
149. Reinsch N, Neuhaus K, Esser S, Potthoff A, Hower M, Mostardt S, Neumann A, Brockmeyer NH, Gelbrich G, Erbel R, Neumann T: **Are HIV patients undertreated? Cardiovascular risk factors in HIV: results of the HIV-HEART study.** *Eur J Prev Cardiol* 2012, **19**:267–274.
150. Lundgren JD, Battegay M, Behrens G, De Wit S, Guaraldi G, Katlama C, Martinez E, Nair D, Powderly WG, Reiss P, *et al*: **European AIDS Clinical Society (EACS) guidelines on the prevention and management of metabolic diseases in HIV.** *HIV Med* 2008, **9**:72–81.
151. Melzi S, Carenzi L, Cossu MV, Passerini S, Capetti A, Rizzardini G: **Lipid Metabolism and Cardiovascular Risk in HIV-1 Infection and HAART: Present and Future Problems.** *Cholesterol* 2010, **2010**:271504.
152. Madruga JR, Cassetti I, Suleiman JM, Etzel A, Zhong L, Holmes CB, Cheng AK, Enejosa J, Study ET: **The safety and efficacy of switching stavudine to tenofovir df in combination with lamivudine and efavirenz in hiv-1-infected patients: three-year follow-up after switching therapy.** *HIV Clin Trials* 2007, **8**:381–390.
153. Negredo E, Cruz L, Paredes R, Ruiz L, Fumaz CR, Bonjoch A, Gel S, Tuldra A, Balague M, Johnston S, *et al*: **Virological, immunological, and clinical impact of switching from protease inhibitors to nevirapine or to efavirenz in patients with human immunodeficiency virus infection and long-lasting viral suppression.** *Clin Infect Dis* 2002, **34**:504–510.
154. Soriano V, Garcia-Gasco P, Vispo E, Ruiz-Sancho A, Blanco F, Martin-Carbonero L, Rodriguez-Novoa S, Morello J, de Mendoza C, Rivas P, *et al*: **Efficacy and safety of replacing lopinavir with atazanavir in HIV-infected patients with undetectable plasma viraemia: final results of the SLOAT trial.** *J Antimicrob Chemother* 2008, **61**:200–205.
155. Mallolas J, Podzamczer D, Milinkovic A, Domingo P, Clotet B, Ribera E, Gutierrez F, Knobel H, Cosin J, Ferrer E, *et al*: **Efficacy and safety of switching from boosted lopinavir to boosted atazanavir in patients with virological suppression receiving a LPV/r-containing HAART: the ATAZIP study.** *J Acquir Immune Defic Syndr* 2009, **51**:29–36.
156. Gatell J, Salmon-Ceron D, Lazzarin A, Van Wijngaerden E, Antunes F, Leen C, Horban A, Wirtz V, Odeshoo L, Van den Dungen M, *et al*: **Efficacy and safety of atazanavir-based highly active antiretroviral therapy in patients with virologic suppression switched from a stable, boosted or unboosted protease inhibitor treatment regimen: the SWAN Study (AI424-097) 48-week results.** *Clin Infect Dis* 2007, **44**:1484–1492.
157. Colafigli M, Di Giambenedetto S, Bracciale L, Tamburrini E, Cauda R, De Luca A: **Cardiovascular risk score change in HIV-1-infected patients switched to an atazanavir-based combination antiretroviral regimen.** *HIV Med* 2008, **9**:172–179.
158. Eron JJ, Young B, Cooper DA, Youle M, Dejesus E, Andrade-Villanueva J, Workman C, Zajdenverg R, Fatkenheuer G, Berger DS, *et al*: **Switch to a raltegravir-based regimen versus continuation of a lopinavir-ritonavir-based regimen in stable HIV-infected patients with suppressed viraemia (SWITCHMRK 1 and 2): two multicentre, double-blind, randomised controlled trials.** *Lancet* 2010, **375**:396–407.
159. Martinez E, Larrousse M, Llibre JM, Gutierrez F, Saumoy M, Antela A, Knobel H, Murillas J, Berenguer J, Pich J, *et al*: **Substitution of raltegravir for ritonavir-boosted protease inhibitors in HIV-infected patients: the SPIRAL study.** *AIDS* 2010, **24**:1697–1707.

160. Masia M, Martinez E, Padilla S, Gatell JM, Gutierrez F: **Endothelial function in HIV-infected patients switching from a boosted protease inhibitor-based regimen to raltegravir: a substudy of the SPIRAL study.** *J Antimicrob Chemother* 2013, **68:**409–413.
161. Gandhi RT, Zheng L, Bosch RJ, Chan ES, Margolis DM, Read S, Kallungal B, Palmer S, Medvik K, Lederman MM, *et al*: **The effect of raltegravir intensification on low-level residual viremia in HIV-infected patients on antiretroviral therapy: a randomized controlled trial.** *PLoS Med* 2010, **7:**8.
162. Hatano H, Hayes TL, Dahl V, Sinclair E, Lee TH, Hoh R, Lampiris H, Hunt PW, Palmer S, McCune JM, *et al*: **A randomized, controlled trial of raltegravir intensification in antiretroviral-treated, HIV-infected patients with a suboptimal CD4+ T cell response.** *J Infect Dis* 2011, **203:**960–968.
163. Yukl SA, Shergill AK, McQuaid K, Gianella S, Lampiris H, Hare CB, Pandori M, Sinclair E, Gunthard HF, Fischer M, *et al*: **Effect of raltegravir-containing intensification on HIV burden and T-cell activation in multiple gut sites of HIV-positive adults on suppressive antiretroviral therapy.** *AIDS* 2010, **24:**2451–2460.
164. Dahl V, Lee E, Peterson J, Spudich SS, Leppla I, Sinclair E, Fuchs D, Palmer S, Price RW: **Raltegravir treatment intensification does not alter cerebrospinal fluid HIV-1 infection or immunoactivation in subjects on suppressive therapy.** *J Infect Dis* 2011, **204:**1936–1945.
165. Llibre JM, Buzon MJ, Massanella M, Esteve A, Dahl V, Puertas MC, Domingo P, Gatell JM, Larrouse M, Gutierrez M, *et al*: **Treatment intensification with raltegravir in subjects with sustained HIV-1 viraemia suppression: a randomized 48-week study.** *Antivir Ther* 2012, **17:**355–364.
166. Vallejo A, Gutierrez C, Hernandez-Novoa B, Diaz L, Madrid N, Abad-Fernandez M, Dronda F, Perez-Elias MJ, Zamora J, Munoz E, *et al*: **The effect of intensification with raltegravir on the HIV-1 reservoir of latently infected memory CD4 T cells in suppressed patients.** *AIDS* 2012, **26:**1885–1894.
167. Byakwaga H, Kelly M, Purcell DF, French MA, Amin J, Lewin SR, Haskelberg H, Kelleher AD, Garsia R, Boyd MA, *et al*: **Intensification of antiretroviral therapy with raltegravir or addition of hyperimmune bovine colostrum in HIV-infected patients with suboptimal CD4+ T-cell response: a randomized controlled trial.** *J Infect Dis* 2011, **204:**1532–1540.
168. Hatano H, Strain MC, Scherzer R, Bacchetti P, Wentworth D, Hoh R, Martin JN, McCune JM, Neaton JD, Tracy RP, *et al*: **Increase in 2-LTR Circles and Decrease in D-dimer After Raltegravir Intensification in Treated HIV-Infected Patients: A Randomized: Placebo-Controlled Trial.** *J Infect Dis* 2013, **208**(9):1436–1442.
169. Massanella M, Negredo E, Puig J, Puertas MC, Buzon MJ, Perez-Alvarez N, Carrillo J, Clotet B, Martinez-Picado J, Blanco J: **Raltegravir intensification shows differing effects on CD8 and CD4 T cells in HIV-infected HAART-suppressed individuals with poor CD4 T-cell recovery.** *AIDS* 2012, **26:**2285–2293.
170. Buzon MJ, Massanella M, Llibre JM, Esteve A, Dahl V, Puertas MC, Gatell JM, Domingo P, Paredes R, Sharkey M, *et al*: **HIV-1 replication and immune dynamics are affected by raltegravir intensification of HAART-suppressed subjects.** *Nat Med* 2010, **16:**460–465.
171. Cuzin L, Trabelsi S, Delobel P, Barbuat C, Reynes J, Allavena C, Peytavin G, Ghosn J, Lascoux-Combe C, Psomas C, *et al*: **Maraviroc intensification of stable antiviral therapy in HIV-1-infected patients with poor immune restoration: MARIMUNO-ANRS 145 study.** *J Acquir Immune Defic Syndr* 2012, **61:**557–564.
172. Wilkin TJ, Lalama CM, McKinnon J, Gandhi RT, Lin N, Landay A, Ribaudo H, Fox L, Currier JS, Mellors JW, *et al*: **A pilot trial of adding maraviroc to suppressive antiretroviral therapy for suboptimal CD4+ T-cell recovery despite sustained virologic suppression: ACTG A5256.** *J Infect Dis* 2012, **206:**534–542.
173. Gutierrez C, Diaz L, Vallejo A, Hernandez-Novoa B, Abad M, Madrid N, Dahl V, Rubio R, Moreno AM, Dronda F, *et al*: **Intensification of antiretroviral therapy with a CCR5 antagonist in patients with chronic HIV-1 infection: effect on T cells latently infected.** *PLoS One* 2011, **6:**e27864.
174. Hunt PW, Shulman NS, Hayes TL, Dahl V, Somsouk M, Funderburg NT, McLaughlin B, Landay AL, Adeyemi O, Gilman LE, *et al*: **The immunologic effects of maraviroc intensification in treated HIV-infected individuals with incomplete CD4+ T-cell recovery: a randomized trial.** *Blood* 2013, **121:**4635–4646.
175. Berenguer J, Alvarez-Pellicer J, Martin PM, Lopez-Aldeguer J, Von-Wichmann MA, Quereda C, Mallolas J, Sanz J, Tural C, Bellon JM, Gonzalez-Garcia J: **Sustained virological response to interferon plus ribavirin reduces liver-related complications and mortality in patients coinfected with human immunodeficiency virus and hepatitis C virus.** *Hepatology* 2009, **50:**407–413.
176. Berenguer J, Rodriguez E, Miralles P, Von Wichmann MA, Lopez-Aldeguer J, Mallolas J, Galindo MJ, Van Den Eynde E, Tellez MJ, Quereda C, *et al*: **Sustained virological response to interferon plus ribavirin reduces non-liver-related mortality in patients coinfected with HIV and Hepatitis C virus.** *Clin Infect Dis* 2012, **55:**728–736.
177. Jennings CL, Sherman KE: **Hepatitis C and HIV co-infection: new drugs in practice and in the pipeline.** *Curr HIV/AIDS Rep* 2012, **9:**231–237.
178. Hunt PW, Martin JN, Sinclair E, Epling L, Teague J, Jacobson MA, Tracy RP, Corey L, Deeks SG: **Valganciclovir reduces T cell activation in HIV-infected individuals with incomplete CD4+ T cell recovery on antiretroviral therapy.** *J Infect Dis* 2011, **203:**1474–1483.
179. Yi TJ, Walmsley S, Szadkowski L, Raboud J, Rajwans N, Shannon B, Kumar S, Kain KC, Kaul R, Tan DH: **A randomized controlled pilot trial of valacyclovir for attenuating inflammation and immune activation in HIV, HSV-2 co-infected adults on suppressive antiretroviral therapy.** *Clin Infect Dis* 2013, **57**(9):1331–1338.
180. Baigent C, Keech A, Kearney PM, Blackwell L, Buck G, Pollicino C, Kirby A, Sourjina T, Peto R, Collins R, Simes R: **Efficacy and safety of cholesterol-lowering treatment: prospective meta-analysis of data from 90,056 participants in 14 randomised trials of statins.** *Lancet* 2005, **366:**1267–1278.
181. Jain MK, Ridker PM: **Anti-inflammatory effects of statins: clinical evidence and basic mechanisms.** *Nat Rev Drug Discov* 2005, **4:**977–987.
182. Aslangul E, Fellahi S, Assoumou LK, Bastard JP, Capeau J, Costagliola D: **High-sensitivity C-reactive protein levels fall during statin therapy in HIV-infected patients receiving ritonavir-boosted protease inhibitors.** *AIDS* 2011, **25:**1128–1131.
183. De Wit S, Delforge M, Necsoi CV, Clumeck N: **Downregulation of CD38 activation markers by atorvastatin in HIV patients with undetectable viral load.** *AIDS* 2011, **25:**1332–1333.
184. Ganesan A, Crum-Cianflone N, Higgins J, Qin J, Rehm C, Metcalf J, Brandt C, Vita J, Decker CF, Sklar P, *et al*: **High dose atorvastatin decreases cellular markers of immune activation without affecting HIV-1 RNA levels: results of a double-blind randomized placebo controlled clinical trial.** *J Infect Dis* 2011, **203:**756–764.
185. Moore RD, Bartlett JG, Gallant JE: **Association between use of HMG CoA reductase inhibitors and mortality in HIV-infected patients.** *PLoS One* 2011, **6:**e21843.
186. Overton ET, Kitch D, Benson CA, Hunt PW, Stein JH, Smurzynski M, Ribaudo HJ, Tebas P: **Effect of statin therapy in reducing the risk of serious non-AIDS-defining events and nonaccidental death.** *Clin Infect Dis* 2013, **56:**1471–1479.
187. Rasmussen LD, Kronborg G, Larsen CS, Pedersen C, Gerstoft J, Obel N: **Statin therapy and mortality in HIV-infected individuals; a Danish nationwide population-based cohort study.** *PLoS One* 2013, **8:**e52828.
188. Ben-Zvi I, Kivity S, Langevitz P, Shoenfeld Y: **Hydroxychloroquine: from malaria to autoimmunity.** *Clin Rev Allergy Immunol* 2012, **42:**145–153.
189. Savarino A, Gennero L, Sperber K, Boelaert JR: **The anti-HIV-1 activity of chloroquine.** *J Clin Virol* 2001, **20:**131–135.
190. Sperber K, Chiang G, Chen H, Ross W, Chusid E, Gonchar M, Chow R, Liriano O: **Comparison of hydroxychloroquine with zidovudine in asymptomatic patients infected with human immunodeficiency virus type 1.** *Clin Ther* 1997, **19:**913–923.
191. Murray SM, Down CM, Boulware DR, Stauffer WM, Cavert WP, Schacker TW, Brenchley JM, Douek DC: **Reduction of immune activation with chloroquine therapy during chronic HIV infection.** *J Virol* 2010, **84:**12082–12086.
192. Paton NI, Goodall RL, Dunn DT, Franzen S, Collaco-Moraes Y, Gazzard BG, Williams IG, Fisher MJ, Winston A, Fox J, *et al*: **Effects of hydroxychloroquine on immune activation and disease progression among HIV-infected patients not receiving antiretroviral therapy: a randomized controlled trial.** *JAMA* 2012, **308:**353–361.
193. Piconi S, Parisotto S, Rizzardini G, Passerini S, Terzi R, Argenteri B, Meraviglia P, Capetti A, Biasin M, Trabattoni D, Clerici M: **Hydroxychloroquine drastically reduces immune activation in HIV-infected, antiretroviral therapy-treated immunologic nonresponders.** *Blood* 2011, **118:**3263–3272.
194. Harris SG, Padilla J, Koumas L, Ray D, Phipps RP: **Prostaglandins as modulators of immunity.** *Trends Immunol* 2002, **23:**144–150.

195. Pettersen FO, Torheim EA, Dahm AE, Aaberge IS, Lind A, Holm M, Aandahl EM, Sandset PM, Tasken K, Kvale D: **An exploratory trial of cyclooxygenase type 2 inhibitor in HIV-1 infection: downregulated immune activation and improved T cell-dependent vaccine responses.** *J Virol* 2011, **85:**6557–6566.

196. Kvale D, Ormaasen V, Kran AM, Johansson CC, Aukrust P, Aandahl EM, Froland SS, Tasken K: **Immune modulatory effects of cyclooxygenase type 2 inhibitors in HIV patients on combination antiretroviral treatment.** *AIDS* 2006, **20:**813–820.

197. Cannon CP, Cannon PJ: **Physiology. COX-2 inhibitors and cardiovascular risk.** *Science* 2012, **336:**1386–1387.

198. Baigent C, Blackwell L, Collins R, Emberson J, Godwin J, Peto R, Buring J, Hennekens C, Kearney P, Meade T, *et al*: **Aspirin in the primary and secondary prevention of vascular disease: collaborative meta-analysis of individual participant data from randomised trials.** *Lancet* 2009, **373:**1849–1860.

199. O'Brien M, Montenont E, Hu L, Nardi MA, Valdes V, Merolla M, Gettenberg G, Cavanagh K, Aberg JA, Bhardwaj N, Berger JS: **Aspirin attenuates platelet activation and immune activation in HIV-1-infected subjects on antiretroviral therapy: a pilot study.** *J Acquir Immune Defic Syndr* 2013, **63:**280–288.

200. Read SW, DeGrezia M, Ciccone EJ, DerSimonian R, Higgins J, Adelsberger JW, Starling JM, Rehm C, Sereti I: **The effect of leflunomide on cycling and activation of T-cells in HIV-1-infected participants.** *PLoS One* 2010, **5:**e11937.

201. Andrieu JM, Lu W: **Long-term clinical, immunologic and virologic impact of glucocorticoids on the chronic phase of HIV infection.** *BMC Med* 2004, **2:**17.

202. Ulmer A, Muller M, Bertisch-Mollenhoff B, Frietsch B: **Low dose prednisolone reduces CD4+ T cell loss in therapy-naive HIV-patients without antiretroviral therapy.** *Eur J Med Res* 2005, **10:**105–109.

203. McComsey GA, Whalen CC, Mawhorter SD, Asaad R, Valdez H, Patki AH, Klaumunzner J, Gopalakrishna KV, Calabrese LH, Lederman MM: **Placebo-controlled trial of prednisone in advanced HIV-1 infection.** *AIDS* 2001, **15:**321–327.

204. Wallis RS, Kalayjian R, Jacobson JM, Fox L, Purdue L, Shikuma CM, Arakaki R, Snyder S, Coombs RW, Bosch RJ, *et al*: **A study of the immunology, virology, and safety of prednisone in HIV-1-infected subjects with CD4 cell counts of 200 to 700 mm^3.** *J Acquir Immune Defic Syndr* 2003, **32:**281–286.

205. Da Silva JA, Jacobs JW, Kirwan JR, Boers M, Saag KG, Ines LB, de Koning EJ, Buttgereit F, Cutolo M, Capell H, *et al*: **Safety of low dose glucocorticoid treatment in rheumatoid arthritis: published evidence and prospective trial data.** *Ann Rheum Dis* 2006, **65:**285–293.

206. Miller KD, Masur H, Jones EC, Joe GO, Rick ME, Kelly GG, Mican JM, Liu S, Gerber LH, Blackwelder WC, *et al*: **High prevalence of osteonecrosis of the femoral head in HIV-infected adults.** *Ann Intern Med* 2002, **137:**17–25.

207. Gori A, Tincati C, Rizzardini G, Torti C, Quirino T, Haarman M, Ben Amor K, van Schaik J, Vriesema A, Knol J, *et al*: **Early impairment of gut function and gut flora supporting a role for alteration of gastrointestinal mucosa in human immunodeficiency virus pathogenesis.** *J Clin Microbiol* 2008, **46:**757–758.

208. Roberfroid M: **Prebiotics: the concept revisited.** *J Nutr* 2007, **137:**830S–837S.

209. Sanders ME: **Probiotics: definition, sources, selection, and uses.** *Clin Infect Dis* 2008, **46**(Suppl 2):S58–S61.

210. Gori A, Rizzardini G, Van't Land B, Amor KB, van Schaik J, Torti C, Quirino T, Tincati C, Bandera A, Knol J, *et al*: **Specific prebiotics modulate gut microbiota and immune activation in HAART-naive HIV-infected adults: results of the "COPA" pilot randomized trial.** *Mucosal Immunol* 2011, **4:**554–563.

211. Irvine SL, Hummelen R, Hekmat S, Looman CW, Habbema JD, Reid G: **Probiotic yogurt consumption is associated with an increase of CD4 count among people living with HIV/AIDS.** *J Clin Gastroenterol* 2010, **44:**e201–e205.

212. Gonzalez-Hernandez LA, Jave-Suarez LF, Fafutis-Morris M, Montes-Salcedo KE, Valle-Gutierrez LG, Campos-Loza AE, Enciso-Gomez LF, Andrade-Villanueva JF: **Synbiotic therapy decreases microbial translocation and inflammation and improves immunological status in HIV-infected patients: a double-blind randomized controlled pilot trial.** *Nutr J* 2012, **11:**90.

213. Schunter M, Chu H, Hayes TL, McConnell D, Crawford SS, Luciw PA, Bengmark S, Asmuth DM, Brown J, Bevins CL, *et al*: **Randomized pilot trial of a synbiotic dietary supplement in chronic HIV-1 infection.** *BMC Complement Altern Med* 2012, **12:**84.

214. Floren CH, Chinenye S, Elfstrand L, Hagman C, Ihse I: **ColoPlus, a new product based on bovine colostrum, alleviates HIV-associated diarrhoea.** *Scand J Gastroenterol* 2006, **41:**682–686.

215. Plettenberg A, Stoehr A, Stellbrink HJ, Albrecht H, Meigel W: **A preparation from bovine colostrum in the treatment of HIV-positive patients with chronic diarrhea.** *Clin Investig* 1993, **71:**42–45.

216. Rump JA, Arndt R, Arnold A, Bendick C, Dichtelmuller H, Franke M, Helm EB, Jager H, Kampmann B, Kolb P, *et al*: **Treatment of diarrhoea in human immunodeficiency virus-infected patients with immunoglobulins from bovine colostrum.** *Clin Investig* 1992, **70:**588–594.

217. Jiang ZD, DuPont HL: **Rifaximin: in vitro and in vivo antibacterial activity–a review.** *Chemotherapy* 2005, **51**(Suppl 1):67–72.

218. Festi D, Mazzella G, Orsini M, Sottili S, Sangermano A, Li Bassi S, Parini P, Ferrieri A, Falcucci M, Grossi L: **Rifaximin in the treatment of chronic hepatic encephalopathy; results of a multicenter study of efficacy and safety.** *Curr Ther Res* 1993, **54:**598–609.

219. Bass NM, Mullen KD, Sanyal A, Poordad F, Neff G, Leevy CB, Sigal S, Sheikh MY, Beavers K, Frederick T, *et al*: **Rifaximin treatment in hepatic encephalopathy.** *N Engl J Med* 2010, **362:**1071–1081.

220. Ambizas EM, Ginzburg R: **Lubiprostone: a chloride channel activator for treatment of chronic constipation.** *Ann Pharmacother* 2007, **41:**957–964.

221. Moeser AJ, Nighot PK, Engelke KJ, Ueno R, Blikslager AT: **Recovery of mucosal barrier function in ischemic porcine ileum and colon is stimulated by a novel agonist of the ClC-2 chloride channel, lubiprostone.** *Am J Physiol Gastrointest Liver Physiol* 2007, **292:**G647–G656.

222. Manns B, Stevens L, Miskulin D, Owen WF Jr, Winkelmayer WC, Tonelli M: **A systematic review of sevelamer in ESRD and an analysis of its potential economic impact in Canada and the United States.** *Kidney Int* 2004, **66:**1239–1247.

223. Stinghen AE, Goncalves SM, Bucharles S, Branco FS, Gruber B, Hauser AB, Pecoits-Filho R: **Sevelamer decreases systemic inflammation in parallel to a reduction in endotoxemia.** *Blood Purif* 2010, **29:**352–356.

224. Navarro-Gonzalez JF, Mora-Fernandez C, Muros de Fuentes M, Donate-Correa J, Cazana-Perez V, Garcia-Perez J: **Effect of phosphate binders on serum inflammatory profile, soluble CD14, and endotoxin levels in hemodialysis patients.** *Clin J Am Soc Nephrol* 2011, **6:**2272–2279.

225. Burger D, Travis S: **Conventional medical management of inflammatory bowel disease.** *Gastroenterology* 2011, **140:**1827–1837. e1822.

6

A study of the prevalence and risk factors leading to HIV infection among a sample of street children and youth

Dibesh Karmacharya[1*], Dongmei Yu[2], Sameer Dixit[1], Rajesh Rajbhandari[1], Bhawana Subedi[1], Sonu Shrestha[1], Sulochana Manandhar[1] and Susan L Santangelo[3]

Abstract

Background: The true prevalence of HIV and other sexually transmitted diseases among street children in Nepal is virtually unknown while information on related behavioural risk factors in this population is non-existent. The risk of HIV infection among street children and adolescents may be especially high due to their marginalized social and economic conditions. This study was conducted to determine the prevalence of HIV infection among a sample of street children and youth of Kathmandu and to identify risk factors associated with HIV infection in this group. A sample of street children and youth was recruited based on the purposive sampling of ten streets in Kathmandu, Nepal, known to have a high density of street children and youth. A total of 251 street children (aged 11–16 years) and youth (aged 17–24 years) were enrolled, with informed consent, from November, 2008 through June, 2009. Most of the participants (95%) were male. Case status was determined by serological assessment of HIV status; data on risk factors were obtained using structured survey interviews. HIV prevalence and rates of a number of behavioural risk factors suspected to play a role in HIV transmission among street children and youth were determined, including unprotected sex, intravenous drug use, and other risky sex and substance use behaviours.

Results: Among the 251 children and youth, we found an overall HIV prevalence of 7.6%. As the sample size of females was small (n = 13) and the behavioural risk factors are likely to be quite different for boys and girls, we conducted separate analyses by gender. As our small sample of females is unlikely to be representative and lacks power for statistical testing, our report focuses on the results for the males surveyed.The strongest behavioural risk factor to emerge from this study was intravenous drug use; 30% of the male subjects were injecting drug users and 20% of those were HIV positive. Furthermore, frequency of drug injection was a highly significant predictor with a dose–response relationship; males reporting occasional injection drug use were nearly 9 times more likely to be HIV positive than never users, while weekly drug injectors had over 46 times the risk of non-users, controlling for exposure to group sex, the only other significant risk factor in the multivariate model.

Conclusions: This sample of street children and youth of Kathmandu has a nearly 20-fold higher prevalence of HIV infection than the general population of Nepal (0.39%). The children and youth engage in number of high risk behaviours, including intravenous drug use, putting them at significant risk of contracting HIV and other sexually transmitted infections.

Keywords: HIV prevalence, Behavioural risk factors, Intravenous drug use, Street children, Kathmandu, Nepal

* Correspondence: dibesh@cmdn.org
[1]Center for Molecular Dynamics Nepal, Sawraj Sadan, Thapathali-11, Kathmandu, Nepal

Background

Nepal is a Low-Income Country, situated in South Asia, with a history of political and economic instability. Poverty and lack of education appear to be some of the factors that lead children and youth to leave their homes and come to the city centers in hopes of better living conditions. More often than not, however, such children are often forced to live on the street, which exposes them to many risks and dangers. Street children have been primarily grouped into three categories: children of the street, children on the street, and abandoned children [1,2]. The first category encompasses children whose entire time is spent living on the streets, including eating and sleeping. These children may have minimal contact with family or relatives. The second category describes children who spend most of the time on the streets but spend time with their families at the end of the day. Abandoned children are those who have been left to live on the streets and have no contact with their family.

The street children and youth are commonly referred to as "Khate" in Nepali, and they are known to roam around in particular areas of the city, where they engage in begging and loitering. A previous study [3] estimated the national population of street children in Nepal at about 5000; of these, 500–600 are thought to reside in Kathmandu. There has been no official census carried out on the population of street children in Kathmandu for the last decade.

There are approximately 71,250 people living with HIV and AIDS in Nepal and the estimated national HIV prevalence rate is 0.39% [4]. The risk of HIV infection among children and adolescents, especially those living on the streets, may be especially high due to their marginalized social and economic situations, as well as the existence of commercial sex and exchange sex (for food, shelter and other needs), along with intravenous drug use and other high risk behaviors in this population [5]. However, there has been no official study carried out to ascertain the actual prevalence of HIV infection in this population.

The National HIV & AIDS Strategy (2006–2011) [6] developed by the National Center for AIDS and STI Control, Government of Nepal, defines Intravenous Drug Users (IDUs), Men having sex with Men (MSM), Male Sex Workers (MSWs), Female Sex Workers (FSWs), Migrants, and Spouses of Prison inmates as the Most At-Risk Populations (MARPs) for developing HIV/AIDS. Similarly, young adults, uniformed service men and women, street children, and trafficked girls are categorized as At Risk Populations (ARPs) as per the government of Nepal, National HIV/AIDS Strategy (2006–2011) [6]. The street children and youth of Nepal may be vulnerable to sexual abuse and exploitation, such as pedophilia. The probability of these children and youth becoming involved in commercial sex and injecting drug use is high, which may increase their risk of HIV infection [5].

The true prevalence of HIV and other sexually transmitted diseases among street children in Nepal is virtually unknown, while information on behavioral risks in this population is non-existent. Worldwide, IDU accounts for 30% of HIV infection [7]. Because many of the street children and youth engage in intravenous drug use [8,9], transmission of HIV in this population is expected to be high. Unprotected sex, usually as exchange sex, is known to be common among street children worldwide [5] and may also be the case for street children and youth of Kathmandu. Furthermore, there are certain other behavioral risk factors (BRFs) which are suspected to play a role in HIV transmission among street children and youth. These include group sex, sex with male and female sex workers, anal sex, alcohol use/abuse, and glue sniffing, all of which may play a role in a street child becoming exposed to and potentially infected with HIV [10]. This study was designed to assess HIV prevalence in a sample of street children and youth from Kathmandu, as well as the BRFs associated with HIV infection in this population.

Methods

Study Sampling

There are an estimated 500–600 street children and youth living on the streets of Kathmandu [3]. The study sample included street children in the age range of 11–16 years, and youth in the age range of 17–24 years. A sample of 251 street children and youth were recruited for the study, based on purposive sampling frames developed within each selected cluster, targeting 10 streets of Kathmandu using information gathered through Focused Group Discussion (FGD); consultation with group leaders of the street children helped ensure an equal sampling probability across the 10 streets. Based on initial information gathered from FGDs, two to four group leaders from among the street children were selected as the main seeds. The seed leaders' main referral list of study participants was used for random sampling. Only street children and youth in the selected areas who had lived on the streets for more than 3 months and did not return home at end of day were recruited for the study (children of the street and abandoned children). Children who were 11 years of age or less were not recruited due to concern about their ability to provide informed consent. Youth above 24 years of age who were street children and youth group leaders participated in the interview but were not recruited into the study; data of the group leaders over the age of 24 were not included in the analyses. The study team consisted of field researchers who have had experience working with the street children of

Kathmandu; they were able to recruit motivators within the population of street children to encourage and facilitate the participation of study subjects.

Data collection

The survey interviews were conducted in confidential settings by the field researchers using a questionnaire developed in the Nepali language. Data on the demographic, social, economic and living conditions of the street children and youth were collected by means of a structured KABP (Knowledge, Attitude, Behavior and Practices) survey questionnaire designed for this study. A blood sample was collected from all study subjects by trained phlebotomists and transported the same day to the laboratory facility of Intrepid Nepal Pvt., Ltd. for serological testing (November 2008-June 2009). Additional qualitative information was also gathered through FGDs conducted by trained field researchers.

The survey questionnaire and FGD guides were developed and pretested for accuracy and effectiveness in an adjoining town, which was not part of the sampling area. The tools were approved as part of the overall proposal approval process by the Nepal Health Research Council (NHRC), the ethical regulatory body of Nepal that insures the protection of human subjects in research. Written and/or verbal consent was obtained from all participants prior to the survey interview and blood sampling. Pre- and post-test counseling were done by trained counselors. The serological test results were distributed to participants in a confidential setting at a Voluntary Testing and Counseling Center (STI and AIDS Care and Treatment Services, Kathmandu, Nepal) where participants were able to receive comprehensive HIV and STI related services, if desired.

Data were collected on general demographic and family status, education, medical and health- related issues, sexual behaviors, drug injecting behaviors and other drug use, knowledge and awareness of HIV and AIDS, and media habits. Male and female participants were interviewed by investigators of the same gender. All interviews were conducted in quiet, private areas designed to make the participant feel comfortable. Altogether nine focus group discussions (FGDs) were held. Each group consisted of eight street children and youth participants. In FGDs, the participants provided information about life on the streets of Kathmandu and their knowledge and behavior related to HIV vulnerability; this greatly helped us understand the overall situation of street children and youth of Kathmandu and develop the survey questionnaire for this study.

Serological testing

HIV serological testing was carried out using the WHO evaluated Enzyme Linked Immuno-Absorbent Assay (ELISA) (HIV1-2 ELISA Diagnostic Kit, Shanghai Kehua Bio-Engineering Co., Ltd.) at the laboratory facility of Intrepid Nepal Pvt., Ltd. Tests were performed using the WHO recommended algorithm for HIV testing and screening. All samples were tested in triplicate with ELISA. If the first test result was positive a second ELISA test was performed on that sample. If the second result was positive, further testing was not carried out, and the test result was considered "Confirmed Positive." If the second test result yielded negative results, a third test was carried out as a "tie breaker."

Statistical analysis

Tests of association between the categorical/descriptive variables and HIV status were investigated via Fisher's exact test and were applied separately in males and females; odds ratios and confidence limits were calculated to assess strength of associations. Association between the quantitative variables and HIV status was investigated by the two sample t-test and logistic regression was used to conduct multivariate analyses. In the multivariate logistic regression analyses, a fully saturated model was first established by including all the variables having a p-value < 0.1 in the univariate tests. The saturated model was then simplified by a backwards elimination stepwise procedure, using 0.05 as the p-value elimination threshold.

Because age was strongly and significantly associated with several other risk factors, we included these risk factors and excluded age itself in the fully saturated model, which resulted in a final model that included frequency of drug injection in the past month, and number of individuals involved in group sex (Table 1). All analyses were carried out using R, an open-source freely available programming language and environment for statistical computing [11].

Results

A total of 251 street children and youth aged 11–24 were surveyed; 19 of these subjects were positive for HIV, yielding an overall prevalence of HIV infection of

Table 1 Multivariate analysis of high risk behaviors leading to HIV infection among the Street Children and Youth of Kathmandu, Nepal

		OR (95% CI)	P
Frequency of drug injection in last month	Never	1.0 (Ref)	
	Sometimes	8.47 (1.27, 56.35)	0.03
	Weekly	46.32 (8.19, 261.95)	<0.001
Number of individuals involved in group sex	0	1.0 (Ref)	
	2~4	6.54 (1.38, 31.01)	0.02
	> 4	0.36 (0.041, 3.23)	0.36

7.6% in this sample. This is over 19 times higher than the estimated HIV prevalence of the general population of Nepal at 0.39% [4].

Our sample of street children in Kathmandu consisted of mostly males (95% or 238: See Table 2). Please note that because the sample of females was so small (n = 13) and because the behavioural risk factors for girls are likely to be different from those for boys, we conducted separate analyses for girls and boys (see Table 2). The remainder of this report will focus on the results for the males surveyed, as our small sample of females is unlikely to be representative and lacks power for statistical testing.

Nearly half the male children and youth interviewed (48%) had been living on the streets for more than 5 years and the majority had living parents (63%), while some (11%) reported that both parents were deceased. Nearly half the male participants (48%) left home when they were between 6 and 11 years old, while 24% were younger than 6 when they left home. Some level of formal education had been attained by 80% of the male children and youth interviewed (and only 62% of the females), with 14% of the males reporting to have studied until at least grade 5. Among boys with no formal education, HIV prevalence (11%) was significantly higher than among those with some education (5.8%). It is noteworthy that among the 5/13 girls with no formal education, 60% (3/5) were HIV positive, while none of the 8 girls with some education were infected.

The vast majority of the male children and youth (94%) reported to have had vaginal intercourse; 64% of those boys had their first sexual intercourse between the age of 12 and 16 years while 24% first experienced sexual intercourse before age 12. Anal sex was experienced by 39% of the boys and 61% of the boys interviewed had had sex with a female sex worker while 12% had had sex with a male sex worker. Furthermore, 37% of the boys

Table 2 Univariate analyses on behavioural risk factors leading to HIV infection on the street children and youth of Kathmandu, Nepal

Variable		Male (N=238)				Female (N=13)		
		HIV+	HIV-	Univariate OR (CI)	p-value	HIV+	HIV-	Univariate p-value
Age (mean)		21.2	15.9	1.7 (1.4, 2.0)	<0.001	22	18.5	0.13
Formal education	Yes	11	180	1.0 (Ref)		0	8	
	No	5	42	1.9 (0.50, 6.5)	0.32	3	2	0.035
Alcohol Use	No	8	55	1.0 (Ref)		0	4	
	Yes	8	167	0.33 (0.12, 0.92)	0.03	3	6	0.50
Sniffing Glue	No	6	43			0	6	
	Yes	10	179	0.40 (0.12, 1.4)	0.11	3	4	0.19
Intravenous Drug Use	No	2	164	1.0 (Ref)		1	7	
	Yes	14	57	20 (4.4, 185)	<0.001	2	3	0.51
Ever shared syringe for drug injection	No	2	167	1.0 (Ref)		1	7	
	Yes	14	53	22 (4.8, 203)	<0.001	2	3	0.51
Frequency of drug injection in last month	Never	2	164	1.0 (Ref)		1	7	
	Sometimes	3	27	9.1 (1.5, 57)	0.02	0	1	
	Weekly	10	26	32 (6.5, 152)	<0.001	2	1	0.24
Subject has regular sex partners	No	6	126	1.0 (Ref)		1	2	
	Yes	10	95	2.2 (0.70, 7.7)	0.19	2	8	1.0
Number of non-regular sex partners within a month of interview	None	6	126	1.0 (Ref)		1	2	
	1	2	15	2.8 (0.52, 15)	0.23	0	2	
	> 1	8	80	2.1 (0.70, 6.3)	0.18	2	6	1.0
Subject participates in group sex	No	9	141	1.0 (Ref)		0	7	
	Yes	7	81	1.4 (0.41, 4.3)	0.60	3	3	0.070
Frequency of anal sex	Never/Rarely	10	138	1.0 (Ref)		1	5	
	Sometimes/Frequently	6	84	0.99 (0.28, 3.1)	1	2	5	1.0

Data for this integarted bio-behavioral HIV study were collected from 251 street children and youth of Kathmandu, Nepal from November, 2008 through June, 2009.

had participated in group sex, with some (32%) engaging in group sex with four or more participants. Many of the street children admitted to having sexual partners other than their regular partners (44% of male participants), and more than 37% of the boys reported having had sexual intercourse with more than 1 partner other than their regular partner in the last month alone. Regular use of condoms appeared to be low in the majority of the street children and youth who were sexually active, with 59% responding that they did not regularly use condoms during sexual intercourse. A total of 87% of the boys reported they had not used condoms during their last sexual encounter despite the fact that 97% reported to have heard of HIV/AIDS, and 91% reported to understand that unsafe sexual practices can lead to HIV infection (data not shown). The vast majority (91%) interviewed stated that they were aware such unsafe sexual practices put them at increased risk of contracting HIV. However, none of these sexual behaviours significantly discriminated between cases with HIV infection and non-cases.

Thirty percent of this sample of male street children (and 38% of the females) were self-reported intravenous drug users and 20% (14/71) of male IDUs were HIV positive ($p < 0.001$), (as were 2/5 or 40% of female IDUs) (Table 2). Boys reporting occasional injection drug use were 9 times more likely to be HIV positive than never users, while weekly drug injectors were at 32 times the risk of non-users. Among the male IDUs, 28% shared needles with their peers and 21% of those sharing needles were HIV positive ($OR = 21.7$; $p < 0.001$).

A significant, but unexpected association was identified between alcohol consumption and HIV status among the boys in the univariate analyses. Alcohol use appeared to be protective, conferring about 1/3 the risk of HIV infection as compared to non-drinkers. Alcohol use was uncorrelated with IDU (data not shown).

Multivariate analysis

In the final multivariate model, which included only the data on boys, number of individuals involved in group sex was a significant risk factor, controlling for drug injection frequency, and was associated with a 6.5-fold increased risk for the boys who endorsed having 2–4 group sex partners as compared with boys who did not participate in group sex.

Intravenous drug use remained a very strong risk factor in the multivariate analyses. The odds of HIV infection were nearly 9 times greater ($OR = 8.5$; 95% CI: 1.3, 56.4) among boys who 'sometimes' injected drugs compared to those who never injected, adjusted for number of group sex partners, while the risk increased to over 46 times that of non IDUs ($OR = 46.3$; 95% CI: 8.2, 262) for the boys who injected drugs at least weekly, adjusting for group sex exposure. Alcohol use was not a significant predictor of risk in the multivariate model.

Discussion

This study, the first of its kind in Nepal, was designed to a) assess the HIV status of a pilot sample of street children and youth of Kathmandu and b) identify risk factors associated with HIV infection among these children and youth. The serological tests revealed an HIV prevalence rate of nearly 8% among the sample of street children and youth surveyed. This is nearly 20 times greater than the estimated HIV prevalence of 0.39% for the general population of Nepal [4]. A similar study carried out in India reported a prevalence rate for HIV infection of 1% in street children of Kolkata [12].

We found significant associations between HIV status and intravenous drug use, and sharing needles. Furthermore, frequency of drug injection was a highly significant predictor with a dose–response relationship; while the risk of HIV infection increased nearly 9-fold among those who occasionally injected drugs, it rose to more than 46 times the baseline risk of those who never engaged in IV drug use for those injecting on at least a weekly basis. These results are similar to findings from other studies where IDUs have been statistically linked to HIV [13]. However, this sample may be unique in that, unlike many/most studies of HIV risk factors for children and youth, it was characterized by a fairly high prevalence of drug injection behaviour, involving 30% of boys and 38% of girls.

In addition, both age and number of group sex partners were found to be independent risk factors for HIV infection among this sample of street children of Kathmandu. As noted above, and in Table 3, age was both significantly associated with the outcome, HIV infection, and significantly associated with several of the other putative risk factors, or exposures, thus meeting the requirements for the classical definition of a confounder, thus we cannot rule out the possibility that age may act as a modifier of some of these other risk factors. Boys engaging in group sex with 2–4 partners carried a more than 6-fold increased risk for HIV infection.

Potential Weaknesses of the Study

We have concerns regarding the validity of some of the answers given by the children on questions that were especially sensitive; the children may not have always provided accurate responses, as the stigma associated with HIV is high. A study carried out on children affected by AIDS in Nepal reported that children reported increased fear and discomfort associated with their HIV status being known in the community [14]. As a result, it may be assumed that street children and youth may not always have been forthright when

Table 3 Associations between Age and Other HIV related risk behaviors among Street Children and Youth of Kathmandu, Nepal

Risk behaviors		Age (mean)	p-value
Formal education	Yes	15.98	
	No	17.23	0.03
Whether have regular sex partners	No	15.78	
	Yes	16.75	0.02
Number of non-regular sex partners within a month of interview	None	15.78	
	1	16.53	
	> 1	16.80	0.070
Group sex	No	15.87	
	Yes	16.84	0.03
Frequency of anal sex	Never/Rarely	16.29	
	Sometimes/Frequently	16.12	0.71
Alcohol use	No	16.14	
	Yes	16.26	0.82
Sniffing Glue	No	18.12	
	Yes	15.74	<0.001
Intravenous Drug Use	No	15.52	
	Yes	17.87	<0.001
Ever shared syringe for drug injection	No	15.51	
	Yes	18.03	<0.001
Frequency of drug injection in last month	Never	15.52	
	Sometimes	16.83	
	Weekly	18.72	<0.001

p-value, generated by a t-test, reflects significance of association between Mean Age and Risk behavior catogories.

answering sensitive questions, such as those concerning condom use and anal and group sex. This may be one reason why this study did not find a clear correlation between condom use or anal sex and HIV, although unprotected anal sex with multiple sex partners has been linked to increased incidence of HIV in adults in prior research [15].

Program Intervention

The concerned stakeholders, including UNICEF/Nepal, were presented with the findings of the study. Participating NGOs and government agencies that have harm reduction programs targeted to street children and youth participated in the dissemination event. Some of the NGOs pledged to work on HIV prevention and awareness in this population, including the initiation of HIV service oriented programs.

Conclusions

This sample of street children and youth of Kathmandu has a nearly 20-fold higher prevalence of HIV infection than the general population of Nepal (0.39%). The children and youth engage in a number of high risk behaviours, including intravenous drug use and sharing needles, putting them at a significant risk of contracting HIV and other sexually transmitted infections. Lack of formal education was a risk factor, albeit not the strongest one, highlighting the need for more education and prevention outreach in a population where formal education is not compulsory and illiteracy is even now, not uncommon.

If this male sample can be used as an indicator of risk among the rest of the street children and youth of Kathmandu, then many of these children are vulnerable and at high risk for HIV infection. Among the most vulnerable street children and youth, those who inject drugs and share needles, there is a danger of increased prevalence of HIV infection without targeted interventions for this at-risk group. Although a much larger study would be required for a more comprehensive picture of the problem throughout Nepal, we hope the findings of this study will raise awareness among concerned health policy makers and ultimately lead to effective intervention programs to address the high prevalence of HIV infection among the street children and youth of Kathmandu before it becomes an epidemic.

Abbreviations

AIDS: Acquired Immune Deficiency Syndrome; ARP: At Risk Population; BRF: Behavioural Risk Factors; ELISA: Enzyme Linked Immuno-Absorbent Assay; FGD: Focused Group Discussion; FSW: Female Sex Worker; HIV: Human Immunodeficiency Virus; IDU: Intravenous Drug Use; KABP: Knowledge Attitude, Behaviour and Practices; MARP: Most At Risk Population; MSW: Male Sex Worker; NHRC: Nepal Health Research Council; OR: Odds Ratio; STI: Sexually Transmitted Infection; WHO: World Health Organization.

Competing interests

The authors declare no conflicts of interest related to this study.

Authors' contributions

The overall study was designed by DK, SD, RR and BS with input from SLS. The field data collection was led by BS and supported by RR and SD. The lab work was done by SM under the supervision of SS. DY carried out all data analyses; DY and SLS interpreted results of statistical testing and made inferences. The manuscript was prepared by DK, SLS, DY and SD. All authors read and approved the final manuscript.

Acknowledgements

This study was supported by financial contributions from the NRN (Non-Nepalese Residents) Community of North America, Friends of Nepal-Los Angeles, Friends of Nepal-New Jersey and UNICEF/Nepal. We will be forever grateful for their support, and for the participation of the street children and youth of Kathmandu, without which this study would not have been possible. We would also like to thank the District AIDS Coordination Committee (DACC) of Kathmandu City for their support, the National Center for AIDS and STD Control (NCASC) for technical and logistical support and all the stakeholders that are involved in the fight against HIV/AIDS in Nepal. We would also like to thank Ms. Rupa Sharma of the Arkansas Department of Health (USA) and Mr. Ganesh Sharma for their valuable input on the study design and analysis.

Author details

[1]Center for Molecular Dynamics Nepal, Sawraj Sadan, Thapathali-11, Kathmandu, Nepal. [2]Massachusetts General Hospital, Psychiatric and

Neurodevelopmental Genetics Unit, Center for Human Genetic Research, Boston, MA, USA. [3]Harvard Medical School, Psychiatry, Harvard School of Public Health, Epidemiology, and Massachusetts General Hospital, Psychiatric and Neurodevelopmental Genetics Unit, Center for Human Genetic Research, Boston, MA, USA.

References

1. Barker G, Knaul F: *Exploited entrepreneurs: Street and working children in developing countries*. Childhope: Working Paper 1; 1991.
2. Campos RRM, Ude W, *et al*: **Social networks and daily activities of street youth in Belo Horizonte, Brazil. Street Youth Study Group.** *Child Dev* 1994, **65:**319–330.
3. *Child Workers in Nepal Concerned Centre (CWIN) HIV/AIDS and Street Children archived report. ref. CAR-60 2579*. Kathmandu: CWIN; 2002.
4. National Estimates of HIV infections, 2009 Nepal: *National Estimates of HIV infections, 2009*. Nepal. Kathmandu: National Center for AIDS and STD Control (NCASC); 2010.
5. Towe VL, ul H, Zafar ST, Sherman SG: **Street life and drug risk behaviors associated with exchanging sex among male street children in Lahore, Pakistan.** *J Adolescent Health* 2009, **44:**222–228.
6. National HIV/AIDS Strategy (2006–2011): Kathmandu: National Center for AIDS and STD Control (NCASC); 2007.
7. *Report on the global AIDS epidemic*. UNAIDS; 2008.
8. Dmirty MK, Lauren Z, *et al*: **HIV seroprevalence in street youth, St Petersburg, Russia.** *AIDS* 2007, **21:**2333–2340.
9. Robbins CL, Zapata L, *et al*: **Multicity HIV seroprevalence in street youth, Ukraine.** *Int J STD AIDS* 2010, **21**:489–496.
10. Rooyen L, Hartell CG: **The health of the street child - The whole says more a synergy of research.** *Int J Adolescence and Youth* 2001, **10:**297–317.
11. R Foundation for Statistical Computing: *A language and environment for statistical computing, reference index version 2.x.x*. Vienna: 14: Development Core Team; 2005.
12. Bal BMR, Mallick AH, Chakraborti S, Sarkar K: **Nontobacco substance use, sexual abuse, HIV, and sexually transmitted infection among street children in Kolkata, India.** *Substance Use Misuse* 2010, **45:**1668–1682.
13. Kral AH BR, Booth RE, Watters JK: **HIV seroprevalence among street-recruited injection drug and crack cocaine users in 16 US municipalities.** *Am J Public Health* 1998, **88:**108–113.
14. *A Situation Assessment of Children Affected by AIDS in Nepal*. Kathmandu: NCASC/Save the Children-Nepal/CREHPA; 2009.
15. Koblina BA HM, Colfaxc G, *et al*: **Risk factors for HIV infection among men who have sex with men.** *AIDS* 2006, **20:**731–739.

7

Hyperlactatemia in a group of HIV patients living in Yaounde-Cameroon

Corinne Tchoula Mamiafo[3], Vicky Jocelyne Ama Moor[1,2*], Jobert Richie N Nansseu[4], Constant Anatole Pieme[2], Claude Tayou[5] and Jeanne Ngogang Yonkeu[1,2]

Abstract

Background and aim: Prolonged exposure to highly active antiretroviral therapy (HAART) is associated with adverse effects such as hyperlactatemia. We determined the prevalence and risk factors for developing hyperlactatemia among human immunodeficiency virus (HIV)-infected cameroonians on antiretroviral therapy (ART).

Methods: We conducted a cross-sectional study from January to April 2012 involving 91 HIV-infected patients receiving ART for at least 12 months and 30 HIV-infected patients who have never received ART (ART-naïve patients). Plasma lactate levels were determined after at least 12 hours of overnight fasting and hyperlactatemia defined as lactate concentrations ≥ 3 mmol/L. The prevalence of hyperlactatemia was determined and the risk factors were analyzed by a multivariate logistic regression model.

Results: The mean lactataemia was significantly higher in the group of HIV patients currently taking ART than in the ART-naïve one (2.3 ± 1.3 and 1.7 ± 0.7 mmol/L respectively, p = 0.002). Patients on first line ART regimens had significantly higher lactatemia than those on second line regimens (2.5 ± 1.5 and 1.9 ± 0.7 mmol/L respectively, p = 0.014). The prevalence of hyperlactatemia in HIV patients receiving ART and in ART-naïve HIV patients was respectively 18.7 and 6.7% (p = 0.095). ART-exposure (adjusted odds ratio (aOR) 5.44, 95% confidence interval (CI) 1.06 – 27.84; p = 0.042) and being on a first line regimen (aOR 16.22, 95% CI 1.57 – 167.91; p = 0.019) were independent strong predictors of hyperlactatemia.

Conclusion: Hyperlactatemia was not rare in our study population. Being on a first line regimen constitutes an important risk factor for developing hyperlactatemia. Measurement of plasma lactate may be useful in optimizing the management of HIV-positive persons on ART.

Keywords: Hyperlactatemia, Antiretroviral therapy, HIV, First line regimen

Introduction

AIDS remains one of the major public health hazards in Africa. The advent and widespread use of HAART in clinical practice has profoundly modified the natural history of HIV infection by significantly improving the prognosis and quality of life of people living with the infection, with a drastic reduction in mortality and morbidity related to HIV and its complications [1]. Unfortunately, the need for permanent medication has led to increasingly more numerous descriptions of new adverse metabolic effects, this being explained by mitochondrial toxicity [2]. It has been demonstrated that this mitochondrial toxicity is associated with hyperlactatemia, lactic acidosis, hepatic steatosis, pancreatitis, lipodystrophy, and peripheral neuropathy [3].

Hyperlactatemia characterized by mild to moderate increases in blood lactate levels in the absence of acidosis has been reported in 8–36% of patients receiving HAART in developed countries, although the majority of cases are asymptomatic or have very mild symptoms [4-8]. Only a small number of patients develop the most severe form of hyperlactatemia, which

* Correspondence: movicky@yahoo.fr
[1]Laboratory of Biochemistry, Yaounde University Teaching Hospital, Yaounde, Cameroon
[2]Department of Biochemistry and Physiological Sciences, University of Yaounde I, Yaounde, Cameroon

presents as metabolic acidosis and is associated with a high mortality rate.

A variety of NRTIs, including stavudine, zidovudine and didanosine, have been associated with hyperlactatemia because of their potential for mitochondrial toxic effects [2,6,9-14]. While stavudine is rarely used in resource-rich settings and is no longer recommended by WHO for initial treatment of HIV-1 infection [14], it remains an important component of standard ART regimens in many resource-limited countries, mainly due to its lower cost [15,16]. Some observational studies have suggested that specific risk factors associated with the development of hyperlactatemia include female sex [17-23], elevated weight or BMI [17,20-23], older age (> 40 years) [17,20], and lower CD4 cell counts [17].

There are limited data on hyperlactatemia caused by prolonged exposure to ART in resource-limited settings like Cameroon. The present study sought at determining the prevalence and determinants related to the development of hyperlactatemia in HIV-infected Cameroonians currently on ART.

Patients and methods

Study participants

This cross-sectional survey was carried out at the HIV out-patient clinic of the Yaounde University Teaching Hospital and the Yaounde Central Hospital. These centers are located in the political capital of Cameroon, and receive a large number of HIV-infected patients living in Yaounde and surrounding town. A convenient sample of 91 HIV-infected patients aged 18 years and above , currently on ART for at least 12 months and regularly followed-up were consecutively enrolled in the study during January – April 2012. These patients were receiving either first line regimen consisting of 2 NRTIs + 1 NNRTI, or second line regimen comprising 2 NRTIs + 1 PI. The choice of a particular regimen was irrespective of potential factors that could induce hyperlactatemia but depended mainly on the availability of ARTs. For quality control purpose, a subset of 30 HIV-infected and ART-naïve patients was also recruited. All the participants were confirmed to be positive for HIV antibody through laboratory detection, and the diagnosis was in line with national HIV/AIDS diagnosis criteria. They were free of alcoholism, chronic hepatitis and were also required not to be on plasma lactate modifying therapies at their enrolment. All the procedures used in this study were in accordance with the current revision of the Helsinki Declaration. A Written and signed informed consent was provided by all the subjects. Consent forms and procedures, as well as survey protocol, were approved by the Cameroon National Ethics Committee (**Reference number: 234/CNE/SE/2011**).

Interview data

At enrollment standardized data collection forms were completed, including sociodemographic characteristics, medical history (AIDS events, CDC/WHO clinical classification, signs and symptoms of symptomatic hyperlactatemia such as nonspecific gastrointestinal symptoms nausea, vomiting, abdominal pain, discomfort or distension, anorexia, peripheral neuropathy, tiredness, muscle weakness, and dyspnea [24]), laboratory markers (CD4 cell counts, FBS (Fasting Blood Sugar), AST (Aspartate Amino Transferase) and ALT (Alanine Amino Transferase) levels), and antiretroviral used.

Sample collection and biochemical assays

After at least 12 hours of overnight fasting and a 30 minutes rest, blood was aseptically collected from each participant by venipuncture in a 5 ml EDTA tube, without a tourniquet or fist clenching. Samples were put on ice and immediately transported to the biochemistry laboratory where plasma specimens were separated by centrifugation at 3000 rpm within 5 min for analyses without delay. Plasma lactate concentrations were determined on an automated clinical chemistry analyzer (BA-88A, MINDRAY laboratory, China) using kits (BIOREX diagnostics, UK) based on the enzymatic conversion of L-lactate to pyruvate by L-lactate oxidase [25].

End point definitions

Concentrations of plasma lactate less than 3 mmol/L were defined as normolactatemic, while those equal or above 3 mmol/L, were consider as hyperlactatemic.

Statistical analysis

Data were coded, entered, and analyzed using SPSS version 20.0 (SPSS Inc., Chicago, Ilinois, USA). Qualitative and quantitative variables were analysed and compared with χ^2 test and Student's **t**-test respectively. Results are expressed as proportion or mean ± SD. The Pearson correlation was used to established the correlation between the variables. ORs with 95% CIs were used to appreciate the impact of different variables on the occurrence of hyperlactatemia, and were calculated by both univariate and multivariate logistic regression analyses while adjusting for confounders. A p value < 0.05 was used to characterize significant results.

Results

A total of 121 patients were included in this study including 91 HIV patients currently taking ART, and 30 ART-naïve HIV patients. Table 1 presents the whole patient clinical characteristics and biochemical determinations. The age ranged from 25 to 67 years old (Mean = 40.3) for patients under ART and between 24 to 64 years old (Mean = 38) for naive ART patients. All the parameters recorded

Table 1 Clinical and biochemical characteristics of the study participants

	Mean ± SD			p
	Patients on ART (n = 91)	ART-naïve patients (n = 30)	Overall (n = 121)	
Age (years)	40.3 ± 9.9	38.5 ± 11.8	39.8 ± 10.4	0.327
Sex (Male/Female)	22/69	6/24	28/93	0.638
CDC Clinical Classification (A/C)	90/1	30/0	120/1	0.752
CD4 count (cells/mm^3)	410.4 ± 231.9	261.8 ± 173.0	373.2 ± 226.9	0.192
AST (IU/L)	27.8 ± 15.9	25.6 ± 10.1	27.3 ± 14.6	0.171
ALT (IU/L)	25.6 ± 20.8	23.1 ± 8.3	24.9 ± 18.4	0.104
FPG (g/L)	0.9 ± 0.2	0.9 ± 0.2	0.9 ± 0.2	0.564
LDH (IU/L)	441.1 ± 138.1	485.1 ± 168.6	452.0 ± 146.8	0.253
Lactataemia (mmol/L)	2.3 ± 1.3	1.7 ± 0.7	2.2 ± 1.2	**0.002***
Hyperlactatemic patients (%)	18.7	6.7	15.7	0.095

FBS: Fasting Blood Sugar; ALT: Alanine Amino Transférase, AST: Aspartate Amino Transférase, LDH: Lactate Dehydrogenase; * p<0.05.

were higher in the group of patients on ART therapy compare to ART naïve except the level of LDH. There was no statistically significant difference between the two groups regarding all these parameters except lactatemia which was significantly (p < 0.005) higher in the group of patients on ART (Table 1). Only classes A and C of the CDC/WHO clinical classification of the HIV infection were noticed. Figure 1 depicts the different therapeutic regimens with the combination AZT – 3TC - NVP being the most recorded (32.97%). The first line ART regimens was the most encountered (66%). However 25.27% of the patients were on LVP/r- TDF-3TC (second line regimen). The mean lactataemia was significantly higher in the group of HIV patients currently taking ART than in the ART-naïve one (2.3 ± 1.3 and 1.7 ± 0.7 mmol/L respectively) (Table 1). Nineteen over the one hundred and twenty one participants (15.70%) presented with hyperlactatemia; among them 17 were HIV patients currently taking ART (18.7%) and the 2 others (6.7%) being ART-naïve patients (Table 1).

Table 2 compares clinical and biochemical parameters between normolactatemic and hyperlactatemic patients taking ART. We did not observe any statistically significant difference between the two groups according to age, sex, CD4+ T-cells count at time of hyperlactatemia, duration of cumulative ART exposure prior to

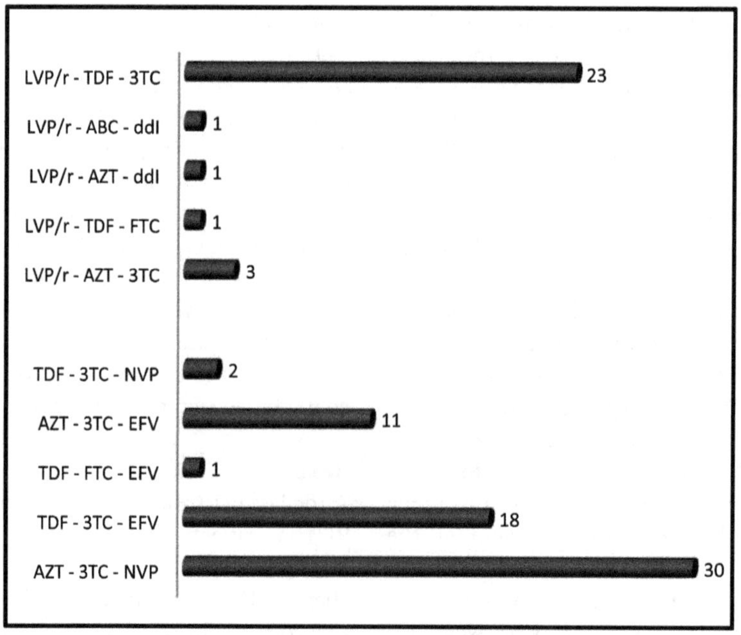

Figure 1 Different therapeutic regimens the 91 ART-receiving subjects were placed on: up are represented second line regimens and down the first line ones and the numbers refer to the number of subjects on each regimen.

Table 2 Characteristics of patients on ART with regard to the occurrence of hyperlactatemia

	Normolactatemic n = 74 (Mean ± SD)	Hyperlactatemic n = 17 (Mean ± SD)	p
Age (years)	40.3 ± 9.4	39.9 ± 12.2	0.865
Sex (Male/Female)	16/58	6/11	0.189
CD4 count at time of hyperlactatemia (cells/mm^3)	414.5 ± 230.8	392.8 ± 239.6	0.730
Duration of cumulative ART exposure prior to hyperlactatemia (years)	5.2 ± 2.9	4.5 ± 3.2	0.382
ART regimens			
First line	44	16	**0.007***
Second line	30	1	
CDC/WHO Class			
A	73	17	0.813
C	1	0	
FPG (g/L)	0.9 ± 0.1	0.9 ± 0.2	0.220
AST (IU/L)	26.7 ± 12.0	32.8 ± 27.4	0.396
ALT (IU/L)	23.1 ± 11.4	36.6 ± 41.8	0.221
LDH (IU/L)	419.7 ± 107.9	534.3 ± 207.0	**0.040***
Lactataemia (mmol/L)	1.8 ± 0.6	4.2 ± 1.8	**< 0.001***

* p<0.05.

hyperlactatemia, FBS, AST and ALT. On contrary, the mean serum LDH (Lactate Dehydrogenase), as well as lactatemia, were significantly higher in the hyperlactatemic group ($p = 0.040$ and $p < 0.001$ respectively). Sixteen patients (25.8%) on first line regimens significantly develop hyperlactatemia ($p = 0.007$). Only one patient on second line regimen (1.1%) presented with severe hyperlactatemia.

Figure 2 is representative of the regimens that have led to hyperlactatemia. There was no statistically significant difference when comparing the mean plasma lactate levels between these regimens. There was no correlation between lactatemia and age ($r = 0.023$, $p = 0.825$), CD4+ T-cells count ($r = 0.071$, $p = 0.506$), FBS ($r = 0.151$, $p = 0.126$), and between lactatemia and serum LDH ($r = 0.181$, $p = 0.085$). On the contrary, there was a positive and significant correlation between lactatemia and AST ($r = 0.439$, $p < 0.001$), and ALT ($r = 0.544$, $p < 0.001$) (Table 3).

While undertaking univariate logistic regression analyses, we did not find any statistically significant association between the occurrence of hyperlactatemia and the sex (OR 2.25, 95% CI 0.789 – 6.42; $p = 0.123$), the duration of cumulative ART exposure (OR 2.59, 95% CI 0.87 – 7.72; $p = 0.089$), and between the occurrence of hyperlactatemia and ART exposure (OR 3.22, 95% CI 0.70 – 14.93; $p = 0.134$) (Table 4). Nevertheless, this latter association became significant after adjusting for age, sex and duration of ART exposure with a coefficient of

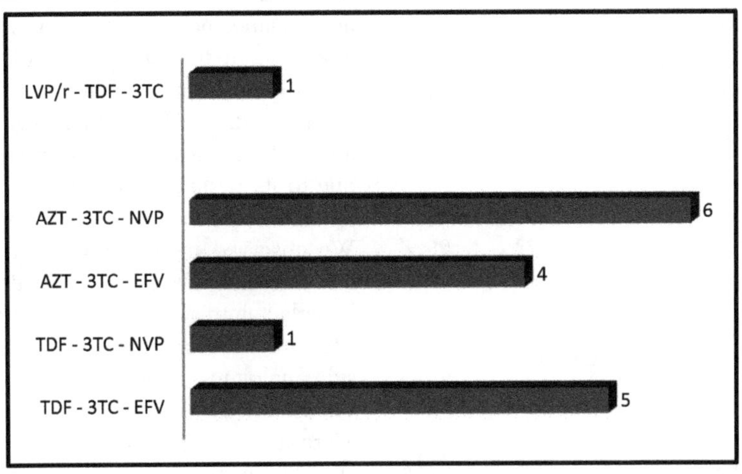

Figure 2 Regimens that have given rise to hyperlactatemia.

Table 3 Correlation between lactatemia and others parameters

Variable	P	Pearson's correlation coefficient (r)
Age	0,825	0,023
CD4 count	0,506	0,071
Fasting Plasma Glucose	0,126	0,151
LDH	0,085	0,181
AST	**<0,001***	**0,439**
ALT	**<0,001***	**0,544**

* p<0.05.

Table 4 Factors likely to influence the occurrence of hyperlactatemia

	Odds ratio	95% CI	p
Sex			
Male	1.00		
Female	2.25	0.79 - 6.42	0.130
Age groups (years)			
20 - 29	1.00		
30 - 39	0.42	0.07 - 2.57	0.347
40 - 49	0.67	0.11 - 4.15	0.664
≥ 50	0.21	0.02 - 2.84	0.243
Duration of cumulative ART exposure			
< 5 years	1.00		
≥ 5 years	2.59	0.87 - 7.72	0.089
ART exposure			
No	1.00		
Yes	3.22	0.70 - 14.93	0.134
CDC clinical stage			
A	1.19	1.1 - 1.28	0.843
C	1.00		
ART regimen			
First line	**10.91**	**1.37 - 86.70**	**0.024***
Second line	1.00		
First line AZT-regimens			
No	1.00		
Yes	1.02	0.32 - 3.32	0.969
First line TDF-regimens			
No	1.00		
Yes	1.17	0.35 - 3.97	0.797
First line 3TC-regimens			
No	1.00		
Yes	0.98	0.94 - 1.02	0.742

* p<0.05.

determination of 0.2 (aOR 5.44, 95% CI 1.06 – 27.84; p = 0.042), but after removing the duration of ART exposure from the model, the last-mentioned association was no more significant (aOR 4.09, 95% CI 0.82 – 20.33; p = 0.085). Being on a first line ART regimen increased more than 10 times the risk of developing hyperlactatemia (OR 10.91, 95% CI 1.37 – 86.70; p = 0.024), this risk becoming more important after adjusting for age, sex, and duration of ART exposure (aOR 16.22, 95% CI 1.57 – 167.91; p = 0.019) with a coefficient of determination of 0.32. We finally observe no significant association between the occurrence of hyperlactatemia and zidovudine-containing regimens, lamivudine-containing regimens, and with tenofovir-containing regimens (Table 4).

Discussion

Lactate is the final product of anaerobic glycolysis, which in a normal state does not accumulate in the body. However, under circumstances such as oxygen deprivation of tissue or impaired oxidative phosphorylation, hyperlactatemia occurs. Lactic acidosis in the absence of tissue ischemia is the hallmark of type B lactic acidosis [26]. Among all anti-HIV medications, it is the NRTIs that have been implicated in type B lactic acidosis [26]. In fact, the pharmacologically active triphosphate moieties of NRTIs act as substrates for human mitochondrial DNA-polymerase gamma, thereby having the potential for incorporation into mitochondrial DNA (mtDNA). As well, mitochondrial exonuclease is inefficient at removing the nucleoside triphosphates [27,28]. The combination of nucleoside triphosphate incorporation and inadequate removal disrupts mtDNA synthesis and results in the arresting of mtDNA-encoded protein synthesis. Eventually, a disruption of oxidative phosphorylation ensues, and lactate accumulates [2].

Stavudine, zidovudine and didanosine are the most frequent NRTIs incriminated in the occurrence of hyperlactatemia [2,6,9-14,29]. The combination of stavudine and didanosine is associated with the greatest relative risk [24]. In this study we had no patient placed on a stavudine-containing regimens because stavudine has been withdrawn from ART regimens recommended for anti-HIV medications in Cameroon since 2011, mainly due to its dyslipidemic effects proven in this milieu [30] and in accordance with the latest WHO guidelines [14]. We observed in our study that zidovudine, lamivudine and tenofovir were not implicated in the occurrence of hyperlactatemia, probably because of the small sample size and probably, the combination of all these nucleoside analogues would increase risk of adverse event development. These findings concur with those from Marceau et al. [29] where increased lactate was not associated with treatment containing lamivudine, zidovudine, abacavir, zalcitabine, efavirenz, nevirapine, and interferon and/or ribavirin. After regrouping regimens in first and second line regimen, we found lactatemia of patients on first line regimens being significantly higher than that of the ones on second line regimen. Furthermore, first line regimen use may confer a sixteen-fold increased risk of developing hyperlactatemia when controlling for other risk factors. These findings can be explained by the fact that PIs, which are part of second line regimen, have not been reported to cause any mitochondrial toxicity [7] given their lack of selectivity for HIV reverse transcriptase [14]. It has been also shown that the incidence and prevalence of hyperlactatemia may vary depending on the number and choice of NRTIs present in an antiretroviral regimen. In fact, in a longitudinal cohort study involving 2144 patients receiving NRTI therapy, the risk of symptomatic hyperlactatemia increased more than 2-fold for each additional NRTI used in a given regimen [31]. Different combinations of NRTIs were also associated with different rates of symptomatic hyperlactatemia [31].

We found significantly elevated plasma lactate levels in patients currently taking ART compared to ART-naïve ones, with an independent five-fold increased risk for the subjects on ART for developing hyperlactatemia when controlling for other covariates. But contrary to John et al. [7] we did not observe any relationship between the occurrence of hyperlactatemia and duration of cumulative ART exposure (especially stavudine in their case). The Lactic Acidosis International Study group [17], as well as Marceau et al. [32], showed an association of older age (age > 40 years) with the development of hyperlactatemia. This was not seen in our study nor in some other ones [7,29,33] probably because our study had a little bit younger age distribution than theirs (mean of 40 years vs. 42 and 44 years respectively). Moreover we found no relationship between the female sex and the occurrence of hyperlactatemia. The same results were reported in others studies [7,29,33]. By contrast, some relevant studies have clearly demonstrated that the female sex constitutes a strong independent risk factor for developing hyperlactatemia [17-20,22,23,34,35], even though the reasons for the observed sex differences in rates of toxicity remain uncertain. As shown in other studies, we observed no association between CD4+ T-cells count, CDC/WHO clinical classification and the occurrence of hyperlactatemia [7,29,33].

There is no consensus on the different thresholds for defining normolactatemia, mild to moderate hyperlactatemia (either symptomatic or not), and severe hyperlactatemia. It has been proposed, from a clinical point of view, that clinically relevant hyperlactatemia may be defined as a lactate concentration of 2.25 – 5 mmol/L, and severe lactic acidosis, as a lactate concentration > 5 mmol/L with a pH < 7.3 or bicarbonate < 20 mmol/L and clinical signs of multiorgan failure [36]. In their study, Marceau et al. [32], based on a previous determination of the reference interval for plasma lactate obtained from 200 healthy venous blood samples (range: 1.5 – 2.25 mmol/L; mean ± SD: 1.4 ± 0.3 mmol/L) [32], defined concentrations of plasma lactate < 2.25 mmol/L as normolactatemic, those between 2.25 and 5 mmol/L as moderately increased, and plasma lactate > 5 mmol/L was considered highly increased. With these definitions, 75.2% of their patients were normolactatemic, 23% had moderately increased serum lactate, and 1.8% had high serum lactate giving thus an overall prevalence of hyperlactatemia (plasma lactate ≥ 2.25 mmol/L) of 24.8% [32]. We had a little bit more normolactatemic subjects than them (81.3% vs. 75.2%) and less hyperlactatemic patients (18.7% vs. 24.8%) assumedly because our definition of normolactatemia was less restrictive than theirs (i.e. < 3 mmol/L vs. < 2.25 mmol/L). As we, they found that the mean value of plasma lactate was significantly higher in the hyperlactatemic group than in the normolactatemic one [32].

The prevalence of asymptomatic hyperlactatemia reported in resource-rich settings varies from one area to another 8.3% [33], 8.7% [37], 18.3% [7] and 21% [4]. As a matter of fact, the lack of a standard biochemical definition for lactic acidosis and symptomatic hyperlactatemia causes confusion and affects incidence and prevalence rates.

Nevertheless, it has been hypothesized that a lactate measurement > 5 mmol/L is defined as severe hyperlactatemia and therefore includes lactic acidosis [17,35]. Fabian et al. in South Africa [35] reported a prevalence of severe hyperlactatemia of 1.3% corroborating our 1.1% even though a huge number of their patients were on stavudine-based regimens.

Unfortunately, the cross-sectional design of the present study could not permit us to determine the incidence and time to onset of hyperlactatemia. Menezes et al. [29] reported a median time to the development of lactic acidosis of 10.8 months while Wester et al. [20] reported a median time of 7.5 months. Moreover we were unable to investigate for other risk factors incriminated or not in the development of hyperlactatemia such as higher baseline BMI (> 30 kg/m^2), lower initial CD4+ T-cells count, higher baseline serum creatinine levels at ART-initiation, this because these informations were lacking in the majority of our patients' files. It is unclear whether and what extent symptomatic hyperlactatemia might progress to lactic acidosis or whether they are two completely separate disorders [7,37]. In fact, routine monitoring of serum lactate levels does not appear to be warranted [7]. Mild, asymptomatic elevations in lactate levels have not been predictive of progression to lactic acidosis [4,7], and a positive predictive value of only 39% for the confirmation of lactic acidosis following a single elevated value has been reported [37]. Taking into account that lactic acidosis can present quite precipitously and progress in a fulminant manner and those patients can be relatively asymptomatic even with high lactate concentrations, lactate levels should be measured as soon as clinical manifestations suggestive of possible symptomatic hyperlactatemia occur in patients currently taking ART. Marceau et al. [32] have proposed that lactate measurements might be performed every 6 months under standardized conditions in asymptomatic patients to detect a trend of increasing lactate concentrations.

Conclusion

Our results showed that chronic compensated and moderated hyperlactatemia is common in ART-exposed HIV infected Cameroonians. Even though stavudine is no more part of ART-regimens, being on a first line regimen constitutes a strong and important risk factor for developing hyperlactatemia. Early diagnosis of symptomatic hyperlactatemia by measurement of plasma lactate under standardized conditions may allow safe outpatient care and optimize the management of these HIV-infected patients on ART.

Competing interest

There is no conflict of interest regarding any of the authors.

Authors' contributions

Study Concept and design: JNY, VJAM, CTM, CAP, CT. Data collection and performing experiments: CTM, VJAM. Statistical Analysis: JRNN. Drafting: JRNN, CTM, CAP. Manuscript Revision: TCM, JRNN, VJAM, CAP, CT, JNY. Study Supervision: JNY. All authors read and approved the final manuscript.

Acknowledgements

The authors gratefully acknowledge all the patients who have accepted to take part in this study.

Author details

[1]Laboratory of Biochemistry, Yaounde University Teaching Hospital, Yaounde, Cameroon. [2]Department of Biochemistry and Physiological Sciences, University of Yaounde I, Yaounde, Cameroon. [3]Department of Biochemistry, Faculty of Sciences, University of Yaounde I, Yaounde, Cameroon. [4]Intensive Care Unit, Mother and Child Centre, Chantal Biya Foundation, Yaounde, Cameroon. [5]Laboratory of Hematology, Yaounde University Teaching Hospital, Yaounde, Cameroon.

References

1. Palella FJJ, Delaney KM, Moorman AC, Loveless MO, Fuhrer J, Satten GA, *et al*: **Declining morbidity and mortality among patients with advanced immunodeficiency virus infection. HIV Outpatient Study Investigators.** *N Engl J Med* 1998, **338**:853–860.
2. Brinkman K, ter Hofstede HJM, Burger DM, Smeitink J, Koopmans PP: **Adverse effects of reverse transcriptase inhibitors: mitochondrial toxicity as common pathway.** *AIDS* 1998, **12**:1735–1744.
3. Dieterich DT: **Long-term complications of nucleoside reverse transcriptase inhibitor therapy.** *AIDS Reader.* 2003, **13**:176–178.
4. Vrouenraets SME, Treskes M, Regez RM, *et al*: **Hyperlactatemia in HIV-infected patients: the role of NRTI-treatment.** *Antivir Ther* 2002, **7**:239–244.
5. Carr A, Miller J, Law M, Cooper DA: **A syndrome of lypoatrophy, lactic acidemia and liver dysfunction associated with HIV nucleoside analogue therapy: contribution to protease inhibitor-related lipodystrophy syndrome.** *AIDS* 2000, **14**:F25–F32.
6. Gérard Y, Maulin L, Yazdanpanah Y, De La Tribonniere X, Amiel C, Maurage CA, *et al*: **Symptomatic hyperlactataemia: an emergency complication of antiretroviral therapy.** *AIDS* 2000, **14**:2723–2730.
7. John M, Moore CB, James IR, Nolan D, Upton RP, McKinnon EJ, *et al*: **Chronic hyperlactatemia in HIV-infected patients taking antiretroviral therapy.** *AIDS* 2001, **15**:717–723.
8. Scalzini A, Tomasoni D, Gattuso G, Fibbia G: *Prevalence of asymptomatic hyperlactatemia in HIV patients treated with nucleoside analogues*, 6th International Congress on Drug Therapy in HIV infection. Glasgow, UK; 2002:116. Abstract available: http://ww1.aegis.org/conferences/hiv-glasgow/2002/hiv6.pdf.
9. Brinkman K, Smeitink JA, Romijin JA, Reiss P: **Mitochondrial toxicity induced by nucleoside-analogue reverse transcriptase inhibitors is a key factor in the pathogenesis of antiretroviral-therapy-related lipodystrophy.** *Lancet* 1999, **354**:1112–1115.
10. Sundar K, Suarez M, Banogon PE, Shapiro JM: **Zidovudine induced fatal lactic acidosis and hepatic failure in patients with acquired immunodeficiency syndrome: report of two patients and review of the literature.** *Crit Care Med* 1997, **25**:1425–1430.
11. Bissuel F, Bruneel F, Habersetzer F, Chassard D, Cotte L, Chevalier M, *et al*: **Fulminant hepatitis with severe lactate acidosis in HIV-infected patients on didanosine therapy.** *J Intern Med* 1994, **235**:337–342.
12. Lonergan JT, Behling C, Pfander H, Hassanein TI, Mathews WC: **Hyperlactatemia and hepatic abnormalities in 10 human immunodeficiency virus-infected patients receiving nucleoside analogue combination regimens.** *Clin Infect Dis* 2000, **31**:162–166.
13. Delgado J, Harris M, Tesiorowski A, Montaner JSG: **Symptomatic elevations of lactic acid and their response to treatment manipulation in human immunodeficiency virus-infected persons: a case series.** *Clin Infect Dis* 2001, **33**:2072–2074.
14. World Health Organization: *Antiretroviral therapy for HIV infection in adults and adolescents: recommendations for a public health approach-2010 revision.* Geneva: World Health Organization; 2010.
15. Murphy RA, Sunpath H, Kuritzkes DR, Venter F, Gandhi RT: **Antiretroviral therapy-associated toxicities in the resource-poor world: the challenge of a limited formulary.** *J Infect Dis* 2007, **196**:S449–S456.
16. Rosen S, Long L, Fox M, Sanne I: **Cost and cost-effectiveness of switching from stavudine to tenofovir in first-line antiretroviral regimens in South Africa.** *J Acquir Immune Defic Syndr* 2008, **48**:334–344.
17. Lactic Acidosis International Study Group: **Risk factors for lactic acidosis and severe hyperlactataemia in HIV-1-infected adults exposed to antiretroviral therapy.** *AIDS* 2007, **21**:2455–2464.
18. Bolhaar MG, Karstaedt AS: **A high incidence of lactic acidosis and symptomatic hyperlactatemia in women receiving highly active antiretroviral therapy in Soweto.** *South Africa. Clin Infect Dis.* 2007, **45**:254–260.
19. Geddes R, Knight S, Moosa MY, Reddi A, Uebel K, Sunpath H: **A high incidence of nucleoside reverse transcriptase inhibitor (NRTI)-induced lactic acidosis in HIV-infected patients in a South African context.** *S Afr Med J* 2006, **96**:722–724.
20. Wester CW, Okezie OA, Thomas AM, Bussmann H, Moyo S, *et al*: **Higher-than-expected rates of lactic acidosis among highly active antiretroviral therapy-treated women in Botswana: preliminary results from a large randomized clinical trial.** *J Acquir Immune Defic Syndr* 2007, **46**:318–322.
21. van Griensven J, Zachariah R, Rasschaert F, Mugabo J, Atte EF, Reid T: **Stavudine- and nevirapine-related drug toxicity while on generic fixed-dose antiretroviral treatment: incidence, timing and risk factors in a three-year cohort in Kigali, Rwanda.** *Trans R Soc Trop Med Hyg* 2010, **104**:148–153.
22. Boulle A, Orrel C, Kaplan R, Van Cutsem G, McNally M, Hilderbrand K, *et al*: **Substitutions due to antiretroviral toxicity or contraindication in the first 3 years of antiretroviral therapy in a large South African cohort.** *Antivir Ther* 2007, **12**:753–760.
23. Osler M, Stead D, Rebe K, Meintjes G, Boulle A: **Risk factors for and clinical characteristics of severe hyperlactataemia in patients receiving antiretroviral therapy: a case–control study.** *HIV Med* 2009, **11**:121–129.

24. Ogedegbe AE, Thomas DL, Diehl AM: **Hyperlactataemia syndromes associated with HIV therapy.** *Lancet Infect Dis* 2003, **3:**329–337.
25. Gutmann I, Wahlefeld A: **Lactate measurements in biological fluids.** In *Methods of enzymatic analysis.* 2nd edition. Edited by Bergmeyer HV. New York: Academic Press; 1974:1461–1465.
26. Ritz E: *Heidland A. Lactic acidosis. Clin Nephrol.* 1977, **7:**231–240.
27. Johnson AA, Ray AS, Hanes J, Suo Z, Colacino JM, Anderson KS, *et al*: **Toxicity of antiviral nucleoside analogs and the human mitochondrial DNA polymerase.** *J Biol Chem* 2001, **276:**40847–40857.
28. Lim SE, Copeland WC: **Differential incorporation and removal of antiviral deoxynucleotides by human DNA polymerase gamma.** *J Biol Chem* 2001, **276:**23616–23623.
29. Menezes CN, Maskew M, Sanne I, Crowther NJ, Raal FJ: **A longitudinal study of stavudine-associated toxicities in a large cohort of South African HIV infected subjects.** *BMC Infect Dis* 2011, **11:**244.
30. Pefura Yone EW, Betyoumin AF, Kengne AP, Kaze Folefack FJ, Ngogang J: **First-line antiretroviral therapy and dyslipidemia in people living with HIV-1 in Cameroon: a cross-sectional study.** *AIDS Res Ther* 2011, **8:**33.
31. Lonergan JT, Havlir D, Barber E, Mathews WC: *Incidence of symptomatic hyperlactatemia in HIV-infected adults on NRTIs*, 9th Conference on Retroviruses and Opportunistic Infections. Seattle; 2002. Abstract available: http://www.retroconference.org/2002/Abstract/13202.htm.
32. Marceau G, Sapin V, Jacomet C, Ughetto S, Cormerais L, Regagnon C, *et al*: **Frequency, risk factors, and outcome of hyperlactatemia in HIV-positive persons: implications for the management of treated patients.** *Clin Chem* 2003, **49:**1154–1162.
33. Boubaker K, Flepp M, Sudre P, Furrer H, Haensel A, Hirschel B, *et al*: **Hyperlactatemia and antiretroviral therapy: the Swiss HIV Cohort Study.** *Clin Infect Dis* 2001, **33:**1931–1937.
34. Matthews LT, Giddy J, Ghebremichael M, Hampton J, Guarino AJ, Ewusi A, *et al*: **A risk-factor guided approach to reducing lactic acidosis and hyperlactatemia in patients on antiretroviral therapy.** *PLoS One* 2011, **6:**e18736.
35. Fabian J, Venter WD, Mkhabela L, Levin JB, Baker L, Naicker S: **Symptomatic hyperlactataemia in adults on antiretroviral therapy: a single-centre experience.** *S Afr Med J* 2008, **98:**795–800.
36. Brinkman K: **Management of hyperlactatemia: no need for routine lactate measurements.** *AIDS* 2001, **15:**795–797.
37. Moyle GJ, Datta D, Mandalia S, Morlese J, Asboe D, Gazzard BG: **Hyperlactataemia and lactic acidosis during antiretroviral therapy: relevance, reproducibility and possible risk factors.** *AIDS* 2002, **16:**1341–1349.

8

Incidence and risk factors for first line anti retroviral treatment failure among Ugandan children attending an urban HIV clinic

Robert Sebunya[1*], Victor Musiime[1,2], Sabrina Bakeera Kitaka[1] and Grace Ndeezi[1]

Abstract

Background: Early recognition of antiretroviral therapy (ART) failure in resource limited settings is a challenge given the limited laboratory facilities and trained personnel. This study aimed at describing the incidence, risk factors and the resistance associated mutations (RAMs) of first line treatment failure among HIV-1-infected children attending the Joint Clinical Research Centre (JCRC), Kampala, Uganda.

Methods: A retrospective cohort of 701 children who had been initiated on ART between January 2004 and September 2009 at the JCRC was studied. Data of children aged 6 months up to 18 years who had been started on ART for at least 6 months was extracted from the clinic charts. The children who failed the first-line ART were taken as cases and those who did not fail as the controls. Data was analysed using STATA version10.

Results: Of 701 children, 240(34%) failed on first line ART (cases) and 461(66%) did not fail (controls). The overall median time (IQR) to first line ART failure was 26.4 (18.9 – 39.1) months. The factors associated with treatment failure were poor adherence [(OR = 10, 95 CI: 6.4 – 16.7) $p < 0.001$], exposure to single dose nevirapine (sdNVP) [(OR = 4.2, 95% CI:1.8-9.4), $p = 0.005$] and a NVP containing regimen [(OR = 2.2,95% CI:1.4-3.6), $p < 0.001$]. Of 109 genotypic resistance profiles analyzed, the commonest non nucleoside reverse transcriptase inhibitor (NNRTI) resistance associated mutations (RAM) were: K103N (59; 54%)), Y181C (36; 27%)) and G190A (26; 24%)) while the commonest nucleoside reverse transcriptase inhibitor (NRTI) RAM was the M184V (89; 81%). Thymidine analogue- mutations (TAMs) were detected in 20% of patients.

Conclusions: One in three children on first-line ART are likely to develop virological treatment failure after the first 24 months of therapy. Poor adherence to ART, a NVP based first-line regimen, prior exposure to sdNVP were associated with treatment failure.

Introduction

Antiretroviral therapy (ART) has been shown to reduce human immunodeficiency virus (HIV) associated morbidity and mortality by restoring and preserving the immunological function [1-6]. Globally, there has been a pronounced increase in scaling up ART services notably in sub-Saharan Africa [7,8], with Uganda being among the pioneering countries [9]. However, ART is long term treatment with the potential of drug toxicity and probable emergency of resistance which results into treatment failure. Treatment failure is suboptimal response or a lack of sustained response to therapy using either clinical, immunological and virological criteria [10]. Paediatric antiretroviral therapy cohorts in low income countries have reported that response to ART is as good or comparable to that in high income countries [4,11]. Single dose nevirapine (sNVP) has been widely used for prevention of mother to child transmission (PMTC) in low resource settings and NVP continues to be used as part of the backbone of non-nucleoside reverse transcriptase inhibitors (NNRTI) among HIV infected children [12]. Some of these cohorts have reported occurrence of resistant mutations to sNVP with subsequent treatment failure [13,14]. The incidence and risk factor for first line ART has not been described in Uganda. In this study we describe the incidence, risk factors for the first line treatment failure among children

* Correspondence: robertsebunya3@gmail.com
[1]Department of Paediatrics and child Health Makerere, University college of Health Sciences, Kampala, Uganda

attending one of the largest paediatric ART program in Uganda. We also describe the resistance associated mutations in this cohort.

Whereas viral load is the ideal tool for monitoring ART response, clinical and immunological monitoring are widely used in resource limited settings like Uganda. There is sufficient evidence suggesting a poor correlation between clinical/immunological and virological ART failure [15-17]. In Uganda like many other sub-Saharan countries there is paucity of data regarding paediatric virological treatment failure.

Methods

This was a retrospective cohort (1-5 yr) follow up. We studied children who started ART at the Joint Clinical Research Centre (JCRC), Kampala, Uganda under the Timetable for Regional Expansion of antiretroviral Therapy (TREAT) program between 2004 – 2009 since all children had similar free scheduled laboratory monitoring within this period.

Children who were aged 6 months to 18 years and had been initiated on ART for at least 6 months were included in the study. Those who had confirmed first line ART treatment failure and referred for second line ART were excluded plus those charts of children which had key missing information like treatment history and laboratory results (CD4 counts, viral load) were excluded.

Study setting

The study was conducted at the JCRC Kampala, Lubowa campus, which houses the headquarters of this HIV care and research institution. It is located 10 km off Entebbe road from Kampala, the capital city of Uganda. At the time of this study, the centre cared for over 2000 HIV infected children majority of whom were perinatally infected and over 10,000 adults with respective outpatient clinics opening from Monday to Friday, 8.00a.m to 5p.m, excluding public holidays. The centre provided free services such as ART, opportunistic infections prophylactic medication, adherence counseling, routine laboratory monitoring tests, and nutritional supplementations. Among the routine laboratory monitoring tests performed were CD4 cell counts and CD4 percentages every 6 months, liver and renal function tests, plasma HIV-1(RNA) viral loads, and genotypic resistance testing when treatment failure was confirmed.

The pediatric clinic had over 1500 children under care with approximately 37 staff members namely; six pediatricians, nine nurses, four counsellors, two home visitors, one pharmacist, two pharmacy technicians, two record officers and one data assistant. Others included play room supervisors (2), phlebotomists (2) and support staff(3) with exclusion of the inpatient/ward staffs. At this clinic, treatment seeking children are recruited into care following self referral by caretakers and referral from other health centres. All HIV exposed infants awaiting DNA PCR results and those infected were/are initiated on Co- trimoxazole prophylaxis. Since most children at the clinic have/had resource constraints, most were, recruited under the PEPFAR funded programs Timetable for Regional Expansion of Anti-retroviral Therapy (TREAT).

The criteria for ART initiation and switching, as well as the ART regimens were by the WHO guidelines for ART initiation in infants and children [18]. Most children above 1 year received medication in tablet formulation with doses determined using WHO weight bands (WHO 2004,2006) [18,19]. Infants received medication largely largely in syrup form determined per kilogram body weight.

Cohort description

We reviewed the clinic charts of patients who had been initiated on ART between Jan 2004 to September 2009, as identified from the patient care database at JCRC. This was the period of the TREAT program where all the children had similar scheduled laboratory monitoring tests like the viral loads, resistance testing and CD4 counts. The baseline was taken to be the time children were initiated on ART. The ART regimen consisted of 2 nucleoside reverse transcription inhibitors (NRTIs; lamivudine, zidovudine, stavudine and abacavir) and a non-nucleoside reverse transcription inhibitor (NNRTI, either nevirapine or efavirenz). Infants (children less than 1 year) were given syrups and older children were given tablets. The children below 3 years of age who developed Tuberculosis were put on triple NRTI regimens, to avoid the drug-drug interaction between nevirapine and rifampicin. The dosage depended on the child's weight. In case of virologic failure, the NNRTI could be switched to the boosted protease inhibitor (PI) lopinavir/ritonavir with 2–3 NRTIs as a second-line regimen. Most of the secondline ART was chosen depending on the resistance profiles that had been done in most of the children who had failed firstline. The commonest second line ART used was combivir (lamivudine/zidovudine)didanosine(ddl) and alluvia.

In this cohort Information regarding Pre-exposure to single dose nevirapine or other antiretroviral drugs as part of a prevention of mother-to- child transmission (PMTCT) could not be entirely ascertained, because some children were orphans and brought in by distant relatives and hence the required information was not readily available.

Laboratory assessment at the study site

Laboratory measurements included a complete blood cell count, CD4 lymphocyte count, and quantitative measurement of HIV load. Quality control assurance was done in reference to international accredited laboratories; UK National External Quality Assessment Service (UKNEQAS) and College of American Pathologists (CAP). Viral load count was done with use of Amplicor monitor standard assay, version 1.5 (Roche Molecular Systems),with a minimum detection limit of 400 copies/ml. CD4 lymphocytes were analyzed by flow cytometry (Bendict Dickson, USA). Genotypic resistance sequencing was done using in house primers. The sequences were edited using BioEdit Sequence Alignment Editor (Version 7.0.5) and analyzed using the HIV drug resistance database of Stanford University [20] for children who had a viral load greater than 2000 copies since this was the threshold beyond which mutations could be detected in the laboratory. The CD4 count and viral load were periodically done every 6 months during the routine visit to the out-patient clinic.

Data collection

We extracted the children's demographic and ART treatment information from their medical records at the clinic using a pre tested standardized data extraction form. This information included their gender, age at the time of assessment and ART initiation, WHO clinical staging at the start of ART, CD4 count/percentage and follow up viral loads at the time of switch were abstracted. Data regarding the use of sdNVP in PMTCT, first-line ART and the serial Weight for Height plus the six monthly follow up tests for up to five years till virological failure was first detected were extracted. History of opportunist infections, resistance mutation tests that were done before switching to second line ART tests were also recorded using the same tool. Adherence to ART was the documented adherence level by the then attending clinician during the fellow up visits. It was done by pill counts and self reports especially in the older children. An adherence greater than 95% was considered as good adherence while that less than 95% was taken as poor adherence.

Virological failure was defined as inability to achieve or maintain suppression of HIV replication to non detectable range. For this study we used virological failure as the determinant of treatment failure.

Statistical analysis

The cumulative incidence of first-line ART failure was ascertained from the proportion of children with viral load > 2000 copies per ml at any time during follow up. Kaplan Meier survival curves plus Cox regression were used to estimate the median time to first line ART treatment failure which was the primary outcome. The Wald test was used to compare the incidence rates of ART failure in the different ART first line regimens. Factors associated with treatment failure were ascertained by comparing various variables among children who failed (cases) with those who never failed (controls) using the chi-square test for categorical data and student t test for continuous variables. Logistic regression was done to determine the factors that independently predict ART treatment failure.

All social demographic and clinical characteristics (variables) were subjected to univariate analysis as (shown in Table 1 and 2). And factors whose p-valve was less than 0.02 at univariate analysis were included in multivariate analysis. The model was then built by dropping the most insignificant factor one at a time with factors whose P-valve was (<)0.05 were taken to be the factors that were independently associated with treatment failure (Table 3).

All analyses were done using STATA version 10 (Reference: StataCorp LP, 4905 Lakeway Drive, College Station, Texas 77845, USA).

Ethical consideration

Ethical clearance was obtained from the School of Medicine Research and Ethics committee (SOMREC), Makerere University College of Health Sciences. Waiver of consent was sought from the SOMREC and JCRC Institutional Review Board (IRB) Research and Ethics Committee (REC). Permission to carry out the study was also obtained from JCRC and the Uganda National Council of Science and Technology (UNCST).

Results

We queried 1068 patients' records from the data base who had been initiated on ART between January 1st 2004 and September 30th 2009, at the JCRC paediatric out-patient clinic. Three hundred and sixty seven (367) records were excluded because some had key missing data including CD4 counts, viral loads, weight, height, resistance mutations profile results, and information on first line ART, or had been referred from other centres after documented failure on first line and others lacked baseline characteristics. The remaining 701 children's records were included as shown in (Figure 1). Pre-exposure to single dose nevirapine or other antiretroviral drugs as part of a prevention of mother-to- child transmission (PMTCT) regimen could not be entirely ascertained in all the children though, because some children were orphan and brought in by distant relatives and hence the required information was not readily available. However 31 children had exposure to sdNVP and of those 29 were also started on neviraipne containing firstline regimen. The median baseline CD4 counts absolute and percentage at start of ART for those who failed and never failed were 241 and 313 cells,15% and 16% respectively.. Most of the children were in clinical stage two of the WHO paediatric HIV staging and were above 5 years of age. Pulmonary tuberculosis being the commonest opportunistic infection as shown in Table 4.

Incidence of first line virological treatment failure

Among 701 participants, 240 (34%) cumulatively failed first-line ART. The median time to failure in months was 26.4 IQR (18.9 – 39.1). 140 (58.3%) failed in 24+ months,

Table 1 A comparison of the social demographic and clinical characteristics between the cases and the controls at ART initiation of ART

Characteristic		Cases (n = 240)	Controls (n = 461)	RR (95 % CI)	P- value
Age	<=5 years	91 (37.9)	174 (37.7)	1.00 (0.81 – 1.24)	0.9643
	>5-10 years	61 (25.4)	139 (30.2)	0.85 (0.67 – 1.09)	0.1877
	>10 – 18 years	88 (36.7)	148 (32.1)	1.14 (0.92 – 1.41)	0.2252
Gender	Female	109 (45.4)	221 (47.9)	0.93 (0.76 – 1.15)	0.5255
	Male	131 (54.6)	240 (52.1)	1.07 (0.87 – 1.31)	0.5255
Next of kin	Parents	162 (67.5)	302 (65.5)	1.06 (0.85 – 1.32)	0.5971
	Grandmother	**25 (10.4)**	**81 (17.6)**	**0.65 (0.46 – 0.93)**	**0.0121***
	Other	53 (22.1)	78 (16.9)	1.23 (0.97 – 1.57)	0.0961
Care taker education level	None	63 (26.5)	101 (22.3)	1.15 (0.92 – 1.45)	0.2262
	Primary	76 (31.9)	175 (38.7)	0.82 (0.66 – 1.03)	0.0783
	Secondary	58 (24.4)	102 (22.6)	1.07 (0.84 – 1.35)	0.5937
	Tertiary (not university)	26 (10.9)	43 (9.5)	1.10 (0.80 – 1.52)	0.5570
	University	15 (6.3)	31 (6.9)	0.94 (0.61 – 1.45)	0.7808
Distance from JCRC	**≤10 km**	**104 (44.3)**	**157 (35.4)**	**1.27 (1.03 – 1.56)**	**0.0248***
	11 – 20 km	91 (38.7)	194 (43.8)	0.87 (0.70 – 1.08)	0.2032
	>20 km	40 (17.0)	92 (20.8)	0.85 (0.64 – 1.12)	0.2411
Past hospitalization	Yes	105 (43.8)	198 (43.2)	1.01 (0.82 – 1.25)	0.8955
	No	135 (56.2)	260 (56.8)	0.99 (0.80 – 1.21)	0.8955
Episodes of hospitalization	No hospitalization	2 (2.0)	3 (1.5)	1.16 (0.39 – 3.44)	>0.999†
	1-2 times	68 (66.6)	120 (61.9)	1.15 (0.82 – 1.61)	0.4139
	≥ 3 times	**32 (31.4)**	**71 (36.6)**	**0.86 (0.61 – 1.21)**	**0.3697**
Opportunistic infections	TB	51 (21.3)	90 (19.5)	1.07 (0.84 – 1.37)	0.5883
	Oral Candidiasis	39 (16.3)	64 (13.9)	1.13 (0.86 – 1.48)	0.4009
	Cryptococcal meningitis	3 (1.3)	2 (0.4)	1.76 (0.85 – 3.63)	0.3448†
	Kaposi sarcoma	2 (0.8)	5 (1.1)	0.83 (0.26 – 2.70)	>0.999†
	Pneumocystic pneumonia	3 (1.3)	5 (1.1)	1.01 (0.44 – 2.70)	>0.999†
	Oesophageal candiasis	1 (0.4)	9 (2.0)	0.29 (0.04 – 1.86)	0.1770†
	Chronic diarrhoea	4 (1.7)	18 (3.9)	0.52 (0.21 – 1.28)	0.1165†
	Bacterialmeningitis	2 (0.8)	5 (1.1)	0.83 (0.26 – 2.70)	>0.999†
HAART Regimen	**EFV**	**113(49.3)**	**278 (64.5)**	**0.67 (0.54 – 0.82)**	**0.0002***
	NVP	**116 (50.7)**	**153 (35.5)**	**1.49 (1.21 – 1.84)**	**0.0002***
Prior exposure to sdNVP	Yes	33 (13.8)	45 (9.9)	1.26 (0.95 – 1.67)	0.1253
	No	**207 (86.2)**	**410 (90.1)**	**0.79 (0.60 – 1.05)**	**0.1253**
Adherence	**Poor**	**116 (48.3)**	**56 (12.2)**	**2.88 (2.39 – 3.46)**	**<0.0001***
	Good	124 (51.7)	405 (87.8)	0.35 (0.29 – 0.42)	<0.0001*
	I	37 (15.4)	65 (14.1)	1.07 (0.81 – 1.42)	0.6389
WHO Stage	II	106 (44.2)	198 (42.9)	1.03 (0.84 – 1.27)	0.7578
	III	85 (35.4)	163 (35.4)	1.00 (0.81 – 1.24)	0.9877
	IV	**12 (5.0)**	**35 (7.6)**	**0.73 (0.44 – 1.21)**	**0.1929**

*CI = Confidence interval, * Significant effect, †Fisher's exact test.*

80 (33.3%) failed within 12–24 months, 11(4.6%) failed within 6–12 months and only 9(3.8%) in within the first 6 months. This is also illustrated in Figure 2.

The factor that was independently associated with time to virologcal failure was poor adherence to ART as shown in Table 5 below.

Table 2 Baseline CD4 counts and viral loads of study participants at ART initiation of the 701 children on ART

		Cases	Controls	
		Median (IQR)	Median (IQR)	P value*
Absolute CD4 count	Overall	241 (79–534)	313 (127–625)	0.035
	≤ 5 years	542 (273 – 1214)	728 (461 – 1129)	0.038
	>5-10 years	257 (133–474)	272 (147–382)	0.873
	>10 – 18 years	135 (50–210)	130 (44–262)	0.622
	Mean (SD)	Mean (SD)	P value	
Percentage CD4 count	Overall	15 (10.5)	16 (11.0)	0.223
	≤ 5 years	19 (10.9)	19 (9.5)	0.945
	>5-10 years	15 (8.3)	16 (12.1)	0.406
	>10 – 18 years	11 (10.0)	13 (11.0)	0.283
	Median (IQR)	Median (IQR)	P value*	
Viral load (x10 ^{4})	Overall	12.0 (2.4 – 38.6)	7.8 (2.3 - 35)	0.176
	≤ 5 years	18.8 (2.9 – 75)	17.7 (2.5 – 52.5)	0.283
	>5-10 years	4.4 (1.5 – 17.4)	6.1 (1.8 – 28.6)	0.658
	>10 – 18 years	13.1 (2.4 – 37.0)	7.6 (2.0 – 25.5)	0.183

** P value based on Wilcoxon rank-sum test.*
The baseline CD4 counts, and viral loads were.

Factors associated with treatment failure

Majority of the children who failed first-line ART were under five years of age (n = 91; 37.9%), male (52.5%), were under the care of parents (n = 162; 67.5%). Their caretakers attained primary education as the highest level (31.9%), as shown in Table 1. When compared to the controls, the children who failed first-line ART were more likely to live within 10 km from the ART providing institution (RR = 1.27(95% CI: 1.03-1.56), p = 0.02). Furthermore, the children who never failed were more likely to be under the care of grandmothers [(17.6% versus 10.4%), RR = 0.65 (95% CI: 0.46 -0.93), p = 0.01]. There was no statistical significance between the baseline CD4cell counts of the controls and cases (illustrated in Table 2).

Table 3 Factors independently associated with treatment failure among the children on ART in the cohort at multivariate analysis

Effect		OR (95% CI)	P- value
CD4 counts at start of ART		0.99 (0.99-1.00)	0.027
Viral load at start of ART		0.99 (0.99-1.00)	0.402
NOK (Relationship)‡	Parents	0.9 (0.61 – 1.60)	0.965
	Grandmother	0.8 (0.42 – 1.55)	0.517
HAART Regimen	NVP	2.2 (1.40 – 3.60)	0.006*
Used sdNVP	Yes	4.2 (1.80 – 9.40)	0.001*
Adherence	Poor	10,0 (6.40 – 16.70)	<0.001*
Distance from JCRC‡‡	≤10 km	1.48 (0.88 – 2.49)	0.142
	11 – 20 km	1.21 (0.72 – 2.03)	0.470

*CI = Confidence interval, * Significant effect. ‡ Reference to other caretakers.*

Past hospitalization, opportunist Infections and WHO clinical staging were not associated with treatment failure. However, nevirapine as opposed to efavirenz as NNRTI backbone (OR = 2.2., 95% CI: 1.40 – 3.60, p = 0.001), poor adherence (OR = 10, 95% CI: 6.4 – 16.7), p < 0.0001) and prior exposure to (sdNVP) (OR = 4,2, 95% CI: 1.8 – 9,4, p = 0.002) were the significantly associated with first line ART treatment failure (Table 3). It important to note that the Viral load and CD4 at initiation of first line ART were not associated with treatment failure.

Resistance associated mutation (RAM) in the children with treatment failure

Of the 240 children who failed first line therapy 109 had genotypic resistance profiles prior to switching to second line therapy. The commonest NNRTI RAMs was K103N (n = 59; 54%). Other common NNRTI RAMs were Y181C (n = 30; 27%), G190A (n = 26; 24%) and K101E (n = 11; 10%). The most common NRTI RAMs was the M184V (n = 89; 81%). Other common NRTI RAMs were the K70R (n = 22; 20%), T215Y (n = 36; 24%), M41L (n = 23; 21%), D67N (n = 15; 14%), K219Q/E (n = 14; 13%) and the L210W making 9% of the TAMs.

It's worth noting that some patients had developed more than one resistance mutation at a time.

Discussion

In this study, we have shown that the cumulative incidence of first line ART failure was 34%, with a median time to first line ART failure of 26.4 months of follow up. Varying rates of virological failure have been reported in other

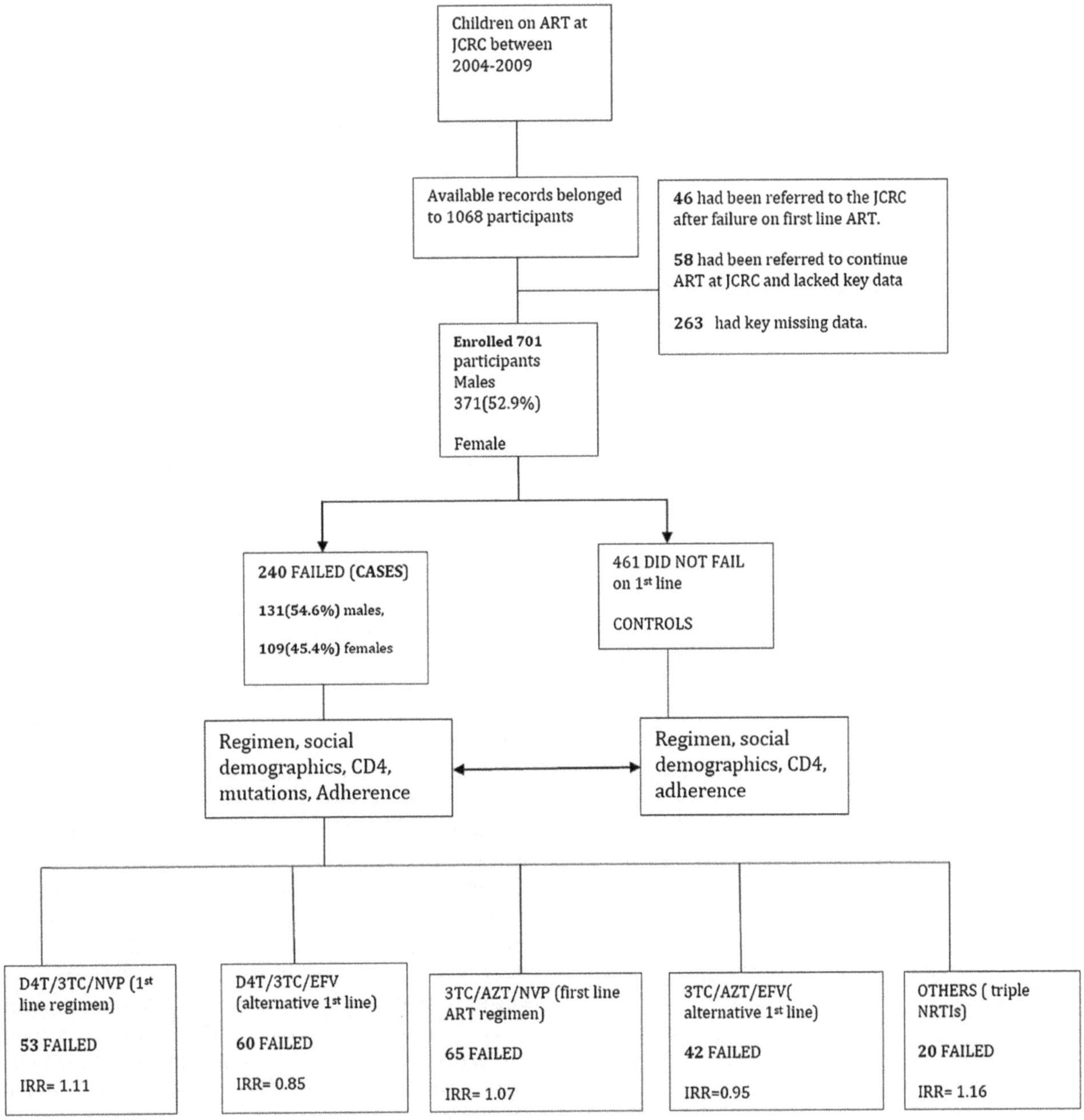

Figure 1 Study profile of the study participants.

studies [15,21,22]. However the treatment failure rate in this study is comparable to other studies in low income countries with a high prevalence of HIV. A similar study done in rural South Africa on 101 HIV infected children reported a slightly higher virological failure rates of 38% compared to ours, with a median duration of NNRTI-based regimen of 31 months of treatment [15]. A comparable rate of 33% was reported among the Thai HIV infected children within 96 weeks of follow up [23].

In our study, patients were more likely to fail on a nevirapine NNRTI regimen compared to an efavirenz based NNRTI backbone regimen. This finding has been documented in similar studies. In the FIRST STUDY [24] by Berg-Wolf et al., the incidence of virological failure in an efavirenz based arm was 41.2 compared to 42.8 in the nevirapine arm per 100 person years after a follow up median time of 5 years. Implying that a NVP based regimen arm was associated with earlier virological failure compared to efavirenz, like our study finding.

Our study showed that treatment failure rate was more in males than the female though the difference was not statistically significant. A cohort of HIV infected children and adults performed in a similar setting (Mulago, Kampala, Uganda) reported that males were more likely to fail on

Table 4 Baseline clinical and demographic characteristics of the study participants at the time of ART initiation

Characteristic		Frequency	%
Age	<=5 years	265	37.80
	>5-10 years	200	28.53
	>10 – 18 years	236	33.67
Gender	Female	330	47.08
	Male	371	52.92
Next of kin	Parents	464	66.19
	Grandmother	106	15.12
	Other	131	18.69
Caretaker education level	None	164	23.77
	Primary	251	36.38
	Secondary	160	23.19
	Tertiary (not university)	69	10.00
	University	46	6.67
Past hospitalization	Yes	303	43.41
	No	395	56.59
Episodes of	0 days	5	1.69
Hospitalization	1-2 days	188	63.51
	≥ 3 days	103	34.80
Opportunistic infections	TB	141	20.11
	Oral Candidiasis	103	14.69
	CCM	5	0.71
	KS	7	1.00
	LIP	2	0.29
	PCP	8	1.14
	Esophageal	10	1.43
	Chronic_diarrhoea	22	3.14
	Bacterial meningitis	7	1.00
HAART regimen	EFV	391	59.24
	NVP	269	40.76
UsedPMTCT services	Yes	31	6.22
	No	617	88.78
Adherence	Poor (<95%)	172	24.54
	Good (>95%)	529	75.46
	I	102	14.55
WHO stage	II	304	43.37
	III	248	35.38
	IV	47	6.70

TB: tuberculosis, *CCM*: cryptococcal meningitis; *KS*, Kaposi'sarcoma; *LIP*, Lymphoid interstitial pnemonitis; *PCP*, pnenocystic carinii pneumonia; *EFV*, efaverenz; *NVP*, niverapine.

ART compared to females [22]. The reason behind this sex difference is not known. Interestingly, there were more male children in our study compared to the Mulago study. Sex differences in response to ART could be biological or

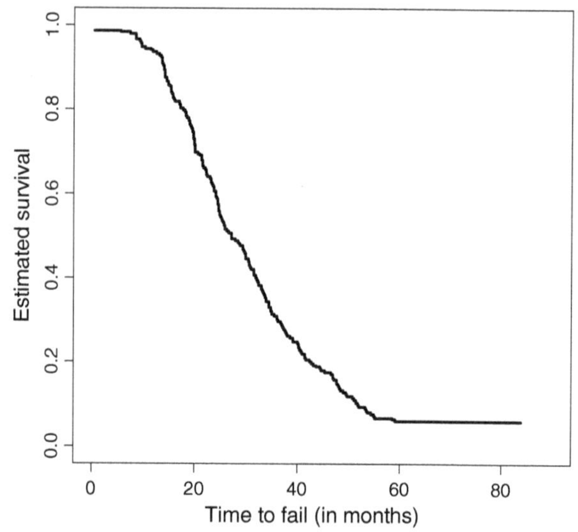

Figure 2 Kaplan Meier survival curve estimating the overall time to failure.

related to provision of care by parents. This is an area that requires further inquiry.

The factors that were independently associated with treatment failure were poor adherence to ART, use of single dose niverapine (sdNVP) in PMTCT and NVP based NNRTIs.

The critical role of adherence in the treatment of HIV has been demonstrated in many clinical trials and clinical care settings [25]. Antiretroviral therapy (ART) adherence is a strong predictor of biological (virological and immunological) and eventual clinical outcome [26-28]. This study findings are consistent with previous studies [25] and further confirms that adherence to ART is critical in the clinical, and biological outcome of ART. Our study further demonstrated that the use of single dose niverapine (sdNVP) as a measure of PMTC of HIV was strongly associated with ART first line treatment failure. This is attributed to the fact that NVP resistance occurs after the use of sdNVP as reported in many studies from all over Sub-Saharan Africa, Uganda inclusive [15,29-31]. A meta analysis to analyze the prevalence of nevirapine resistance after sdNVP was 35.7% in women and 52.6% in children [13]. The landmark HIVNET 012 trial in Uganda revealed a resistance of 46% in children and 25% in women [32]. These findings are also similar to what was reported among Ugandan children who had been exposed to sdNVP that were less likely to achieve virological suppression if initiated on a non nucleoside reverse transcriptase inhibitor (NNRTI) [33] regimen. For a long time in Uganda, NVP was used for PMTCT of HIV and has also been part of the backbone of the NNRTI regimen. It is worth noting that the study participants had been initiated on ART between 2004 to 2009 in which usage of protease Inhibitors (PI) as

Table 5 Factors associated with time to failure among the children who failed ART

Effect		Coefficient (s.e)	Hazard ratio (95% CI)	P- value
Age†	<=5 years	0.11 (0.19)	1.18 (0.82 – 1.69)	0.551
	>5-10 years	−0.05 (0.18)	0.96 (0.67 – 1.38)	0.767
NOK (Relationship) ‡	Parents	0.13 (0.27)	0.42 (0.24 - 0.74)	0.453
	Grandmother	−0.52 (0.59)	0.86 (0.58 – 1.28)	0.053°
HAART regimen††	EFV	−0.11 (0.16)	0.69 (0.44 – 1.08)	0.493
Used PMTCT services	Yes	0.03 (0.23)	0.86 (0.54 – 1.39)	0.888
Adherence	Poor	−0.38 (0.14)	1.06 (0.50 – 1.10)	0.008*
Distance from JCRC	≤10 km	0.37 (0.21)	1.45 (0.97 – 2.18)	0.073
	11 – 20 km	0.36 (0.21)	1.43 (0.95 – 2.16)	0.091

† Reference to age >10 -18 yrs, ‡ Reference to other caretakers.
*°Borderline significance, †† Reference to NVP, * Significant effect.*
NOK next of kin, PMTCT prevention of mother to child transmission.

a backbone of the first line ART if there had been exposure to sdNVP had not been rolled out in Uganda after the recommendation from the World health Organization in 2010. It's possible that some children could have remained on a failing regimen after exposure to sdNVP thus treatment failure.

In this study children who were initiated on a NVP based first line ART were twice as likely to fail compared to those treated with EFV containing one. A prospective longitudinal study in Thailand reported that children on a NVP backbone NNRTI were 3.7 times more likely to develop virological failure compared to efavirenz [21]. These results are also consistent with earlier findings in Kampala, Uganda [22]. The finding in this study could further be explained by the fact that efavirenz is more efficacious than nevirapine [34,35] as reported in some studies. Secondly NVP compared to EFV is commonly associated with adverse side effects and increased morbidity and mortality [36]. In the event that adverse events occur the drugs are stopped and this could contribute to poor adherence with eventual drug resistance and treatment failure.

A grandmother being the primary caretaker was less associated with treatment failure compared to other caretakers at univariate analysis. However this factor did not reach statistical significance at multivariate analysis possibly due to the small numbers of children whose primary caretaker were grandmothers. A recent Ugandan study [37] reported that children in the rural settings of Uganda had better adherence compared to their urban counterparts(91.3% vs 88.2%). Majority of grandparents in Uganda reside in rural settings and often offer more time and parental care to their grand children hence good adherence. This could explain why children whose primary caretaker was a grandmother never failed in big proportions as compared to others with different care takers.

Resistance profiles that were performed prior to switching to second line, revealed the M184V and the K103N being the commonly observed NRTI and NNRTI RAMs, respectively. TAMs occurred in 20% of the resistance profiles. This pattern of RAMs among children with virological failure on reverse transcriptase based therapy is consistent with what has been reported from studies in sub-Saharan Africa [22,38,39], Thailand. In the Thai children [21], Y181C occurred in 58% and K103N in 34% of NNRTIs RAMs. In the same study M184V/I occurred in 84%, K65R in 11%, and Q151M in 5% with TAMs occurring in 18% of the NRTIs resistance mutations. The current study reports more of the K103N as opposed to the Y181C in the NNRTIs while the proportion of M184V was consistent with the previous study. This finding was expected as most of the children at JCRC (current study) were on an efavirenz containing regimen that induces commonly the K103N as opposed to nevirapine that induces commonly the Y181C [34] which occurred in the Thai study. The NNRTIs and 3TC have a low genetic barrier to resistance. So their RAMs are the first to appear. M184V has been shown to emerge in high prevalence among children and adults failing on a 3TC-containing regimen in developed countries [40]. In Uganda, it's been reported in children as early as 1.5 months [38] of ART. Other cross sectional studies have likewise reported a high prevalence of M184Vamong African [41,42] with mutations conferring resistance to NVP and EFV the NNRTIs occurring after 1–6 months of failure. This study showed occurrence of all the major TAMs in 20%. This finding is comparable to what Thai reports of 18% [21]. However this is in contrast to earlier reports from Uganda [20,39] that reported nearly no TAMs. Our finding could have resulted from the fact that our study had a big sample size compared to the above studies. Secondly a possibility of mother to child transmission of the RAMs since baseline resistance testing prior to ART initiation was never done cannot be ruled out. However this study highlights the fact that the thymine analogue mutations are present in our setting and their presence will compromise second line ART options.

Study strength and limitations

We studied a relatively large number of HIV infected children on ART to examine the incidence of and median time to first line ART failure compared to similar studies. We however acknowledge some limitations in our study. Being a retrospective nested case control, we could not control for some of the possible confounders. Secondly baseline resistance testing was not done, so the exact impact of primary drug resistance prior to ART initiation and the accumulation of RAMs is unknown.

Conclusion and recommendations

In a low resource setting where nevirapine still forms a backbone of first-line ART like Uganda, our findings suggest that one in three children on first-line ART are likely to develop virological treatment failure after the first 24 months of therapy.

We recommend that, efavirenz as opposed to nevirapine be used as first-line non-nucleoside backbone. Furthermore that adherence to ART should be emphasized at all levels of care in paediatric ART service providers to prevent the development of treatment failure.

Abbreviations

RS: Robert Sebunya; VM: Victor Musiime; SBK: Sabrina Bakeera Kitaka; GN: Grace Ndeezi; JCRC: Joint clinical resarch centre; ART: Antiretroviral therapy; PMTC: Prevention of mother to child transmission; RAMs: Resistance associated mutations; TAMs: Thymidine analogue mutations; NNRTIs: Non nucleoside reverse transcriptase inhibitors; NRTIs: Nucleotide reverse transcriptase inhibitors; NVP: Nevirapine; EFV: Efavirenz.

Competing interests

The authors declare that they have no competing interests.

Authors' contributions

RS; designed the study, collected data, interpreted study findings and wrote up the primary draft manuscript. GN, VM: Helped with the interpretation of the study findings, reviewed and assisted with the critical revision of the manuscript before submission.SBK: reviewed and commented on first draft manuscript before submission. VM was one of the Paediatricians that offered care for the children at the study site. All authors read and approved the final manuscript.

Acknowledgment

The authors would like to thank the Clinical operation and Health Service Research(CORHE) project for funding the research; the management and staff of the JCRC, Kampala who supported this work, in particular Mathew Odera, Carol Nakachwa, Geoffrey Anguyo, Judith Byaruhanga, Grace Mirembe, Hilda Kizito, Elizabeth Kaudha, Shiba Nahurira Kituuka and and Victoria Nabagereka.

We also thank the case Western Reserve University for their support of the resistance testing laboratory results, the paediatricians of the Department of Paediatrics and Child Health of Makerere University.

Author details

[1]Department of Paediatrics and child Health Makerere, University college of Health Sciences, Kampala, Uganda. [2]Joint Clinical Research Centre, Kampala, Uganda.

References

1. Ciaranello AL, Chang Y, Margulis AV, *et al*: **Effectiveness of pediatric antiretroviral therapy in resource-limited settings: a systematic review and meta-analysis.** *Clin Infect Dis* 2009, **49:**1915–1927.
2. Puthanakit T, Oberdorfer A, Akarathum N, *et al*: **Efficacy of highly active antiretroviral therapy in HIV-infected children participating in Thailand's national access to antiretroviral program.** *Clin Infect Dis* 2005, **41:**100–107.
3. Patel K, Hernan MA, Williams PL, *et al*: **Long-term effectiveness of highly active antiretroviral therapy on the survival of children and adolescents with HIV infection: a 10-year follow-up study.** *Clin Infect Dis* 2008, **46:**507–515.
4. Musoke PM, Mudiope P, Barlow-Mosha LN, *et al*: **Growth, immune and viral responses in HIV infected African children receiving highly active antiretroviral therapy: a prospective cohort study.** *BMC Pediatr* 2010, **10:**56.
5. Aboulker J, Babiker A, Chaix M, *et al*: **Highly active antiretroviral therapy started in infants under 3 months of age: 72-week follow-up for CD4 cell count, viral load and drug resistance outcome Paediatric European Network for Treatment of AIDS (PENTA).** *AIDS* 2004, **18:**237–245.
6. Reddi A, Leeper SC, Grobler AC, *et al*: **Preliminary outcomes of a paediatric highly active antiretroviral therapy cohort from KwaZulu-Natal, South Africa.** *BMC Pediatr* 2007, **7:**13.
7. UNAIDS: *2010 report on the global AIDS epidemic.* World Health organization; 2010.
8. Katabira ET, Oelrichs RB: **Scaling up antiretroviral treatment in resource-limited settings: successes and challenges.** *AIDS* 2007, **21**(4):S5–S10.
9. WHO: *Uganda leads the way in innovative AIDS treatment*; 2005. www.who.int/bulletin/volumes/83/4/infocus.pdf. Accessed December 15, 2005.
10. WHO: *Manual on paediatric HIV care and treatment for district hospitals.* Geneva, Switzerland: WHO; 2011.
11. Peacock-Villada E, Richardson BA, John-Stewart GC: **Post-HAART outcomes in pediatric populations: comparison of resource-limited and developed countries.** *Pediatrics* 2011, **127:**e423–e441.
12. Katabira ET, Kamya MR, Kalyesubula I, Namale A: *National antiretroviral treatment and care guideline for adults, adolescents and children.* Kampala, Uganda; 2009.
13. Arrivé E, Newell M-L, Ekouevi DK, *et al*: **Prevalence of resistance to nevirapine in mothers and children after single-dose exposure to prevent vertical transmission of HIV-1: a meta-analysis.** *Int J Epidemiol* 2007, **36:**1009–1021.
14. Hunt GM, Coovadia A, Abrams EJ, *et al*: **HIV-1 drug resistance at antiretroviral treatment initiation in children previously exposed to single-dose nevirapine.** *AIDS* 2011, **25:**1461–1469.
15. Barth RE, Tempelman HA, Smelt E, Wensing AM, Hoepelman AI, Geelen S: **P.0 Long-term outcome of children receiving antiretroviral treatment in rural South Africa: substantial virologic failure on first-line treatment.** *Pediatr Infect Dis J* 2011, **30:**52–56.
16. Reynolds SJ, Nakigozi G, Newell K, *et al*: **Failure of immunologic criteria to appropriately identify antiretroviral treatment failure in Uganda.** *AIDS* 2009, **23:**697–700.
17. Emmett SD, Cunningham CK, Mmbaga BT, *et al*: **Predicting virologic failure among HIV-1-infected children receiving antiretroviral therapy in Tanzania: a cross-sectional study.** *J Acquir Immune Defic Syndr* 2010, **54:**368–375.
18. *Antiretroviral therapy of HIV infection in infants and children: recommendations for a public health approach (2006 revision).* WHO; 2006. http://www.who.int/hiv/pub/guidelines/WHOpaediatric.pdf.
19. Sharland M, Blanche S, Castelli G, Ramos J, Gibb D: **PENTA guidelines for the use of antiretroviral therapy, 2004.** *HIV Med* 2004, **5:**61–86.
20. Standford University: *HIV drug resistance database*, hivdb.stanford.edu. Accessed september 30. ; 2011.
21. Jittamala P, Puthanakit T, Chaiinseeard S, Sirisanthana V: **Predictors of virologic failure and genotypic resistance mutation patterns in thai children receiving non-nucleoside reverse transcriptase inhibitor–based antiretroviral therapy.** *Pediatr Infect Dis J* 2009, **28:**826–830.
22. Kamya MR, Mayanja-Kizza H, Kambugu A, *et al*: **Predictors of long-term viral failure among ugandan children and adults treated with antiretroviral therapy.** *J Acquir Immune Defic Syndr* 2007, **46:**187–193.
23. Bunupuradah T, Puthanakit T, Kosalaraksa P, *et al*: **Immunologic and virologic failure after first-line NNRTI-based antiretroviral therapy in Thai HIVinfected children.** *AIDS Res Ther* 2011, **8:**40.
24. Berg-Wolf M, Hullsiek KH, Peng G, *et al*: **Virologic, immunologic, clinical, safety, and resistance outcomes from a long-term comparison of efavirenz-based versus nevirapine- based antiretroviral regimens as initial therapy in HIV-1– infected persons.** *HIV Clin Trials* 2008, **9**(5):324–336.

25. Sharon M, Friedland G, Matts J, Child C, Margaret Chesney TB, AIDS CPfCRo: **The consistency of adherence to antiretroviral therapy predicts biologic outcomes for human immunodeficiency virus-infected persons in clinical trials.** *Clin Infect Dis* 2002, **34:**1115–1121.
26. McNabb JC, Ross JW, Abriola K, Turley C, Nightingale CH, Nicolau DP: **Adherence to highly active antiretroviral therapy predicts virologic outcome at an inner-city human immunodeficiency virus clinic.** *Clin Infect Dis* 2001, **33:**700.
27. Ford N, Darder M, Spelman T, Maclean E, Mills E, Boulle A: **Early adherence to antiretroviral medication as a predictor of long-term HIV virological suppression: five-year follow up of an observational cohort.** *PLoS One* 2010, **5:**e10460.
28. Bangsberg DR, Perry S, Charlebois ED, *et al*: **Non-adherence to highly active antiretroviral therapy predicts progression to AIDS.** *AIDS* 2001, **15:**1181.
29. Eshleman SH, Hoover DR, Chen S, *et al*: **Resistance after single-dose nevirapine prophylaxis emerges in a high proportion of malawian newborns.** *AIDS* 2005, **19:**2167–2169.
30. Eshleman S, Guay L, Mwatha A, *et al*: **Comparison of nevirapine (NVP) resistance in Ugandan women 7 days vs. 6–8 weeks after single-dose NVP prophylaxis: HIVNET 012.** *AIDS Res Hum Retroviruses* 2004, **20:**595–599.
31. Eshleman SH, Guay LA, Mwatha A, *et al*: **Characterization of nevirapine resistance mutations in women with subtype A vs. D HIV-1 6–8 weeks after single-dose nevirapine (HIVNET 012).** *J Acquir Immune Defic Syndr* 2004, **35:**126.
32. Guay LA, Musoke P, Fleming T, *et al*: **Intrapartum and neonatal single-dose nevirapine compared with zidovudine for prevention of mother-to-child transmission of HIV-1 in Kampala, Uganda: HIVNET 012 randomised trial.** *Lancet* 1999, **354:**795–802.
33. Musiime V, Ssali F, Kayiwa J, *et al*: **Response to nonnucleoside reverse transcriptase inhibitor-based therapy in HIV-infected children with perinatal exposure to single-dose nevirapine.** *AIDS Res Hum Retroviruses* 2009, **25:**989–996.
34. Bannistera WP, Ruizb L, Alessandro C-L, *et al*: **Comparison of genotypic resistance profiles and virological response between patients starting nevirapine and efavirenz in EuroSIDA.** *AIDS* 2008, **22:**367–376.
35. Manfredi R, Calza L, Chiodo F: **Efavirenz versus nevirapine in current clinical practice: a prospective, open-label observational study.** *J Acquir Immune Defic Syndr* 2004, **35:**492–502.
36. van Leth PP F, Ruxrungtham K, Baraldi E, Miller S, Gazzard B, Cahn P, Lalloo UG, van der Westhuizen IP, 2NN Study team: **Comparison of first-line antiretroviral therapy with regimens including nevirapine, efavirenz, or both drugs, plus stavudine and lamivudine: a randomised open-label trial, the 2NN Study.** *Lancet* 2004, **363:**1253–1263.
37. Musiime V, Kayiwa J, Kiconco M, *et al*: **Response to antiretroviral therapy of HIV type 1-infected children in urban and rural settings of Uganda.** *AIDS Res Hum Retroviruses* 2012, **28:**00.
38. Ruel TD MRK, Pelin Li M, *et al*: **Early virologic failure and the development of antiretroviral drug resistance mutations in HIV-infected Ugandan children.** *J Acquir Immune Defic Syndr* 2011, **56:**44–50.
39. Reynolds SJ, Kityo C, Mbamanya F, *et al*: **Evolution of drug resistance after virological failure of first-line active antiretral viral therapy regimen in Uganda.** *Int Med Press* 2009, **14:**293.
40. Gibb DM, Walker AS, Kaye S, *et al*: **Evolution of antiretroviral phenotypic and genotypic drug resistance in antiretroviral-naive HIV-1 infected children treated with abacavir/lamivudine, zidovudine/lamivudine or abacavir/zidovudine, with or without nelfinavir (the PENTA 5 trial).** *Int Med Press* 2002, **7:**293–304.
41. Germanaud D, Derache A, Traore M, *et al*: **Level of viral load and antiretroviral resistance after 6 months of non-nucleoside reverse transcriptase inhibitor first-line treatment in HIV-1-infected children in Mali.** *J Antimicrob Chemother* 2010, **65:**118–124.
42. Gody J, Charpentier C, Mbitikon O: **High prevalence of antiretroviral drug resistance mutations in HIV-1 Non-B subtype strains from African children receiving antiretroviral therapy regimen according to the 2006 revised WHO recommendations.** *J Acquir Immune Defic Syndr* 2008, **49:**566–569.

9

Drug resistance in children at virological failure in a rural KwaZulu-Natal, South Africa

Sureshnee Pillay[1], Ruth M Bland[1,2], Richard J Lessells[1,3], Justen Manasa[1], Tulio de Oliveira[1,4] and Sivapragashini Danaviah[1,5*]

Abstract

Background: Better understanding of drug resistance patterns in HIV-infected children on antiretroviral therapy (ART) is required to inform public health policies in high prevalence settings. The aim of this study was to characterise the acquired drug resistance in HIV-infected children failing first-line ART in a decentralised rural HIV programme.

Methods: Plasma samples were collected from 101 paediatric patients (≤15 yrs of age) identified as failing ART. RNA was extracted from the plasma, reverse transcribed and a 1.3 kb region of the pol gene was amplified and sequenced using Sanger sequencing protocols. Sequences were edited in Geneious and drug resistance mutations were identified using the RegaDB and the Stanford resistance algorithms. The prevalence and frequency of mutations were analysed together with selected clinical and demographic data in STATA v11.

Results: A total of 101 children were enrolled and 89 (88%) were successfully genotyped; 73 on a non-nucleoside reverse-transcriptase inhibitor (NNRTI)-based regimen and 16 on a protease inhibitor (PI)-based regimen at the time of genotyping. The majority of patients on an NNRTI regimen (80%) had both nucleoside reverse-transcriptase inhibitor (NRTI) and NNRTI resistance mutations. M184V and K103N were the most common mutations amongst children on NNRTI-based and M184V among children on PI-based regimens. 30.1% had one or more thymidine analogue mutation (TAM) and 6% had ≥3 TAMs. Only one child on a PI-based regimen harboured a major PI resistance mutation.

Conclusions: Whilst the patterns of resistance were largely predictable, the few complex resistance patterns seen with NNRTI-based regimens and the absence of major PI mutations in children failing PI-based regimens suggest the need for wider access to genotypic resistance testing in this setting.

Background

Globally and within South Africa, access to paediatric antiretroviral therapy (ART) has increased significantly and this in turn has impacted on mortality and morbidity among HIV-infected children [1-5]. The face of paediatric HIV is, thus, now that of a chronic disease rather than one that will necessarily result in death or serious morbidity [6]. The challenge of long-term adherence to ART in children gives rise to the potential for the emergence of drug resistance leading to treatment failure [7,8]. In resource–limited settings, there are challenges to the implementation, long-term effectiveness and sustainability of ART programmes where limited laboratory capacity to monitor treatment effectiveness and a lack of paediatric antiretroviral (ARV) formulations are notable restrictions [9]. There is some evidence that outcomes for children in rural areas of South Africa are poorer than those in urban areas [10]. In addition, socio-economic and psychosocial factors impact on optimal adherence and access to ART which in turn accelerate the development of drug resistance [11]. Without optimal management, patients can remain on failing regimens for long periods leading to the accumulation of drug resistance mutations, which can then confer cross-resistance to drugs in the same class and compromise future therapy [7,8]. The number of drugs available in South

* Correspondence: sdanaviah@africacentre.ac.za
[1]Africa Centre for Health and Population Studies, College of Health Sciences, University of KwaZulu-Natal, Durban, South Africa
[5]Rm 135, 1st Floor, DDMRI, 719 Umbilo Road, Congella 4013, South Africa

Africa is limited and there are currently no third-line options available to children failing therapy.

The data on ARV resistance in children in South Africa are relatively limited and have largely been restricted to urban hospital-based programmes, which may not be representative of all programmes [12-18]. Of the seven published studies in South Africa that used genotyping to determine the level of resistance the largest study included 51 genotypes and none was from a rural setting [12-18]. Continuing surveillance of drug resistance is important not only to guide paediatric ART policies but also to explore whether there might be a role for genotypic resistance testing within clinical care of HIV-infected children in this region. This is important because evidence-based management of children will ensure the longevity of their ART regimens. We have previously reported high levels of drug resistance in adults failing first-line ART in our decentralised, primary health care programme [19]. The primary objective of this study was to determine the frequency and patterns of resistance mutations in children failing first-line ART.

Results

Participants

Of the approximately 1653 children (≤15 years) who were initiated in and are currently active in the ART program, we identified a total of 101 children with evidence of virological failure on first-line ART and enrolled them between August 2011 and December 2012. The median time between last viral load result and genotyping was 3.1 months (IQR 1.4 - 7.0). Of the 101 samples, genotyping using the SATuRN genotyping method was successful in 89 cases (88.1%) (Figure 1). The mean viral load of the successful genotypes was 4.92 $\log_{10}$ copies/ml ± 5.3 (2.35-6.18$\log_{10}$ copies/ml). Twelve samples (11.9%) failed to amplify by PCR and were subsequently submitted for viral load quantification. Of these, six patients had a viral load at the time of genotyping of >1000copies/ml (mean = 3.77$\log_{10}$ copies/ml; range = 3.0-4.4 $\log_{10}$ copies/ml) but failed to amplify while five were suppressed with viral loads <1000copies/ml. There was insufficient sample to perform viral load quantification for one patient's sample.

The characteristics of the children with a genotype are shown in Table 1. Sixteen children (18.0%) were on a first-line protease inhibitor-based regimen and 73 (82.0%) were on an NNRTI-based regimen at the time of genotyping. The overall median duration of ART was 3.3 years (IQR 2.5 - 4.4) and the median duration of ART failure was 1.8 years (IQR 0.8 - 2.4).

Of the 89 children genotyped, 41 (46.1%) had, on at least one occasion, successfully suppressed viremia to <1000 copies/ml. The median duration on ART was slightly longer for those children on an NNRTI-based regimen compared to those on a PI-based regimen (3.4 years vs. 2.7 years) but the duration of ART failure was broadly similar between the same two groups (Table 2). We noted that the clinical and demographic characteristics of patients who suppressed compared with those that never suppressed (n = 48) was comparable (Table 3). The majority of patients in both groups were on 3TC-D4T-EFV both at initiation and at the time of genotyping (Table 3). Patients who had not suppressed were on a failing regimen for a statistically shorter (p = 0.04) period of time (median = 1.6 yrs; IQR = 1.4 yrs) compared with those that did suppress viremia (median = 1.9 yrs; IQR = 1.8 yrs). In addition, children who managed to suppress their viremia during treatment were older at the time of genotyping (p = 0.02) compared with those that never suppressed (Table 3). As expected, the median viral load at the time of genotyping of patients who never suppressed (median = 4.7 $\log_{10}$ cp/ml; IQR = 0.9

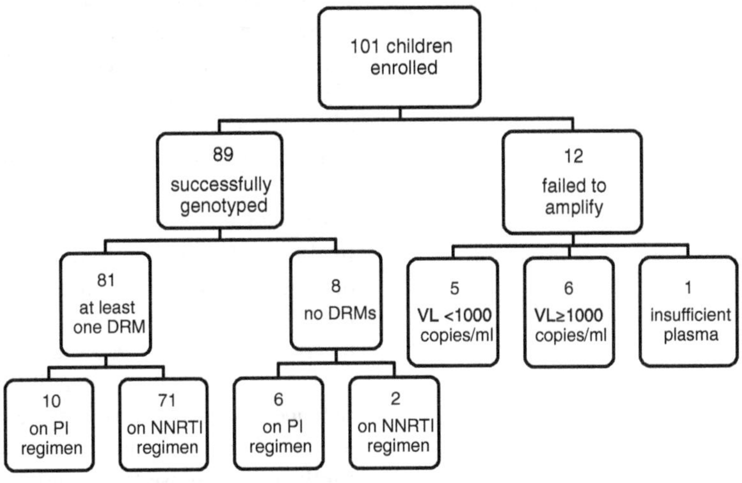

Figure 1 Flow chart showing children enrolled at PHC clinics and outcomes of genotyping.

Table 1 Demographic and clinical characteristics of the 89 children with a genotype

Characteristic	Outcome
Gender, male, *n* (%)	53 (59.6)
At ART initiation	
Age, years, median (IQR)	7 (3.7-9.6)
Number of children per age group n(%)	
0-3 years	17 (23)
4-9 years	37 (50)
10-15 years	20 (27)
Viral load, log_{10} copies/ml, median (IQR)	4.0 (3.7-4.7)
CD4+ cell count, cells/µl, median (IQR)	286 (112–560)
By Age category:	
0 - 2 yrs (n = 3)	817 (31–1564)
>2 – 5 yrs (n = 29)	469 (194–619)
>5 yrs (n = 38)	200 (69–363)
ART regimen, *n* (%)	
d4T/3TC/EFV	64 (71.9)
d4T/3TC/LPVr	12 (13.5)
ABC/3TC/EFV	8 (8.9)
ABC/3TC/LPVr	4 (4.5)
AZT/3TC/EFV	1 (1.1)
At genotyping	
Age, years, median (IQR)	10.2 (7.7 – 12.9)
Number of children per age group n(%)	
0-3 years	4 (4.5)
4-9 years	38 (42.7)
10-15 years	47 (52.8)
Viral load prior to genotyping*, log_{10} copies/ml, median (IQR)	4.2 (3.8-4.8)
CD4+ cell count prior to genotyping*, cells/µl,	460 (228–769)
median (IQR)	
By Age category:	2339 (1621–2538)
0 - 2 yrs (n = 4)	685 (442–956)
2 – 5 yrs (n = 37)	295 (147–564)
>5 yrs (n = 47)	
ART regimen at time of genotyping, *n* (%)	
d4T/3TC/EFV	58 (65.2)
d4T/3TC/LPVr	8 (8.9)
ABC/3TC/EFV	14 (15.7)
ABC/3TC/LPVr	8 (8.9)
AZT/3TC/EFV	1 (1.1)
Duration of ART, years, median (IQR)	3.3 (2.5-4.4)
Duration of ART failure[†], years, median (IQR)	1.8 (0.8-2.4)

Table 1 Demographic and clinical characteristics of the 89 children with a genotype *(Continued)*

Time between last viral load and genotype, months, median (IQR)	3.1 (1.4-7.0)
History of ART substitution[#], yes, n (%)	12 (13.5)

Key:
d4T, stavudine; 3TC, lamivudine; EFV, efavirenz; LPVr, lopinavir/ritonavir; ABC, abacavir; AZT, zidovudine; ART, antiretroviral therapy; IQR, interquartile range.
*Last measurements recorded prior to date of genotype.
[†]Duration of antiretroviral failure was estimated from the date of the first viral load >1000 copies/ml to date of genotype, unless there was a viral load <50 copies/ml in-between, in which case the time was estimated from the next viral load >1,000 copies/ml. If there was no viral load ≤1,000 copies/ml then time was calculated from date of ART initiation.
[#]Substitutions included changes of single drugs due to toxicity or guideline changes.

log_{10} cp/ml) was significantly higher ($p = 0.02$) than those that did (median = 3.9 log_{10} cp/ml; IQR = 4.7 log_{10} cp/ml).

Drug resistance mutations (DRM)

All of the sequences accepted for analysis were deemed of high quality having passed all quality and contamination tests as described. The HIV isolates from all patients successfully genotyped were identified as HIV-1 subtype C variants. Of the 89 genotypes, 81 (91.0%) demonstrated at least one DRM while 8 (9.0%) had no DRM (Table 4). For those on an NNRTI-based regimen, the majority of genotypes had both NRTI and NNRTI mutations. Thymidine analogue mutations (TAMs) were detected in 22 (24.7%) genotypes, while three or more TAMs were detected in only four of 89 genotypes (4.5%). The Q151M complex (a multinucleoside resistance mutation) was present in two genotypes, one from a child on an NNRTI-based regimen and one from a child on a PI-based regimen. Only one child on a PI-based regimen (1/16, 6.3%) harbored a major protease mutation and the most common pattern for children on PI-based regimens was the M184V mutation alone (Table 4).

An analysis of the genotypic susceptibility scores (GSS) of patients revealed that the median GSS for patients on a PI regimen (median = 2.0, IQR = 1.25) was higher as compared with those on an NNRTI-regimen (median = 1.0, IQR = 0.5). The majority (n = 12, 75%) of the patients on a PI-regimen, had GSS scores ≥2 while only 10 (14%) of those on an NNRTI-based regimen had comparable scores.

Discussion

In this study, we determined the frequency and patterns of drug resistance mutations in children failing first-line ART in a rural primary health care ART programme where care is delivered largely by nurses and counselors. For older children on NNRTI-based regimens, drug resistance mutations were detected in the majority. Whilst in most cases the mutations would be unlikely to significantly compromise a second-line regimen based on a ritonavir-boosted PI, five patients had complex mutation

Table 2 Characteristics of children on NNRTI-based and PI-based regimens (based on regimen at time of genotype)

	NNRTI ($n = 73$)	PI ($n = 16$)
At ART initiation		
Age, years, median (IQR)**	7.6 (5.2-10)	1.5 (0.7-3.8)
CD4+ cell count, cells/μl, median (IQR)*	256 (108–477)	647 (112–817)
Viral load, log_{10} copies/ml, median (IQR)	3.9 (3.7-4.2)	4.7 (4.7-4.7)
At Genotyping		
Age at genotyping, years, median (IQR)	11.4 (8.9-13.4)	5.0 (2.7-7.5)
CD4+ cell count prior to genotyping, cells/μl, median (IQR)**	379 (167–668)	762 (603–1123)
Viral load prior to genotyping, log_{10} copies/ml, median (IQR)	4.3 (3.8-4.8)	4.3 (3.8-5.2)
Comparative measures		
Duration of ART, years, median (IQR)	3.4 (2.6-4.5)	2.7 (1.6-4.0)
Duration of ART failure, years, median (IQR)	1.8 (0.9-2.4)	1.6 (0.8- 2.3)
Time between last viral load and genotyping, months, median (IQR)	3.3 (1.6-7.1)	3.0 (1.1-4.85)

Key: Difference in means at a 1% (**) or 5% (*) level of significance using the Student's T-Test.

patterns (three or more TAMs or Q151M complex) that might substantially limit the future activity of the NRTI class of drugs. In contrast, the younger children on PI-based regimens more often had no drug resistance mutations (six of 16 cases) and all but one had an absence of major protease mutations. This suggests a potential need for drug resistance genotyping, particularly in this group on PI-based regimens, to determine the appropriateness of regimen switch and to preserve first-line regimens where possible.

Table 3 Comparison of outcomes for patients who successfully suppressed viremia to <1000cp/ml with patients who were unable to suppress viral replication while on treatment

	Suppressed (n = 41)	Never suppressed (n = 48)
Gender:		
Male	23	30
At initiation:		
Age, years, median (IQR)	6.9 (4.4-9.8)	7.1 (3.2-9.6)
Viral load, log_{10} cp/ml, median (IQR)	3.8 (3.4-4.7)	4.2 (3.7-4.7)
CD4, cells/μl, median (IQR)	290 (136–563)	281 (89–560)
Regimen		
3TC-D4T-EFV	33	31
3TC-D4T-LPV/r	6	6
3TC-ABC-EFV	1	7
3TC-ABC-LPV/r	0	4
3TC-AZT-EFV	1	0
At genotyping:		
Age, years, median (IQR)*	11.1 (8.5-13.1)	9.8 (5.6-12.3)

Key: *Statistical significance (T-test, P<0.05).

These data represent one of the largest drug resistance studies of paediatric patients failing ART undertaken thus far in South Africa [12-18]. In addition, this study was unique in being from a rural decentralized primary health care programme where the delivery of ART to adults and children has scaled up rapidly. The characteristics of the children included in the study highlight some of the challenges of ART delivery in this setting, with very long time spent on failing regimens, a finding also reported amongst our adults on ART [19]. This suggests not only challenges to long-term adherence but also deficiencies in following the protocol for virological monitoring and switch to second-line ART guidelines. Problems with delayed switching have been well documented in South Africa [1,9,17] and these may be particularly problematic with children as many nurses and counselors are not confident managing paediatric ART and receive insufficient support and training in these issues. Some of the barriers to adherence in this setting are complex and difficult to address with the resources available within the health system. Furthermore, in rural areas with largely paper-based systems, results may simply be lost or misfiled and therefore overlooked.

First-line ART in South Africa using NNRTI-based regimens is challenging given the low genetic barrier of currently available drug options such as efavirenz and nevirapine and the fact that only one or two key DRMs are required to confer high-level resistance or cross-resistance to a drug class [20]. High-level resistance mutations and cross-resistance severely compromises future ART options, a dire consequence for paediatric patients who require lifelong ART. We detected high levels of drug resistant mutations in the group failing NNRTI-based regimens. The majority (80%) had both NRTI and NNRTI resistance mutations. The proportion that had complex

Table 4 The frequency of major drug resistance mutations and resistance complexes associated with PIs, NRTIs and NNRTIs of the 89 genotyped patients

	NNRTI-based regimen (n = 73)		PI-based regimen (n = 16)	
NNRTI mutations	Number	Percentage	Number	Percentage
Any NNRTI DRM	60	82.2	4	25.0
L100I	5	6.9	0	0
K101EP	6	8.2	0	0
K103NRS	46	63.0	2	12.5
V106M	23	31.5	2	12.5
V108I	7	9.6	1	6.3
Y181C	2	2.7	0	0
Y188HCL	7	9.6	1	6.3
G190AS	9	12.3	1	6.3
P225H	14	19.2	0	0
M230L	3	4.1	0	0
NRTI mutations				
Any mutation	63	86.3	10	62.5
M41L	7	9.6	0	0
K65NR	4	5.5	1	6.3
D67NG	8	11.0	0	0
K70ER	7	9.6	0	0
L74VI	4	5.5	1	6.3
Y115F	3	4.1	2	12.5
M184VI	60	82.2	10	62.5
L210W	1	1.4	0	0
T215FYI	9	12.3	0	0
K219QREN	5	6.9	0	0
Any TAMS	22	30.1	0	0
1 TAM	11	15.1	0	0
2 TAMs	7	9.6	0	0
≥3 TAMs	4	5.5	0	0
Q151M complex	1	1.4	1	6.3
PI mutations				
Any PI mutation	0	0	1	6.3
V82A	0	0	1	6.3

NRTI resistance patterns, such as three or more TAMs or Q151M complex, was lower (5.5%) than another recent study of 38 children on ART from the same province where 39% had three or more TAMs [17] despite a shorter duration (median = 2.8 yrs; IQR = 1.9- 2.3 yrs) on ART compared with our cohort (median = 3.3 yrs; IQR = 2.5-4.4 yrs). This suggests that the majority of children failing first-line NNRTI-based regimens in our cohort should retain susceptibility to a second-line regimen consisting of two alternative NRTIs and a ritonavir-boosted PI.

It was noteworthy that only one of 17 children on a PI-based regimens had a major PI resistance mutation. The low prevalence of PI mutations has been previously described in a number of manuscripts [17,21,22] This does raise the possibility of differential adherence to different components of the ART regimen (lopinavir/ritonavir syrup can be poorly tolerated), to problems with dosing of lopinavir/ritonavir syrup or possibly to drug-drug interactions particularly for those co-infected with TB, all issues we were unable to explore in detail for this study but which are subject to on-going research.

The finding that around nine in ten children with virological failure had at least one drug resistance mutation is consistent with other studies from South Africa [22-24] and a systematic review of studies from low- and middle-income countries, which reported a pooled proportion of 90% of children on ART with any DRM [8] The proportion with TAMs (23%) was similar to that seen in a similar paediatric programme in the Western Cape (19%) [22], although lower than the 56% reported in a systematic review of first-line failure of paediatric patients [8]. The proportion with TAMs was surprisingly low given the long duration of virological failure, and was also lower than the 40% reported from adults in our programme with a similar duration of ART and similar time on a failing regimen in an adult cohort from the same region [19]. This might suggest that adherence levels were either too low or too variable for the accumulation of TAMs over time. Alternatively, there was differential adherence to components of the regimen, with avoidance or suboptimal dosing of stavudine (d4T). The lack of major PI mutations in the young children on LPV/r-based regimens is consistent with other studies from the region which have shown PI mutations to be much more commonly associated with full dose ritonavir-based regimens [16,21-23].

Currently our genotyping costs are approximately 50 US$ at reagents cost and less than 100US$ when staff and transport costs are added on. The normal cost of genotyping is 250–300 US$ in the public sector. In order to facilitate large-scale genotyping and in the interest of reducing costs, we did not perform a pre-genotype confirmatory viral load, yet we successfully genotyped 88% (89/101) of our cohort. Our genotyping system and reagents are likely to be affordable to upper middle-income countries like South Africa and Botswana but further cost reductions would be required to make drug resistance testing affordable in lower middle-income and low income countries within Africa. An additional feature of our study was that genotypes directed subsequent clinical care where a doctor, social worker and other clinic staff managed patients from enrolment to implementing an intervention post-genotyping as was carried out in an adult cohort from the same area. The results from our study addressed three of the ten goals of the Department of Health 2010 ART Guidelines in that we present a means of achieving the best outcomes for HIV-infected patients receiving ART in a cost-effective manner; we employ existing infrastructure, that of a decentralised rural public health clinic facility for patient management; and by identifying DRMs early we ensure patient retention on lifelong ART by instituting early interventions to halt ART failure and prevent morbidity and mortality.

Interpretation of these data should be subject to some limitations of the study. This was a cross-sectional study and whilst we identified as many children with first-line ART failure as possible, we were unable to accurately estimate what proportion of all children on ART had virological failure and we cannot be certain that we included all children meeting the eligibility criteria. Further, we did not have accurate information on prior exposure to pMTCT regimens either in the mother or infant therefore have no means of assessing its impact on the spectrum of DRMs we observed in this cohort. We can speculate that the patterns of NNRTI mutations we observed are suggestive of and may arise from pMTCT exposure, however we cannot determine with certainty from our data whether DRMs in these children were acquired or transmitted via MTCT. We note this as a limitation of the present study. Although these data represent the largest group of genotypes for children failing first-line ART in South Africa, the numbers remain small. This highlights the need for collaborative studies and surveillance from multiple representative sites in order to inform national policies. The data regarding protease inhibitor resistance mutations could be limited by exploring only the protease gene and it is possible that we missed mutations at other sites, e.g. Gag cleavage sites [25].

Conclusions

In conclusion, this study has demonstrated that the spectrum of drug resistance mutations in this rural cohort is varied. The concerning prevalence of high-level resistance mutations particularly the frequency of TAMs amongst this paediatric cohort is an indicator of the time these patients spent on a failing regimen. This highlights the need for timely identification of patients failing ART and the implementation of early interventions be it drug switches or effective, reinforced, adherence counseling with appropriate follow-up. The use of genotyping, without a concurrent viral load, was efficient at identifying patients failing as a result of resistance mutations, determining the resistance profile of the patients and directing interventions for patient management. In this way, treatment options can be extended, a critical consideration for paediatric patients.

Methods

Setting

The study was conducted in the predominantly rural Hlabisa health sub-district in northern KwaZulu-Natal, South Africa. The programme, delivered by the Department of Health with support from the Africa Centre for Health and Population Studies (www.africacentre.ac.za), has been described previously [1,23,26]. HIV treatment and care is fully devolved to 17 primary health care (PHC) clinics and delivered largely by nurses and counsellors, with medical officers visiting clinics on a weekly or fortnightly basis. The programme adheres to national ART guidelines. At the time of the study, children eligible for ART aged 0–3 years (or weight under 10 kg) were commenced on a protease inhibitor (PI)-based regimen whereas children older than 3 years were commenced on a non-nucleoside reverse-transcriptase inhibitor (NNRTI)-based regimen. Viral load monitoring was scheduled six-monthly, although precise timing of viral load measurements was quite variable. Treatment of HIV-infected children was scaled up from late 2004 but accelerated in 2008 [1,23,27].

Study design

This cross-sectional study enrolled children (≤ 15 years of age) who had been receiving ART for more than 12 months with evidence of virological failure, defined as two consecutive viral loads >1000 copies/ml. Children with virological failure were identified from all 17 clinics both passively, during routine clinic visits, and actively, through interrogation of the programme database, which is housed at the Africa Centre and also by looking at all paediatric case files at the clinics. At the same time, the files of any children not eligible for the study but who were overdue for a routine viral load measurement were noted and a blood sample, to be taken at the next clinic visit, was requested. Single drug substitutions were allowed for toxicity or in the event of guideline changes. Any child meeting the enrolment criteria was subsequently enrolled. A medical officer enrolled all children and, either a parent or guardian provided the written informed consent. Demographic and clinical information were collected from clinical charts at the time of enrolment and a venous blood sample (4 ml EDTA tube) was collected on the same day.

Laboratory methods

Blood specimens, collected at the primary health care clinics, were transported from the Africa Centre to the Durban laboratory (~200 km away) on the same day of collection. Samples were received at the laboratory, recorded in a Laboratory Information Management System (LIMS) and the plasma was harvested and stored at −80°C until use. This blood specimen was collected specifically for resistance genotyping and was not reserved for viral load testing.

We used the affordable and open access Southern African Treatment Resistance Network (SATuRN) drug resistance genotyping system [Manasa et al. in preparation]. Briefly, this is an in-house method that costs approximately 50 US$ at reagent price. In order to keep the costs low, no viral load was performed before drug resistance genotyping. Ribonucleic acid (RNA) was extracted using the Qiagen RNA Mini kit (Qiagen N.V., Venlo, Netherlands) and reverse transcribed using the Superscript® III First-Strand Synthesis kit (Life Technologies, Carlsbad, CA) and RT21 specific primer (CTGTATTTCAGCTATCAAGTCCTTTGATGGG). A 1315 bp fragment of the *pol* gene, covering all the 99 protease codons and the first 240 codons of the reverse transcriptase (RT) gene was amplified with the high fidelity proofreading Platinum® Taq DNA polymerase (Life Technologies, Carlsbad, CA) and primers MAW26(TTGG AAATGTGGAAAGGAAGGAC) and RT21 (CTGTATTT CAGCTATCAAGTCCTTTGATGGG) for the first step and PRO1 (TAGAGCCAACAGCCCCACCA) and RT20 (CTGCCAATTCTAATTCTGCTTC) for the second step polymerase chain reaction (PCR). Population sequencing was performed on successfully amplified PCR products that were identified by gel electrophoresis and visualized as a 1.3 kb fragment under ultraviolet (UV) light. The PCR products were cleaned using the PureLink® PCR purification kit (Life Technologies, Carlsbad, CA) and were sequenced using the Sanger BigDye® terminator sequencing protocol (Life Technologies, Carlsbad, CA) and four bidirectional primers (RTC1F-ACCTACACCTGTCAACATAA TTG, RTC2R-TGTCAATGGCCATTGTTTAACCTTTGG, RTC3F-CACCAGGGATTAGATATCAATATAATGTGC, and RTC4R-CTAAATCAGATCCTACATACAAGTCA TCC), and run on an ABI 3130xl genetic analyser (Life Technologies, Carlsbad, CA), finally generating a consensus sequence spanning 300 amino acids of RT and 99 amino acids of the protease gene. The first 240 codons of the RT gene cover all currently recognized RT mutations associated with resistance to available RT inhibitors. Samples that failed to amplify were submitted for viral load testing using the Biocentric HIV RNA Charge Virale method (Biocentric, Bandol, France) with a detection limit of 50 copies/ml.

Sequence assembly and quality analysis

Sequences were imported into Geneious (Biomatters Ltd, Auckland, New Zealand), visually edited and deemed high quality if the quality score was higher than 80% post-trimming. Once trimmed these fragments were mapped to a reference strain (Accession# JN665021.1) to create a contig, which was further assessed for quality and ambiguities before a consensus sequence was extracted. Prior to the detection of drug resistance mutations (DRM) using bioinformatics software applications, we submitted each consensus to the Calibrated Population Resistance Tool (CPR) (http://hivdb.stanford.edu) for a final quality check. Sequences were deemed high quality if they had no ambiguities or insertions/deletions. In order to test for contamination we blasted our sequences against the public dataset using NCBI blast (http://www.ncbi.nlm.nih.gov/blast) and against our local database using a BlastServer application. Sequences were deemed not a contaminant if the identity to previously genotyped samples was lower than 98%. Finally, we constructed a maximum likelihood (ML) phylogenetic tree using phyML with GTR, gamma and percentage of invariable sites estimated from dataset. Trees were evaluated with 100 bootstraps and visualized in FigTree (http://tree.bio.ed.ac.uk/software/figtree/) in order to identify contamination where sequences cluster together with low genetic diversity.

Data analysis

All sequences, laboratory results (viral loads, CD4+ cell counts) and clinical and demographic data were entered into the SATuRN RegaDB database [28,29]. The database first identifies the subtype of each sequence using Rega HIV Subtyping tool version 2 [30,31], and thereafter determines the effect of DRMs on antiretroviral susceptibility using the three primary drug resistance interpretation algorithms, developed at Stanford University, Agence nationale de recherches sur le sida et les hépatitis virales (ANRS) and the Rega Institute. The amino acid positions on the RT gene relevant to the NRTI drug resistance mutations were 41, 62, 65, 67, 69, 70, 74, 75, 77, 115, 116, 151, 184, 210, 215 and 219. For the NNRTI drug class we included the amino acid positions 100, 101, 103, 106, 108, 138, 179, 181, 188, 190, 221, 225, 227 and 230 of the RT gene. Finally, for the PI drug class we interrogated our sequences using the following major drug resistance amino acid positions of the protease gene: 30, 32, 46, 47, 48, 50, 54, 58, 74, 76, 82, 83, 84, 88 and 90. Mutations were coded as DRMs at these positions based on the IAS mutation list of 2013 [32]. Drug resistance mutations, clinical measurements and demographic data were exported from RegaDB for analysis.

Descriptive statistics were used to summarise the demographic and clinical characteristics. Medians and the interquartile range (IQR) were calculated for continuous data. For analysis of drug resistance mutations, frequency distributions of the major DRMs were derived. Duration on ART was defined as the number of months between the date of ART initiation and the date of genotyping. The "duration of ART failure" was defined as the period from the date of the first viral load >1000 copies/ml to date of genotyping, unless there was a viral load <50 copies/ml in between, in which cases the duration was estimated from the time of the next available viral load >1000 copies/ml. If there was no viral load ≤1000 copies/ml then duration was calculated from date of ART initiation.

Abbreviations

ART: Antiretroviral therapy; ARV: Anti-retroviral; CPR: Calibrated population resistance; DRMs: Drug resistance mutations; HIV: Human immunodeficiency virus; LIMS: Laboratory information management system; NRTI: Nucleoside reverse transcriptase inhibitors; NNRTI: Non-nucleoside reverse transcriptase inhibitors; PCR: Polymerase chain reaction; PI: Protease inhibitors; SATuRN: Southern African Treatment Resistance Network; TAMs: Thymidine analogue mutations.

Competing interests

The authors declare no competing interests in relation to this manuscript.

Authors' contributions

SP and JM carried out the laboratory assays. SD and JM performed sequence analysis. SD performed the statistical analysis. SP and SD produced the first draft of the manuscript. TdO, RMB, RJL and SD formulated the design and coordinated the study. All authors contributed to the editing and production of the final manuscript. All authors read and approved the final manuscript.

Acknowledgements

The authors extend our gratitude to the participants of the study as well as their parents/guardians. We are also grateful to the following people who assisted in various capacities: Xolile Kineri, Zakhona Gumede, Lungani Ndwadwa, Carina Herbst, Pretty Nkosi, Nokuthula Sikhosana and the tireless nurses at the Primary Health Care Clinics in our study area.

Author details

[1]Africa Centre for Health and Population Studies, College of Health Sciences, University of KwaZulu-Natal, Durban, South Africa. [2]Royal Hospital for Sick Children, Glasgow, UK. [3]Department of Clinical Research, London School of Hygiene and Tropical Medicine, London, UK. [4]Research Department of Infection, University College of London (UCL), London, UK. [5]Rm 135, 1st Floor, DDMRI, 719 Umbilo Road, Congella 4013, South Africa.

References

1. Janssen N, *et al*: **Successful paediatric HIV treatment in rural primary care in Africa.** *Arch Dis Child* 2010, **95**(6):414–421.
2. Meyers T, *et al*: **Changes in pediatric HIV-related hospital admissions and mortality in Soweto, South Africa, 1996–2011: light at the end of the tunnel?** *J Acquir Immune Defic Syndr* 2012, **60**(5):503–510.
3. Bland RM: **Management of HIV-infected children in Africa: progress and challenges.** *Arch Dis Child* 2011, **96**(10):911–915.
4. Patel SD, *et al*: **Increases in pediatric antiretroviral treatment, South Africa 2005–2010.** *PLoS One* 2012, **7**(9):e44914.
5. Davies MA, *et al*: **Outcomes of the South African National Antiretroviral Treatment Programme for children: the IeDEA Southern Africa collaboration.** *S Afr Med J* 2009, **99**(10):730–737.
6. Mofenson LM, Cotton MF: **The challenges of success: adolescents with perinatal HIV infection.** *J Int AIDS Soc* 2013, **16:**18650.
7. Gupta RK, Gibb DM, Pillay D: **Management of paediatric HIV-1 resistance.** *Curr Opin Infect Dis* 2009, **22**(3):256–263.
8. Sigaloff KC, *et al*: **HIV-1-resistance-associated mutations after failure of first-line antiretroviral treatment among children in resource-poor regions: a systematic review.** *Lancet Infect Dis* 2011, **11**(10):769–779.
9. Meyers T, *et al*: **Challenges to pediatric HIV care and treatment in South Africa.** *J Infect Dis* 2007, **196**(Suppl 3):S474–S481.
10. Fatti G, *et al*: **Increased vulnerability of rural children on antiretroviral therapy attending public health facilities in South Africa: a retrospective cohort study.** *J Int AIDS Soc* 2010, **13:**46.
11. Macdonald P, *et al*: **Paediatric human immunodeficiency virus treatment outcomes from a resource-limited setting in south africa: highly active antiretroviral therapy alone is not enough.** *Vulnerable Child Youth Stud* 2011, **6**(3):208–221.
12. Wallis CL, *et al*: **Emergence of drug resistance in HIV-1 subtype C infected children failing the South African National Antiretroviral roll-out program.** *Paeiatric I nfectious Dis J.* 2009, **38**(12):1123–1125.
13. Barth RE, *et al*: **Long-term outcome of children receiving antiretroviral treatment in Rural South Africa.** *Pediatr Infect Dis J* 2011, **30**(1):52–56.
14. van Zyl G, *et al*: **Protease inhibitor resistance in South African children with virologic failure.** *Pediatr Infect Dis J* 2009, **28**(12):1125–1127.
15. Pillay V, *et al*: **HIV type 1 subtype C drug resistance among pediatric and adult South African patients failing antiretroviral therapy.** *AIDS Res Hum Retroviruses* 2008, **24**(11):1449–1454.
16. Taylor BS, *et al*: **Rapid development of antiretroviral drug resistance mutations in HIV-infected children less than Two years of Age initiating protease inhibitor-based therapy in South Africa.** *AIDS Res Hum Retroviruses* 2011, **27**(9):945–956.
17. Green TN, *et al*: **Drug resistance and coreceptor usage in HIV type 1 subtype C-infected children initiating or failing highly active antiretroviral therapy in South Africa.** *AIDS Res Hum Retroviruses* 2012, **28**(4):324–332.
18. Latinovic O, *et al*: **Pharmacotherapy of HIV-1 infection: focus on CCR5 antagonist maraviroc.** *Clin Med Ther* 2009, **1**:1497–1510.
19. Manasa J, *et al*: **High-levels of acquired drug resistance in adult patients failing first-line antiretroviral therapy in a rural HIV treatment programme in KwaZulu-Natal, South Africa.** *PLoS One* 2013:0. in press.
20. Osterholzer D: **The role of etravirine in the management of treatment-experienced pediatric patients with HIV.** *HIV AIDS (Auckl)* 2013, **5**:67–73.
21. Frange P, *et al*: **Lopinavir/ritonavir-based antiretroviral therapy in human immunodeficiency virus type 1-infected naive children rare protease inhibitor resistance mutations but high lamivudine/emtricitabine resistance at the time of virologic failure.** *PaedPaediatric Infec Dis J* 2011, **30**(8):684–688.
22. Orrel C, *et al*: **Resistance in pediatric patients experiencing virologic failure with first- and second-line antiretroviral therapy.** *Paediatric Infec Dis J* 2013, **32**(6):644–647.
23. Wallis CL, *et al*: **Low rates of nucleoside reverse transcriptase inhibitor (NRTI) resistance detected in a well monitored cohort in South Africa accessing antiretroviral therapy.** *Antivir Ther* 2012, **17**(2):313–320.
24. Pillay D: **Implications of HIV drug resistance on first and second line therapies in resource limited settings :report froma workshop organised by the collaborative HIV and anti-HIV drug resistance network.** *Antivir Ther* 2013, **18**(6):831–836.
25. Doyon L, *et al*: **Second locus involved in human immunodeficiency virus type 1 resistance to protease inhibitors.** *J Virol* 1996, **70**(6):3763–3769.
26. Houlihan CF, *et al*: **Cohort profile: Hlabisa HIV treatment and care programme.** *Int J Epidemiol* 2011, **40**(2):318–326.
27. Cooke GS, *et al*: **Need for timely paediatric HIV treatment within primary health care in rural South Africa.** *PLoS One* 2009, **4**(9):e7101.
28. de Oliveira T, Shafer RW, Seebregts C: **Public database for HIV drug resistance in southern Africa.** *Nature* 2010, **464**(7289):673.
29. Libin P, *et al*: **RegaDB: community-driven data management and analysis for infectious diseases.** *Bioinformatics* 2013, **29**(11):1477–1480.
30. Alcantara LC, *et al*: **A standardized framework for accurate, high-throughput genotyping of recombinant and non-recombinant viral sequences.** *Nucleic Acids Res* 2009, **37**(Web Server issue):W634–W642.
31. de Oliveira T, *et al*: **An automated genotyping system for analysis of HIV-1 and other microbial sequences.** *Bioinformatics* 2005, **21**(19):3797–3800.
32. Johnson VA, *et al*: **Update of the drug resistance mutations in HIV-1: March 2013.** *Top Antivir Med* 2013, **21**(1):6–14.

10

Increasing Hepatitis C treatment uptake among HIV-infected patients using an HIV primary care model

Edward R Cachay[1,3*], Lucas Hill[2], Craig Ballard[2], Bradford Colwell[2], Francesca Torriani[1,3], David Wyles[1,3] and William C Mathews[1]

Abstract

Background: Access to Hepatitis C (HCV) care is low among HIV-infected individuals, highlighting the need for new models to deliver care for this population.

Methods: Retrospective cohort analysis that compared the number of HIV patients who initiated HCV therapy: hepatology (2005–2008) vs. HIV primary care model (2008–2011). Logistic-regression modeling was used to ascertain factors associated with HCV therapy initiation and achievement of sustained viral response (SVR).

Results: Of 196 and 163 patients that were enrolled in the HIV primary care and hepatology models, 48 and 26 were treated for HCV, respectively ($p = 0.043$). The HIV/HCV-patient referral rate did not differ during the two study periods (0.10 vs. 0.12/patient-yr, $p = 0.18$). In unadjusted analysis, predictors ($p < 0.05$) of HCV treatment initiation included referral to the HIV primary care model (OR: 1.7), a CD4+ count ≥400/mm3 (OR: 1.8) and alanine aminotranferase level ≥63U/L (OR: 1.9). Prior psychiatric medication use correlated negatively with HCV treatment initiation (OR: 0.6, $p = 0.045$). In adjusted analysis the strongest predictor of HCV treatment initiation was CD4+ count (≥400/mm3, OR: 2.1, $p = 0.01$). There was no significant difference in either clinic model (primary care vs. hepatology) in the rates of treatment discontinuation due to adverse events (29% vs. 16%), loss to follow-up (8 vs. 8%), or HCV SVR (44 vs. 35%).

Conclusions: Using a HIV primary care model increased the number of HIV patients who initiate HCV therapy with comparable outcomes to a hepatology model.

Keywords: HIV, HCV treatment, Primary care, Hepatology

Introduction

Access to hepatitis C (HCV) treatment remains low in HIV-infected individuals in the USA [1-3], resulting in increased morbidity and cost due to HCV related complications [4,5].

The following factors account in part for the low treatment rates of HCV in the HIV population: increased prevalence of competing medical co-morbidities [6], ongoing substance/alcohol dependence and neuropsychiatric disease [7]. Additional disincentives for patients to seek HCV treatment include: low efficacy and severe side effects associated with conventional HCV therapies (pegylated interferon and ribavirin) [8]; long waiting time prior to HCV intake appointment in sub-specialty clinics [9]; and commuting to a different location from where they routinely receive their HIV care [10,11].

In April 2008, the University of California at San Diego (UCSD) transitioned from a hepatology specialty model to an HIV primary care hepatitis program for the management of HCV in HIV-infected patients without advanced cirrhosis. Many centers around the country with a high burden of HIV/HCV co-infection have implemented similar multidisciplinary co-infection programs, but there is little data describing the structure, processes, and outcomes of these programs. Thus, we sought to compare

* Correspondence: ecachay@ucsd.edu
[1]Department of Medicine, Owen Clinic, University of California at San Diego, 200 W. Arbor Drive, San Diego, CA 92103-8681, USA
[3]Department of Medicine, Division of Infectious Diseases, University of California at San Diego, San Diego, CA, USA

the rates of referral, treatment initiation and completion between a prior hepatology-managed co-infection clinic and a subsequent HIV primary care managed co-infection clinic after the first three years of transition.

Methods

Study design and patients

We compared two adult cohorts: (1) UCSD hepatology specialty model (1 Jan 2005–31 March 2008) and (2) the UCSD Owen hepatitis co-infection clinic (1 April 2008–30 July 2011). Inclusion criteria required: (1) a documented clinical decision regarding HCV treatment eligibility; (2) if treated, HCV treatment consisting of pegylated interferon and ribavirin. The study was approved by the UCSD Human Research Protection Program.

Description of HIV primary care model

The UCSD Owen clinic cares for more than 3,000 HIV-infected patients of whom approximately 20% are co-infected with HCV. Prior to April 2008 a team of hepatologists managed a once weekly clinic for assessment of HIV/HCV patients. There were no explicit inclusion criteria for referral to the traditional hepatology-based clinic. Historically, HIV providers made referral decisions based on their own referral criteria. The new hepatitis co-infection primary care model also operates as one clinic session per week and is staffed by three HIV clinicians with Infectious Diseases certification, a psychiatrist, two clinical pharmacists specialized in HIV care, one health educator and a substance counselor. There was no change in procedures for patient referral to the primary care managed co-infection clinic nor were there any other structural changes to the HIV clinic during the transition process; all HIV patients under care with viral hepatitis co-infection could be referred by their HIV primary care provider for evaluation. Every patient underwent a detailed clinical, laboratory and imaging (ultrasound and/or abdomino-pelvic computer tomography) assessment for staging degree of liver disease according to standard of care and ruling out indirect evidence of advanced liver disease and/or portal hypertension [12]. Patients with HCV genotype 1 or 4 were offered a liver biopsy performed by the interventional radiology service unless patients declined the procedure. Esophagogastroduodenoscopies when required were completed by the gastroenterology service. Our minimal requirements for HCV treatment eligibility were: (1) undetectable HIV viral load and CD4 cell count $\geq 200/cm^3$ if on antiretroviral therapy; (2) CD4 cell count $\geq 500/cm^3$ irrespective of HIV viral load value if naïve to antiretroviral therapy; (3) absence of Child B or C liver cirrhosis; (4) stable concurrent medical co-morbidity; (5) favorable recommendation from the team's psychiatrist; (6) registration in the San Diego needle exchange program in the case of ongoing parenteral drug use with documentation of controlled HIV infection as in (1) and (2), plus documentation of no missed clinic appointments during HCV staging process; and (7) alcohol sobriety for at least 3 months prior to HCV treatment initiation. Homeless patients were required to receive all weekly pegylated interferon injections in clinic.

HCV treatment monitoring strategies and role of pharmacists in the HIV primary care model

Following favorable consideration to initiate HCV therapy, a patient was assigned to one of three groups for HCV treatment monitoring: Group 1 had patients without major significant medical co-morbidity, social barriers and no on-going illicit substance use. Group 2 comprised patients with on-going substance use and/or homelessness, Group 3 included patients with severe neuropsychiatric disease (i.e. prior suicidal attempts) and/or medical co-morbidities (i.e. history of congestive heart failure). Patients were followed by physicians and pharmacist specialized in HIV where frequency of follow-up and laboratory testing was based on monitoring group assignment (Additional file 1: Table S1 and Additional file 2: Table S2). Pharmacists verified: (1) potential medication interactions; (2) HIV antiretroviral adherence; (3) HCV health education; (4) insurance coverage for access to HCV medication; and (5) patient understanding of HCV medication dosing, administration, and possible side effects. During HCV treatment, HIV pharmacists assist in monitoring: (1) adherence to HCV therapy; (2) critical laboratory results; (3) HCV medication and adjunctive therapy access during treatment course; and (4) unexpected medication interactions/clinical complaints not reported by the patient to physicians.

Study outcomes

The primary outcome was the difference in the number of referred patients who initiated HCV therapy in both cohorts during the study period. Secondary outcomes were: (1) referral rates by HIV primary care providers for HCV treatment consideration and (2) proportion of patients that following HCV therapy achieved sustained viral response (SVR).

Independent variables

The following independent variables were assessed: (1) sociodemographic (age, sex, race/ethnicity, HIV risk factor); (2) HIV related (CD4 cell count, HIV viral load and proportion of patients on antiretroviral therapy); (3) HCV viral load and genotype; (4) histological severity of liver disease according to modified Knodell score; (5) neuropsychiatric history, including proportion of patients on any psychotropic medications; (6) history of self-reported illicit substance and/or alcohol use within the last 3 months of HCV treatment evaluation by completion of the ASSIST instrument [13] and subsequent evaluation by the substance abuse counselor and (7) laboratory values [hemoglobin, platelet count, alanine aminotransferase (ALT), international normalized ratio (INR)].

Statistics

Baseline comparison of clinical characteristics between patients referred to the two clinic models was evaluated using exact Wilcoxon tests for continuous and Fisher's test for categorical variables. Among patients referred to each clinic model differences in reasons for deferring HCV therapy were explored using chi-square analyses. Bivariate analyses were used to explore the effect of each independent variable in predicting the decision for HCV treatment initiation. Then, we fitted a multiple logistic regression model to adjust for confounding and effect modification of variables associated with HCV therapy initiation using the co-variates found to be significant in prior bivariate analysis ($p < 0.10$). We estimated referral rates as the number of referrals per patient-year of follow-up during the study period. The beginning of follow-up for the hepatology or primary care group was defined as the later of either the date of first date of each cohort study period or the date of first visit to each co-infection clinic model. The end of follow-up for each group was the earlier of either the date of last visit to the co-infection clinic model or the end of the two respective study periods. The referral rate ratio and 95% confidence interval was estimated with its associated p-value. Analyses were performed using NCCSS version 8.0 (Kaysville, Utah, USA).

Results

From a total of 667 and 616 HIV/HCV co-infected patients during the studied periods, 256 and 203 were referred for HCV treatment evaluation to the HIV primary care and hepatology models, respectively. The HCV prevalence was similar during studied periods, HIV primary care model (17%) and hepatology (18%). The patient referral rate for HCV treatment did not differ during the 2 study periods, 0.12 vs. 0.10/patient-year for HIV primary care and hepatology models [difference −0.02, 95% confidence intervals (CI) −0.03 to 0.06; $p = 0.18$]. Main reasons for exclusion of 100 patients after initial visit are shown in Figure 1. The final study cohorts were composed of 196 and 163 patients for the HIV primary care and the hepatology models, respectively. Of note there was no difference in the proportion of patients excluded in both clinic models due to prior HCV treatment null-response (11/196 vs. 6/163; $p = 0.39$), Figure 1.

Patients referred to the HIV primary care model were older (median 48 vs. 45 years), had a higher proportion of non-hispanics (85 vs. 74%) and reported more frequently heterosexual sex as HIV risk factor (24 vs. 15%) than those referred to the hepatology model. They also had higher median CD4+ cell counts (431 vs. 372/mm^3) and platelet counts (208 vs. 184 × 103/mm^3) at the time of HCV treatment consideration (Table 1). There were

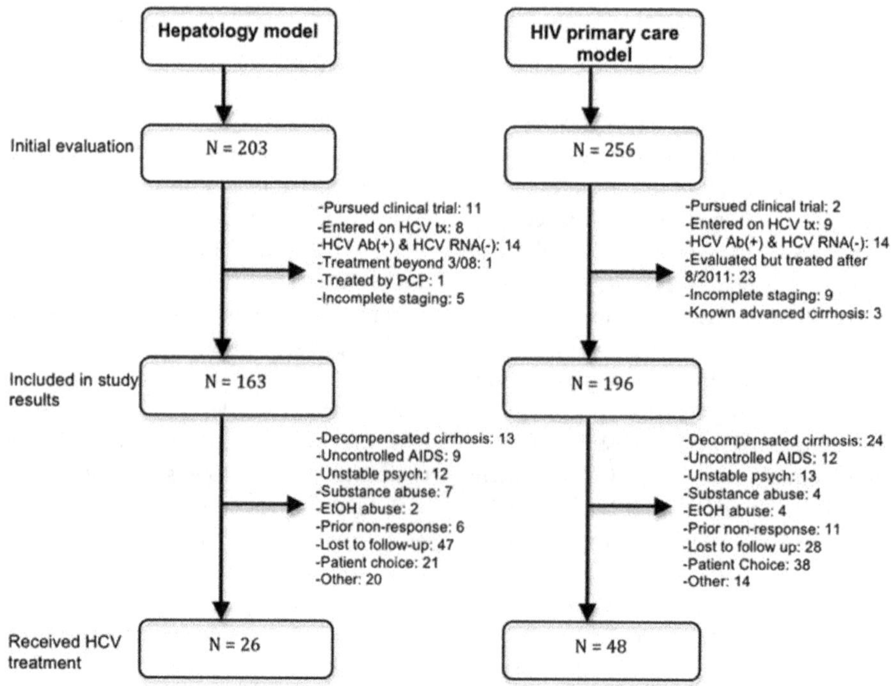

Figure 1 Flow of included patients.

Table 1 Characteristics of the patients assessed for hepatitis C treatment consideration according to clinic model

Clinic model	Hepatology (n = 163)	HIV primary care (n = 196)	*P* value
Median age – years (range)	45(26–73)	48(19–75)	0.02[a]
Sex: Male (%)	137(84)	165(84)	0.97[b]
Race			
White	115	138	0.20[c]
Black	39	50	
Asian	0	3	
Other/unknown	9	5	
Ethnicity			
Hispanic	35	26	0.03[c]
Not-Hispanic	121	167	
Unknown	7	3	
HIV risk factors			
Gay/bisexual	79	78	0.003[c]
Heterosexual	24	46	
Intravenous drug use	3	8	
Hemophilia	8	5	
combination	25	47	
Other/unknown	24	12	
Median CD4+ cell count – cells/mm^3 (range)[1]	372 (29–1179)	431 (38–1612)	0.05[a]
Median HIV load – $\log_{10}$ copies/mL (range)	2.6 (2.6–5.8)	2.6 (2.6–6.6)	0.12[a]
Number on HAART therapy – %	132 (81)	172 (88)	0.08[b]
Hepatitis C genotype[2]			
Genotype 1,4	125	158	0.68[c]
Genotype 2,3	31	35	
Median HCV load – $\log_{10}$ copies/mL (range)[3]	6.29 (1.9–8.4)	6.43 (2.2–8.4)	0.43[a]
Liver biopsy scores [4]			
F0-2	39	42	0.95[c]
F3,4	37	39	
Any neuropsychiatry history – %	100 (61%)	119 (61%)	0.85[b]
On any psychiatry medications – %	75 (46%)	88 (45%)	0.83[b]
Drugs or alcohol use within 3months of HCV treatment consideration			
No	71	115	0.0001[c]
yes	45	72	
unknown	47	9	
Median hemoglobin levels – g/dL (range)	14.7 (9–18.7)	14.3 (7.7–17.6)	0.13[a]
Median platelet count –1000/mm^3 (range)	184 (44–531)	208 (41–548)	0.004[a]
Median ALT – U/L (range)	68 (20–980)	57 (12–1280)	0.51[a]
Median INR (range)	1.1 (0.9–2.3)	1.0 (0.9–2.6)	0.05[a]

ALT = Alanine aminotransferase ; AST = Aspartate aminotransferase; INR = International normalized ratio.
[1] CD4+ counts available in 150 of 163 patients in the hepatology model and in all patients in HIV primary care model.
[2] HCV genotype was not available in seven patients in hepatology model and one in HIV primary care model.
[3] Liver biopsies: 70 in hepatology and 67 in HIV primary care models.
[4] Two patients in the hepatology model had no available HCV viral load.
[a] Wilcoxon Rank-Sum Test.
[b] Chi-square Test.
[c] Fisher's exact Test.

Table 2 Characteristics of the patients treated for hepatitis C according to clinic model and treatment outcomes

Clinic model	Hepatology (n = 26)	HIV primary care (n = 48)	*P* value
Median age – years (range)	44 (27–62)	49 (19–61)	0.18[a]
Sex: Male (%)	23 (88)	38 (79)	0.32[b]
Race			
White	21	32	0.44[c]
Black	4	13	
Other/unknown	1	3	
Ethnicity			
Hispanic	5	7	0.12[c]
Not-Hispanic	19	41	
Unknown	2	0	
HIV risk factors			
Gay/bisexual	8	21	0.008[c]
Heterosexual	5	14	
Intravenous drug use	1	0	
Hemophilia	3	0	
combination	3	11	
Other/unknown	6	2	
Median CD4+ cell count – cells/mm^3 (range)	375 (149–1179)	522 (130–1142)	0.02[a]
Number with undetectable HIV load (%)	22 (85)	29 (83)	0.88[b]
Hepatitis C genotype[2]			
Genotype 1/4	19	39	0.42[b]
Genotype 2/3	7	9	
Median HCV load – $\log_{10}$ copies/mL (range)	6.04 (5.1–7.7)	6.41 (3.0–7.6)	0.88[a]
Liver biopsy scores [1]			
F0-2	8	12	0.37[c]
F3,4	9	23	
Number with relapse after prior HCV treatment (%)	5 (19)	5 (11)	0.29[b]
Any neuropsychiatry history – %	17 (65)	23 (48)	0.15[b]
On any psychiatry medications – %	11 (42)	15 (31)	0.34[b]
Drugs or alcohol use within 3months of HCV treatment consideration			
No	12	32	0.0001[c]
Yes	5	16	
Unknown	9	0	
Median hemoglobin levels – g/dL (range)	14.8 (11.1–16.9)	14.5(12.1–16.6)	0.17[a]
Median platelet count –1000/mm^3 (range)	178 (56–367)	224 (113–418)	0.01[a]
Median ALT – U/L (range)	71 (22–980)	64 (19–1087)	0.48[a]
Median INR (range)	1.1 (0.9–1.4)	1.0 (0.9–1.2)	0.69[a]
HCV treatment outcomes			
№ Patients with rapid viral response (%)	4 (15)	12 (25)	0.34[b]
№ Patients with complete early viral response (%)	9 (35)	26 (54)	0.11[b]
№ Patients with end of treatment response (%)	12 (46)	24 (50)	0.75[b]
№ Patients with sustained viral response (%)	9 (35)	21 (44)	0.45[b]
№ Patients who discontinued HCV therapy due to non-viral response (%)	8 (31)	9 (19)	0.24[b]

Table 2 Characteristics of the patients treated for hepatitis C according to clinic model and treatment outcomes *(Continued)*

№ Patients who discontinued HCV therapy due to treatment-related side effects (%)	4 (15)	14 (29)	0.16[b]
№ Patients lost to follow-up (%)	2 (8)	4 (8)	0.92[b]

[1] Liver biopsies were not performed in 2 and 6 patients with genotype 1 in the hepatology and HIV primary care models respectively.
[a] Wilcoxon Rank-Sum Test.
[b] Chi-square Test.
[c] Fisher's exact Test.

no differences between clinic model cohorts of referred patients in plasma HIV or HCV viral load, HCV genotype distribution, liver fibrosis score, proportion of patients -receiving HIV therapy, -with neuropsychiatric history, -on psychotropic medications. Among patients referred to the HIV primary care model, 37% reported use of drugs or heavy alcohol within 3 months of HCV treatment consideration (Table 1).

While in the HIV primary care model a higher proportion of patients (19 vs. 13%) chose to defer HCV therapy due to personal reasons (e.g. did not want to request time off at work), in the hepatology model more patients failed to initiate HCV therapy due to loss-to-follow up (29 vs. 14%), overall comparison χ^2 15.6, df = 8, p = 0.03 (Figure 1).

Treatment rates and predictors of Hepatitis C treatment

More patients were treated for HCV in the HIV primary care model than in the hepatology model (48 vs. 26, p = 0.043). This difference was more apparent in the second year of implementation of the HIV primary care model, when comparing the proportion of patients treated for HCV by year of study periods: year 1 (9 vs. 13%), year 2 (35 vs. 11%), year 3 (44 vs. 28%), for HIV primary care vs. hepatology models, respectively, χ^2 8.1, df = 2, p =0.02.

Patients treated in the HIV primary care model had a higher median CD4+ cell count (522 vs. 375/mm^3), platelet count (224 vs. 178 × 10^3/mm^3, p = 0.01) and frequency of drugs or alcohol use within 3 months of HCV therapy evaluation (33 vs. 19%). Among those treated for HCV, there were no differences between clinic models in the age, race/ethnicity, HIV/HCV viral load, proportion on HIV therapy, HCV genotype distribution, liver fibrosis score, relapse after prior HCV treatment or prevalence of psychiatric disease (Table 2). When comparing clinical characteristics of HCV treated and untreated patients within each model, in the hepatology model there were no clinical variables associated with the decision to initiate HCV treatment. However, patients treated for HCV under the HIV primary care model had higher CD4+ cell counts, lower rates of psychiatric illness, and were prescribed fewer psychotropic medications (Table 3). Using bivariate categorical analysis, independent predictors of HCV therapy initiation included being referred to the HIV primary care model [odds ratio (OR) 1.8, 95% CI 1.1–2.9, p = 0.04]; having a higher CD4+ count (≥400/mm3, OR: 1.8, 95% CI 1.1–3.0) and ALT levels (> 63 U/L, OR: 1.9, 95% CI 1.2–2.9). Prior psychiatric medication use correlated negatively with HCV treatment initiation (OR: 0.6, 95% CI 0.3–0.99). Logistic regression analysis adjusting for all aforementioned significant variables showed that the strongest predictor of HCV treatment initiation was CD4+ count (≥400/mm3, OR: 2.1, 95% CI 1.2–3.6, p = 0.01) whereas a history of prior psychiatric medication use decreased the chances of HCV treatment initiation (OR: 0.5, 95% CI 0.3–0.9, p = 0.02), (Table 4).

Outcomes of HCV treatment

Similar proportions of patients achieved undetectable HCV viral load -at week 4 (rapid viral response [RVR]), -at week 12 (complete early viral response [cEVR]) and at week 48 (end of treatment response [ETR]) in both models (HIV primary care vs. hepatology): RVR [12/48(25%) vs. 4/26(15%)], cEVR [26/48(54%) vs. 9/26(35%)] and ETR (24/48(50%, vs. 12/26(46%)]. Twenty-one of 48 patients (44%) in the HIV primary care and 9 of 26 patients (35%) in the hepatology model achieved HCV SVR (p =0.45).

When comparing both models (primary care vs. hepatology), there were no differences in the overall HCV treatment discontinuations rates [27/48(56%) vs. 14/26 (54%), p = 0.84] or cause-specific reasons HCV-treatment discontinuation rates: (1) non-viral response [9 /48 (18%) vs. 8/26 (31%), p = 0.24]; (2) HCV therapy-related adverse events [14/48 (29%) vs. 4/26 (16%), p =0.19]; and loss to follow-up (4/ 48 (8%) vs. 2/26 (8%), p = 0.92]. The median time for HCV treatment discontinuation due to adverse events in the HIV primary care model was 12 weeks (range 1–55) and was comparable to the hepatology model (median 8 weeks, range 1–40). The reasons for treatment discontinuation in the hepatology model (n = 4) were hematologic (2) and neuropsychiatric (2) side effects. In the HIV primary care model, main reasons for adverse-events HCV treatment discontinuation (n = 14) were neuropsychiatric (7) and somatic (7) side effects. The somatic side effects included: severe fatigue (3), anorexia /weight loss (2), dizziness (1) and skin rash (1). In the HIV primary care model, 16 (33%) HCV treated patients were actively

Table 3 Comparison of characteristics of the treated vs. untreated patients for hepatitis C according to clinic model

Clinic Model	Hepatology			HIV Primary care		
	Treated (n = 26)	Not treated (n = 137)	*P*	Treated (n = 48)	Not treated (n = 148)	*P*
Median age – years (range)	44 (27–62)	45 (26–73)	0.73[a]	49 (19–61)	48 (23–75)	0.46[a]
Sex: Male (%)	23 (89)	114 (83)	0.50[b]	38 (79)	127 (86)	0.27[b]
Race						
White	21	94	0.46[c]	32	106	0.63[c]
Black	4	35		13	37	
Other/unknown	1	8		2	5	
Ethnicity						
Hispanic	5	30	0.64[c]	7	19	0.59[c]
Not-Hispanic	19	102		41	16	
Unknown	2	5		0	3	
HIV risk factors						
Gay/bisexual	8	71	0.18[c]	21	57	0.33[c]
Heterosexual	5	19		14	32	
Intravenous drug use	1	2		0	8	
Hemophilia	3	5		0	5	
combination	3	22		11	36	
Other/unknown	6	18		2	10	
Median CD4+ cell count – cells/mm^3 (range)	375 (149–1179)	371 (29–1025)	0.68[a]	522 (130–1142)	388 (38–1612)	0.005[a]
Number of patients on HIV therapy (%)	22 (85%)	110 (80%)	0.61[b]	44 (92%)	128 (87%)	0.74[b]
Number with undetectable HIV load (%)	22 (85%)	95 (69%)	0.11[b]	40 (83%)	115 (78%)	0.41[b]
Hepatitis C genotype[1]						
Genotype 1/4	19	106	0.32[c]	39	119	0.90[b]
Genotype 2/3	7	24		9	26	
Median HCV load – $\log_{10}$ copies/mL (range)[2]	6.0 (5.1–7.7)	6.3 (1.9–8.4)	0.71[a]	6.4 (3.01–7.6)	6.4 (2.2–8.4)	0.19[a]
Liver biopsy scores						
F0-2	8	31	0.10[c]	12	30	0.19[c]
F3-4	9	28		13	26	
unknown	9	78		23	92	
Any neuropsychiatry history – %	17 (65%)	83(61%)	0.65[b]	23(48%)	96(65%)	0.04[b]
On any psychiatry medications – %	11 (42%)	64(47)	0.68[b]	15(31%)	73(49)	0.03[b]
Drugs or alcohol use within 3months of HCV treatment consideration						
No	12	59	0.55[c]	32	83	0.15[c]
Yes	5	40		16	56	
Unknown	9	38		0	9	
Median hemoglobin levels – g/dL (range)	14.8 (11.1–16.9)	14.7 (9–18.7)	0.37[a]	14.5 (12.1–16.6)	14.2 (7.7–17.6)	0.67[a]
Median platelet count –1000/mm^3 (range)	178 (56–367)	185 (44–531)	0.47[a]	224 (113–418)	207 (41–548)	0.18[a]

Table 3 Comparison of characteristics of the treated vs. untreated patients for hepatitis C according to clinic model *(Continued)*

Median ALT – U/L (range)	71 (22–980)	67 (20–488)	0.56[a]	64 (19–1087)	56 (12–1280)	0.25[a]
Median INR (range)	1.1 (0.9–1.4)	1.1 (0.9–2.3)	0.33[a]	1.0 (0.9–1.2)	1.0 (0.9–2.6)	0.66[a]

[1] In the hepatology model (7) and HIV primary care model (3) patients had no available genotype, all in untreated group, there were no patients with genotype #4 in treated groups.
[2] Two patients in the untreated group in the hepatology model had no available HCV viral load.
[a] Wilcoxon Rank-Sum Test.
[b] Chi-square Test.
[c] Fisher's exact Test.

using illicit substances of whom 2 were using intravenous drugs and 4 were homeless. None of the treated homeless patients were lost to follow-up.

Among patients treated in the HIV primary care model, 17 were considered high-risk: substance use and/or homelessness (n = 10) and severe psychiatric and/or medical comorbidities (n = 7). The group of 'high-risk' patients was assigned to special HCV treatment monitoring strategies as described in Additional file 1: Table S1. There were no statistical differences between high-risk vs. non high-risk patients in the rates of SVR, discontinuations due to non-viral response or HCV therapy-related adverse events or loss to follow-up (Table 5). However, the difference in point estimates for loss to follow-up (18% vs. 3% [p = 0.08] for high and non-high risk, respectively) partially validates the criteria we used to identify high risk patients.

Discussion

Our comparison of the performance of an HIV primary care model for the treatment of HCV among HIV-infected patients in comparison to a subspecialty hepatology model allows the following conclusions to be made: (1) In the HIV primary care model there were more patients treated for HCV and fewer were lost to follow-up; (2) HCV treatment referral rates did not differ during two study periods; (3) discontinuation rates were similar in both models despite the increased prevalence of ongoing substance use in the HIV primary care model; (4) the rate of HCV cure (SVR) was similar in both clinic models.

The idea of using an HIV primary care model for the treatment of HCV is not new [8,14-17]. However, a novel component of our approach was the integration of HIV clinical pharmacists to enhance protocol adherence and patient safety. Undoubtedly, the role of the pharmacists is becoming more prominent since the introduction of HCV direct acting antivirals in co-infected individuals, where attention to medication interactions is particularly important [18].

The patient referral rate for HCV treatment did not increase during the HIV primary care model, but referred patients had less obvious clinical or laboratory signs of decompensated liver disease such as thrombocytopenia or coagulopathy (Table 2). It is not clear whether this was the result of the increased awareness among HIV providers about importance of HCV treatment in the HIV primary care model. What is known is that in the HIV primary care model, 33% of patients treated for HCV had history of ongoing substance use and 4 patients were homeless. Despite this 'high risk population' treated for HCV by the HIV primary care model, the proportions of HCV treatment discontinuation (either due to adverse events or loss to follow-up) and cure were similar to the hepatology model. Moreover, the treatment outcomes in the high-risk patients were similar to the non-high risk patients treated in the HIV primary care model. In particular there was no difference in the rate of treatment discontinuation due to adverse events (Table 5). We acknowledge that our samples size was small to detect as significant differences between high-risk and non-high risk treated patients. But the message to highlight is that the collaborative monitoring strategy use by the HIV primary care model allowed the HCV cure of patients that may have been rendered unfavorable HCV treatment candidates in other subspecialty models [2]. The finding that patients with unstable psychiatric conditions, higher HIV viral loads and lower CD4 cell counts were less likely to be treated in the HIV primary care model was in line with the Owen Clinic protocol of working prospectively with patients to link them to care and, once they are more stable and engaged, initiate HCV therapy [19]. This contrasted with the lack of association with any of the studied variables to predict HCV therapy initiation in the hepatology model.

The present study found no significant differences in the rates of HCV SVR and discontinuation of HCV therapy due to adverse events, however, the SVR trend was greater in patients treated on the HIV primary care clinic (44 vs. 35%) despite having almost double discontinuations due to adverse events of patients treated by the hepatology clinic (29 vs. 16%), perhaps due our lack of sample size to detect those differences as significant (e.g. current sample size has 10% power to detect a difference of 9% in SVR as significant). In the absence of a difference in the proportion of patients with viral relapse after prior HCV therapy in both treatment models, we believe that this observation may be explained by unmeasured clinical factors such as: 1) potential better interleukin-28B gene polymorphism allele profile in patients treated in the HIV primary care

Table 4 Predictors of Hepatitis C treatment among patients referred to the hepatology (n = 163) and HIV primary care models (n = 196) in unadjusted and adjusted analyses

Covariate	Unadjusted OR (95% CI)	*P* value	Adjusted OR (95% CI)	*P* value
Hepatitis C treatment				
(HIV primary care vs. hepatology model)	1.7 (1.0–2.9)	0.04	1.6 (0.9–2.8)	0.08
CD4+ cell count [1]				
(≥400 vs. < 400 cells/mm^3)	1.8 (1.1–3.03)	0.03	2.1 (1.2–3.6)	0.01
Having detectable HIV load				
(≥400 vs. < 400 copies/mL)	0.5 (0.3–1.1)	0.09	0.6 (0.3–1.1)	0.09
On any psychiatry medications				
(any vs. none)	0.6 (0.3–0.99)	0.04	0.5 (0.3–0.9)	0.02
Alanine aminotransferase levels				
(≥63 vs. < 63U/L)	1.9 (1.2–2.9)	0.002	1.4 (0.8–2.3)	0.3
Any neuropsychiatry history				
(yes vs. no)	0.7 (0.4–1.2)	0.17		
Age – years				
Per year increase	1.0 (0.9–1.03)	0.88		
Sex – biological				
(male vs. female)	1.2 (0.6–2.3)	0.65		
Race				
(white vs. non-white)	1.2 (0.6–2.5)	0.61		
Ethnicity:				
(non-hispanic vs. hispanic)	1.6 (0.2–13.4)	0.68		
HIV risk factors				
Men having sex with men	Reference			
Heterosexual	1.6 (0.9–3.2)	0.14		
Intravenous drug use	0.4 (0.1–3.6)	0.44		
Hemophilia	1.3 (0.3–5.1)	0.68		
Combination	1.1 (0.5–2.1)	0.86		
Hepatitis C genotype [2]				
(1/4 vs. 2/3)	0.8 (0.4–1.5)	0.50		
Liver biopsy scores [3]				
(Proportion F3-4 vs. F0-2)	1.2 (0.6–2.5)	0.55		
Drugs or alcohol use within 3 months of HCV evaluation[4]				
(yes vs. no)	0.7 (0.4–1.3)	0.24		
HCV load – $\log_{10}$ copies/mL[5]				
(>6.33 vs. ≤ 6.33)	0.8 (0.5–1.4)	0.46		
Hemoglobin levels				
(>14.1 vs. ≤ 1 4.1 g/dL)	1.5 (0.8–2.6)	0.13		
Platelet count				

Table 4 Predictors of Hepatitis C treatment among patients referred to the hepatology (n = 163) and HIV primary care models (n = 196) in unadjusted and adjusted analyses *(Continued)*

(>139 vs. ≤ 139 – 1000/mm^3)	1.3 (0.8–2.1)	0.31
INR levels		
(>1.1 vs. ≤1.1)	0.5 (0.2–1.3)	0.16

[1]CD4+ counts available in 150 of 163 patients in the hepatology model and in all patients in HIV primary care model.
[2] HCV genotype was not available in seven patients in hepatology model and one in HIV primary care model.
[3] Liver biopsies: 70 in hepatology and 67 in HIV primary care models.
[4] No data available in 47 patients in the hepatology model and in 9 patients in the HIV primary care model.
[5] Two patients in the hepatology model had no available HCV viral load.

Table 5 Characteristics and outcomes of patients treated for hepatitis C in the HIV primary care model dichotomized according to risk category based on assigned HCV treatment monitoring group*

Clinic model	High-risk (n = 17)	Non-high-risk (n = 31)	*P* value
Median age – years (range)	49 (19–61)	47 (33–61)	0.77[a]
Sex: Male (%)	14 (82)	24 (77)	0.68[b]
Race			
White	13	19	0.14[c]
Black	2	11	
Other/unknown	2	1	
Ethnicity			
Hispanic	2	5	0.68[c]
Not-Hispanic	15	26	
Median T CD4+ cell count – cells/mm^3 (range)	515(130–1136)	529(170–1140)	0.55[a]
Number with undetectable HIV load (%)	14 (82)	26 (84)	0.91[b]
Hepatitis C genotype			
Genotype 1/4	13	26	0.53[b]
Genotype 2/3	4	5	
Median HCV load – $\log_{10}$ copies/mL (range)	6.44(4.05–7.46)	6.40(3.0–7.6)	0.73[a]
Liver biopsy scores [1]			
F0-2	4	8	0.51[c]
F3,4	6	7	
Median Hemoglobin levels – g/dL (range)	14.5(12.9–15.8)	14.4(12.1–16.6)	0.63[a]
Median Platelet count –1000/mm^3 (range)	191(113–418)	227(119–402)	0.38[a]
Median ALT – U/L (range)	85(22–301)	56(19–1087)	0.08[a]
HCV treatment outcomes			
№ Patients with Sustained viral response (%)	5(29)	16(52)	0.14[b]
№ Patients who discontinued HCV therapy due to non-viral response (%)	2(12)	7(23)	0.36[b]
№ Patients who discontinued HCV therapy due to treatment-related side effects (%)	6(35)	8(26)	0.49[b]
№ Patients lost to follow-up (%)	3(18)	1(3)	0.08[b]

* High-risk patients comprised patients with substance use and/or homelessness (n = 10) and severe psychiatry and/or medical comorbidities (n = 7).
[1] Liver biopsies were not performed in 6 patients with genotype 1 in the high-risk (n = 3) and non-high risk (n = 3) respectively.
[a] Wilcoxon Rank-Sum Test.
[b] Chi-square test.
[c] Fisher's exact test.

model [20], since this test was not available in our institution at the time we performed study; 2) a positive effect of HIV primary care model in motivating patients while on HCV therapy that led to improved adherence and hence chances of cure in those who were able to tolerate HCV therapy [21]. This study has important limitations. First, this was not a randomized clinical trial; rather the aim was to compare the performance of 2 clinic-based models with balanced and overall comparable study populations. Second, the HIV primary care model did not treat patients with advanced cirrhosis given that these individuals are more prone to develop severe adverse events. Thus, our findings do not apply to patients with advanced liver disease, who still stand to benefit from specialized care by hepatologists. Third, we cannot rule out that the increasing rates of HCV treatment initiation over time in the HIV primary care model could be the result of secular trends: (a) aging of cohort and more urgency for treatment, (albeit we found no difference in liver fibrosis scores in both cohorts when liver biopsies were performed); (b) concurrent emphasis in the literature of epidemiologic evidence that liver disease is one of the leading causes of death in HIV-infected people, which may have motivated more treatment [22]. It could be argued that HCV treatment uptake rate in the HIV primary care model was not ideal (25%). However, our reported HCV-treatment rates are higher than a recently reported aggressive program to engage HIV/HCV co-infected patients in care sponsored by the United States National Institutes of Health [23] and similar to many European countries,[24] despite the fact we had considerably less accrual time than other clinic-based studies [16]. We believe that our study results underestimate the positive impact of the HIV primary care model in the HCV treatment uptake rate, since 23 patients in this model were excluded from the analysis because: (1) Three patients were still receiving HCV therapy and therefore we could not assess their final outcomes; (2) twenty patients who were staged and eligible for conventional HCV therapy within study period elected to wait for HCV protease inhibitors availability and initiated HCV treatment right before or after 30 July 2011, (Figure 1).

The fact that 10% of patients in both cohorts presented with advanced cirrhosis and were not eligible for HCV therapy highlights the importance of reducing disparities in access to HCV care in the HIV population [3,25]. New HCV therapies offer higher chances of cure, simpler and hopefully less toxic regimens [26,27]. However, to scale up HCV treatment among the HIV infected population, we will need an inclusive collaborative approach that reduces the negative referral bias of physicians when making HCV treatment decisions in vulnerable populations with ongoing barriers to care [22,28,29]. We believe that the HIV primary care model could be useful in other settings and countries burdened by the high prevalence of HCV and difficult to treat urban, poor, marginalized populations that require both more efficacious HCV therapies and newer collaborative models of care such as the one described here [30].

In conclusion, in this exploratory analysis, the use of an HIV primary care model supported by pharmacists specialized in HIV care increased the number of patients who initiate and successfully finish HCV therapy with comparable virological outcomes to a subspecialty hepatology model, highlighting the importance of increasing the absolute number of HIV-infected patients treated for HCV at any given time.

Competing interests

The authors have no conflict of interest.

Authors' contributions

EC Clinical care, IRB request supervision, study design, data collection, data analyses and manuscript preparation. LH, Clinical care, IRB preparation and submission, study design, data collection and data analyses. CB, BC study design, IRB request supervision and clinical care. FT & DW clinical care. Wm CM, study design, IRB submission supervision and data analyses. All authors read and approved the final manuscript.

Acknowledgements

We would like to thank Ms. Susan McQuillen for administrative assistance and Joe Montanez for providing substance counseling to our patients.

Funding

This work was supported in part by the Clinical Investigation Core of the University of California San Diego Center for AIDS Research [AI036214], the CFAR Network of Integrated Clinical Systems (CNICS) [R24 AI067039-01A1], and the Pacific AIDS Education and Training Center (PAETC). The funders had no role in study design, data collection and analysis, decision to publish, or preparation of the manuscript.

Author details

[1]Department of Medicine, Owen Clinic, University of California at San Diego, 200 W. Arbor Drive, San Diego, CA 92103-8681, USA. [2]Skaggs School of Pharmacy and Pharmaceutical Sciences, University of California at San Diego, San Diego, CA, USA. [3]Department of Medicine, Division of Infectious Diseases, University of California at San Diego, San Diego, CA, USA.

References

1. Scott JD, Wald A, Kitahata M, *et al*: **Hepatitis C virus is infrequently evaluated and treated in an urban HIV clinic population.** *AIDS Patient Care STDS* 2009, **23:**925–929.
2. Vellozzi C, Buchacz K, Baker R, *et al*: **Treatment of hepatitis C virus (HCV) infection in patients coinfected with HIV in the HIV Outpatient Study (HOPS), 1999–2007.** *J Viral Hepat* 2011, **18:**316–324.
3. Reiberger T, Obermeier M, Payer BA, *et al*: **Considerable under-treatment of chronic HCV infection in HIV patients despite acceptable sustained virological response rates in a real-life setting.** *Antivir Ther* 2011, **16:**815–824.
4. Gordon S, Pockros P, Terrault N, *et al*: **Impact of disease severity on health care costs in patients with chronic hepatitis C (CHC) virus infection.** *Hepatology* 2012, **56:**1651–1660.
5. Norton BL, Park L, McGrath LJ, Proeschold Bell RJ, Muir AJ, Naggie S: **Health care utilization in HIV-infected patients: assessing the burden of hepatitis C virus coinfection.** *AIDS Patient Care STDS* 2012, **26:**541–545.
6. Goulet JL, Fultz SL, McGinnis KA, Justice AC: **Relative prevalence of comorbidities and treatment contraindications in HIV-mono-infected and HIV/HCV-co-infected veterans.** *AIDS* 2005, **19**(Suppl 3):S99–S105.

7. Golden J, O'Dwyer AM, Conroy RM: **Depression and anxiety in patients with hepatitis C: prevalence, detection rates and risk factors.** *Gen Hosp Psychiatry* 2005, **27**:431–438.
8. Fleming CA, Tumilty S, Murray JE, Nunes D: **Challenges in the treatment of patients coinfected with HIV and hepatitis C virus: need for team care.** *Clin Infect Dis* 2005, **40**(Suppl 5):S349–S354.
9. Lekas HM, Siegel K, Leider J: **Challenges facing providers caring for HIV/HCV-coinfected patients.** *Qual Health Res* 2012, **22**:54–66.
10. Astell-Burt T, Flowerdew R, Boyle P, Dillon J: **Is travel-time to a specialist centre a risk factor for non-referral, non-attendance and loss to follow-up among patients with hepatitis C (HCV) infection?** *Soc Sci Med* 2012, **75**:240–247.
11. Preau M, Protopopescu C, Raffi F, *et al*: **Satisfaction with care in HIV-infected patients treated with long-term follow-up antiretroviral therapy: the role of social vulnerability.** *AIDS Care* 2012, **24**:434–443.
12. Ghany MG, Strader DB, Thomas DL, Seff LB: **Diagnosis, management and treatment of hepatitis C: un update.** *Hepatology* 2009, **49**:1335–1374.
13. WHO ASSIST Working Group: **The Alcohol, Smoking and Substance Involvement Screening Test (ASSIST): development, reliability and feasibility.** *Addiction* 2002, **97**:1183–1194.
14. Curcio F, Di Martino F, Capraro C, *et al*: **Together . . . to take care: multidisciplinary management of hepatitis C virus treatment in randomly selected drug users with chronic hepatitis.** *J Addict Med* 2010, **4**:223–232.
15. Ford N, Singh K, Cooke GS, *et al*: **Expanding access to treatment for hepatitis C in resource-limited settings: lessons from HIV/AIDS.** *Clin Infect Dis* 2012, **54**:1465–1472.
16. Kieran J, Dillon A, Farrell G, *et al*: **High uptake of hepatitis C virus treatment in HIV/hepatitis C virus co-infected patients attending an integrated HIV/hepatitis C virus clinic.** *Int J STD AIDS* 2011, **22**:571–576.
17. Parry J: **HIV groups have much to teach hepatitis doctors about better diagnosis and treatment.** *BMJ* 2012, **344**:e1266.
18. Ingiliz P, Rockstroh JK: **HIV-HCV co-infection facing HCV protease inhibitor licensing: implications for clinicians.** *Liver Int* 2012, **32**:1194–1199.
19. Cachay ER, Wyles DL, Goicoechea M, *et al*: **Reliability and predictive validity of a hepatitis-related symptom inventory in HIV-infected individuals referred for hepatitis C treatment.** *AIDS Res Ther* 2011, **8**:e29.
20. Ge D, Fellay J, Thompson AJ, Simon JS, Shianna KV, Urban TJ, Heinzen EL, Qiu P, Bertelsen AH, Muir AJ, Sulkowski M, McHutchison JG, Goldstein DB: **Genetic variation in IL28B predicts hepatitis C treatment-induced viral clearance.** *Nature* 2009, **461**:399–401.
21. Morse DS, Schiff M, Levit S, Cohen-Moreno R, Williams GC, Neumark Y: **A pilot training program for a motivational enhancement approach to hepatitis C virus treatment among individuals in Israeli methadone treatment centers.** *Subst Use Misuse* 2012, **47**:56–66.
22. Joshi D, O'Grady J, Dieterich D, Gazzard B, Agarwal K: **Increasing burden of liver disease in patients with HIV infection.** *Lancet* 2011, **377**:1198–1209.
23. Moak ZSD, Osinusi A, Silk R, Kotb C, *et al*: **Community engagement in a unique federal-local partnership: A model for hepatitits care and research [Abstract WEPE051].** In *Program and abstracts of the19th International AIDS Conference July 22–27. Washington DC, USA.* 2012.
24. Grint D, Peters L, Vogel M, Beniowski M, Pradier C, Battegay M, Jevtovic D, Soriano V, Lundgren J, Rockstroh J, Kirk O, Mocroft A: **Temporal changes and regional differences in treatment uptake of hepatitis C therapy in EuroSIDA [Abstract 0243].** In *Posters and abstracts of the Eleventh International Congress on Drug Therapy in HIV Infection, Glasgow.* 2012.
25. Rourke SB, Sobota M, Tucker R, *et al*: **Social determinants of health associated with hepatitis C co-infection among people living with HIV: results from the Positive Spaces, Healthy Places study.** *Open Med* 2011, **5**:e120–e131.
26. McHutchison JG, Everson GT, Gordon SC, *et al*: **Telaprevir with peginterferon and ribavirin for chronic HCV genotype 1 infection.** *N Engl J Med* 2009, **360**:1827–1838.
27. Poordad F, McCone J Jr, Bacon BR, *et al*: **Boceprevir for untreated chronic HCV genotype 1 infection.** *N Engl J Med* 2011, **364**:1195 1206.
28. Lambert SM, Page AN, Wittmann J, *et al*: **General practitioner attitudes to prescribing hepatitis C antiviral therapy in a community setting.** *Aust J Prim Health* 2011, **17**:282–287.
29. Hall CS, Charlebois ED, Hahn JA, Moss AR, Bangsberg DR: **Hepatitis C virus infection in San Francisco's HIV-infected urban poor.** *J Gen Intern Med* 2004, **19**:357–365.
30. Poveda E, Vispo E, Barreiro P, de Mendoza C, Labarga P, Fernández-Montero JV, Martin-Carbonero L, Soriano V: **Predicted effect of direct acting antivirals in the current HIV-HCV-coinfected population in Spain.** *Antivir Ther* 2012, **17**:571–575.

11

Highlights from the 2012 International Symposium on HIV & Emerging Infectious Diseases (ISHEID): from cART management to the search of an HIV cure

Alain Lafeuillade[1*], Vicente Soriano[2], Marie Suzan-Monti[3,4,5], Mario Stevenson[6], Jacques Izopet[7] and Hans-Jürgen Stellbrink[8]

Abstract

The 2012 International Symposium on HIV and Emerging Infectious Diseases (ISHEID) provided a forum for investigators to hear the latest research developments in the clinical management of HIV and HCV infections as well as HIV-1 reservoirs and cure research. Combined anti-retroviral therapy (c-ART) has had a profound impact on the disease prognosis of individuals living with HIV-1 infection. However, although these anti-retroviral regimens are able to reduce plasma viremia to below the limits of detection for sustained periods of time, there is a rapid recrudescence in plasma viremia if treatment is interrupted. Therefore, despite this potent anti-retroviral suppression, HIV-1 is able to persist within the infected individual. The main 2012 ISHEID theme was, hence "searching for an HIV cure". In this report we not only give details on this main topic of the 2012 ISHEID but also summarize what has been discussed in the areas of HIV epidemiology, access to care, antiretroviral therapy management and recent progress in the therapy of HCV infection in patients with HIV.

Keywords: HIV pandemic, HIV cure, HIV reservoirs, Antiretroviral therapy, HCV coinfection, Access to care, New anti-HCV drugs

Introduction

The 2012 International Symposium on HIV and Emerging Infectious Diseases (ISHEID) was held in Marseilles, France, on May 23–25. This congress attracted more than 1,000 participants from all over the world (70% outside France) and allowed detailed discussions around current issues in HIV research and care. In this summary, we focus on the epidemiological aspects, the study of HIV reservoirs and the search for an HIV cure, combined antiretroviral therapy (c-ART) management in 2012 and new therapies for patients coinfected by HCV.

Update on HIV epidemic, prevention and progress towards universal access

Anna Mia Ekström reported recent changes in HIV incidence, with a tendency to stability or decrease, except for Eastern Europe and Central Asia [1]. A HIV concentrated epidemic developed in Bulgaria, among most at-risk groups (IVDUs, MSM, prisoners and people from Romania) [2]. Annual new infections dropped by 21% since 1997, but in 2010 new infections (2.7 millions) still exceeded AIDS-related deaths (1.8 millions), 97% of them occurring in low- and middle-income countries (LMIC) [3]. Three points were discussed: i) the difficulty to measure HIV incidence using current methodologies since HIV prevalence became a poor estimate of incidence due to different factors including access to c-ART and variable retention in c-ART programs affecting survival; ii) c-ART coverage is not a sufficient guide to measure the success of scaling up to treatment since the percentage of lost-to-follow up patients (LTFU) 48 months after c-ART initiation varies from 20 to 45% in LMIC. The drop-out problem affected also the success of PMTCT programs, pointing the need to measure completion rather than enrolment into programs; iii) the real-

* Correspondence: alain.lafeuillade@ch-toulon.fr
[1]Department of Infectious Diseases, General Hospital, Toulon, France

effectiveness of c-ART programs in Sub-Saharan Africa is heavily impacted by health system factors resulting in a drop from 90% efficacy to 19% effectiveness.

Yves Souteyrand presented the WHO targets for 2015 and the challenges that need to be addressed [4], including increasing resources for HIV programs while reducing inequities in LMIC. The global resources allocated to HIV programs dropped from 16 to 15 billion USD for the first time in 2010. To achieve universal access to c-ART governments must be consistent with their engagements. Although global c-ART coverage was 47% by the end of 2010, geographic, demographic, socio-economic and vulnerable groups-related inequities produced large variations in coverage, from 10% in North Africa and the Middle East to 63% in Latin America and the Caribbean. Other key challenges consist in improving earlier access to treatment and sustaining long-term treatment. Beside the problem of LTFU, attention must be paid to retention in pre c-ART care where substantial LTFU is reported from HIV-testing to ART initiation [5]. HIV and STDs testing, CD4 cell counting and viral load at the 1st visit in the HIV program in Mexico City resulted in 51% detection increase but 60% of newly HIV-diagnosed people were not linked to care [6].

The Treatment 2.0 framework [7] represents a comprehensive approach to achieve these goals, focused on 5 areas of actions: 1) optimize drug regimens; 2) improve access to a package of simple affordable point-of-care and other simplified diagnostics; 3) reduce treatment costs; 4) improve delivery systems; 5) mobilize communities in HIV prevention, treatment, and human rights-related issues. In the Karnataka province (India), coordination between government and civil society partners resulted in higher decentralization of ART delivery services and increase in HIV diagnoses [8], with positive impacts on reduction in LTFU, on adherence and on strengthening primary and secondary health care service, beneficial for program sustainability [9]. In 2010 in Armenia, 73% of HIV diagnosed people were linked to care, 46% started ART and 14.9% were LTFU. However, 57.7% of newly HIV-infected people were diagnosed lately, pointing the need to reinforce this program for efficient entry into care [10].

Another issue to achieve universal access concerns health policy decisions at governmental levels in the context of financial constraints. YazdanYazdanpanah asked how to best utilize available resources in LIC or HIC. Cost-effectiveness analyses (CEA) are tools to assist decision makers in choosing from among competing alternatives, in situations of uncertainty and limited resources for prioritizing the use of health care services, but they are one component among others including fairness, ethics, and political issues. Most CEAs focus on more effective intervention that are often more expensive and allow to consider whether the additional benefit is worth the additional cost. They can be used to consider optimal timing of ART initiation. Studies in South-Africa [11] and France [12] showed that earlier treatments may significantly reduce HIV burden and costs. CEAs were used to evaluate HIV testing strategies [13] or pre-exposure prophylaxis (PrEP) interventions, showing that high PrEP efficacy in high HIV incidence populations is cost-saving and cost-effective [14].

HIV treatment as prevention (TasP), contrarily to PrEP strategies, is no more controversial today. Based on results from numerous studies demonstrating TasP as a potent tool to reduce HIV transmission, Joep Lange stated that implementation of TasP should not await further efficacy trials and need national plans for TasP roll-out. Although designated as the breakthrough of year 2011[15], TasP will not be enough to end the HIV epidemic [16]. The spectrum of engagement in HIV care in USA showed that only 19% of HIV-infected people had an undetectable viral load [17]. The challenge is to keep everybody in treatment to lower HIV transmission rate and decrease incidence, but also to treat earlier to maximize individual and public health benefits. Moreover TasP should be scaled up in conjunction with other effective HIV prevention interventions.

Mark Wainberg discussed results and controversies about PrEP strategies that appeared to be the hottest point of debate of this meeting [18]. Will the use of ART before sexual exposure prevent HIV acquisition? Efficacy was largely demonstrated in many *in vitro* experiments and in monkey models. Human efficacy trials, based on Tenofovir® treatment versus placebo design, produced inconsistent results.Of the 5 trials using oral daily PrEP, 2 failed to show a benefit (VOICE, Fem-PrEP) while iPrex, TDF-2 and Partners Prep trials reported 44 to 75% reduction of HIV transmission, respectively. The Caprisa trial, based on vaginal Tenofovir® gel, resulted in 39% transmission reduction [19]. Adherence was key issue since detectable drug levels strongly correlated with prophylactic effect. Several questions were raised: is daily PrEP high adherence achievable? Although few resistant viruses were described in these trials, the question of emergence and spread of resistances must be addressed. How to exclude acute infection before starting any PrEP? Is there a risk of change in behavior that could off-set the benefit of PrEP? Similar safer sex practices, fewer sexual partners and no difference in STDs acquisition were observed among iPrex participants. Is oral PrEP safe enough? Adverse events were significantly more frequent in the TDF/FTC arm in the Fem-Prep trial. Evidence for safety needs to be strongly addressed. The PrEP strategies raised rightful fears considering the current situation of the HIV epidemic: treatments are for those who need them; other prevention strategies are much more efficient; they will increase health care-related costs and re-allocate resources from research or prevention fields.

Intermittent PrEP strategies could represent an alternative to daily PrEP. They are based on data from animal models and from the Caprisa trial where intermittent use of TDF gel was effective, whereas its daily use in VOICE was ineffective. They could induce a better adherence with a potentially better efficacy/safety ratio and could be more cost-effective than daily PrEP. This hypothesis will be tested in the ANRS IPERGAY trial [20]. There are not yet clear responses to these challenges and further research to evaluate PrEP strategies is necessary before concluding the debate.

HIV reservoirs & the search of an HIV cure

Animal models are crucial for a better understanding of HIV persistence during therapy and for the development of novel therapeutic strategies in the quest of a cure for HIV/AIDS. While sterilizing cure is defined by complete eradication of HIV infected cells from the body, functional cure is defined by undetectable viremia without antiretroviral therapy, no CD4 loss, no immunological defects and no disease progression. Guido Silvestri reviewed the similarities between HIV and pathogenic SIV infection of macaques including chronic immune activation, mucosal immune dysfunction, microbial translocation and high levels of infection of central-memory CD4+ T cells [21]. These non-human primate models provide real opportunities for several reasons: (i) identity, dose, and route of virus challenge are known (ii) various clinical parameters such time of infection or duration of c-ART can be controlled (iii) active and persistent reservoirs can be fully characterized (iv) testing of "risky" interventions is possible. Longitudinal collections of blood/tissue, as well as elective necropsy are available for determining virologic and immunologic parameters. Among limitations, challenge viruses (SIV, SHIV) are not HIV and obtaining levels of virus suppression similar to these obtained in HIV-infected humans is sometimes hard to achieve. To conclude, Guido Silvestri discussed pros and cons of developing a standardized non-human primate resource and underlined the need of close collaboration between "monkey people" and "human people".

The sources of HIV persistence in c-ART-treated individuals could arise from residual ongoing viral replication or resting $CD4^+$ T cells (and/or other cellular reservoirs) harboring stably integrated, transcriptionally silent but replication-competent proviruses. Carine Van Lint reviewed the multiple mechanisms that control HIV latency at a molecular level [22]. Beside post-transcriptional blockade via inefficient viral mRNA transport and inhibitory miRNAs, several blockades occur at a transcriptional level. Strong preference for proviral integration in protein-encoding transcriptionally active genes has been demonstrated. Recent data indicate a modest preference for integration in the same transcriptional orientation as the host gene, suggesting that transcriptional interference could play a major role in the establishment and maintenance of HIV-1 latency through different mechanisms (enhancer trapping, promoter occlusion, steric hindrance). The chromatin organization of the provirus and the epigenetic control of the promoter region (histone acetylation and methylation, DNA methylation) are also important. However, the high degree of methylation of HIV-1 promoters from infected individuals receiving suppressive antiretroviral therapy was not confirmed in a recent study. The absence of inducible cellular transcription factors, such as NF-KB and NFAT, that are excluded from the nuclei of resting cells, the sequestration of P-TEFb in a HEXIM/75 K sn RNA-bound inactive form and the absence of Tat and Tat-associated factors are the other mechanisms that maintain HIV-1 latency.

Several approaches can be used to reactivate viral latency with the expectation that new cell infections can be blocked *in vivo* by immune surveillance or antiretroviral drugs. IL7 or PKC agonists like prostratin can induce cellular transcription factors (STAT 5, NF-KB). HDACi (Histone deacyltransferase inhibitors) like SAHA (Vorinostat) promote histone acetylation, HMTi (Histone methyltransferase inhibitors) like chaetocin decrease histone methylation and DNA methylation inhibitors like decitabine decrease DNA methylation. HMBA induce the recruitment of the kinase complex P-TEFb (Cyclin T1/CDK9) to the HIV-1 promoter. Synergistic activation of HIV-1 expression by prostratin and vorinostat has been observed *in vitro*. Similarly, synergistic activation of HIV-1 expression by prostratin and HMBA has been obtained. Therefore one of the most promising strategies to target latent reservoirs could reside in combinations of several families of compounds (Figure 1).

Tae-Wook Chun reviewed the main basic and clinical aspects of HIV reservoirs that were discovered during the past two decades [23]. Understanding the mechanisms by which HIV persists in the face of potent antiretroviral therapy is crucial for developing strategies to eliminate reservoirs and ultimately eradicate HIV. Homeostatic expansion of latent viral reservoir is an important issue but recent infections due to residual HIV replication, particularly in the gut lymphoid tissue, have to be taken into account. In addition, cell-to-cell spread of HIV permits ongoing replication despite antiretroviral therapy. The use of HDACi (such as vorinostat) for purging HIV in latently infected, resting $CD4^+$ T cells from infected individuals on ART had a minimal impact compared to prostratin and anti-CD3. Recent data indicate that stimulation of patient CD8+ T cells with HIV gag

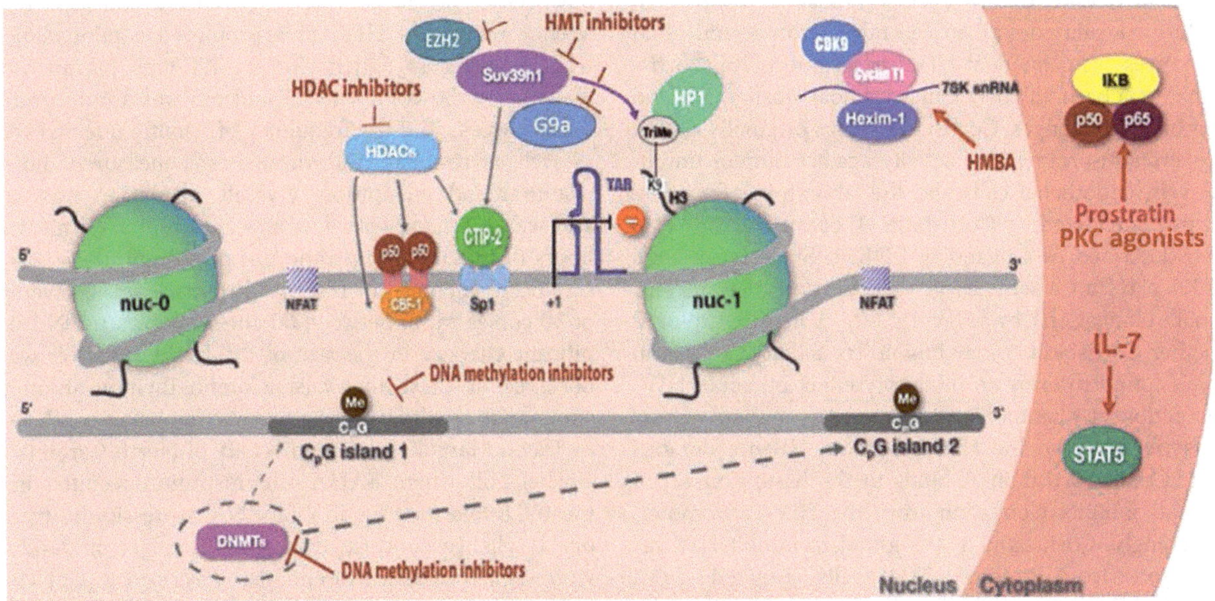

Figure 1 Different targets and drugs to reactivate proviral HIV-1 DNA from latency.

peptides enhanced the cytotoxic T cell (CTL) responses and led to killing of vorinostat-treated cells. Therefore reactivation of viral latency *in vivo* is probably insufficient to accelerate the death of the reactivated cell and will require therapeutic vaccine to boost CTL responses in patients undergoing purging protocols to eliminate the latent reservoir. Gene therapy based on zinc-finger nuclease-mediated elimination of HIV coreceptors and stem cell transplantation from CCR5 delta 32 homozygous donors can generate HIV-resistant CD4$^+$ T cells but important challenges need to be addressed.

Romas Geleziunas [24] discussed progress in the search for small molecule activators of latent HIV. He described a primary cell, HIV latency assay modified from an original assay developed by Planelles of the University of Utah. In this assay, memory CD4$^+$ T cells are generated from naive T cells by antibody and cytokine treatment and then infected with a luciferase encoding HIV-1 variant that undergoes a single cycle of infection. The assay exploits a codon optimized luciferase that increases the sensitivity of the reactivation assay. The assay has been miniaturized to 384 well plates and automated for high throughput screening employing ten thousand cells per 20 uL well and 20 nL of compound. The screening efforts have focused on HDACi. Histone acetylation of the HIV-1 LTR is believed to be a major mechanism through which transcription of the LTR is blocked and inhibitors of histone deacetylases have been demonstrated to activate latent HIV-1 *in vitro*. Vorinostat (SAHA) is an HDAC inhibitor and is a licensed drug for the treatment of cutaneous T cell lymphoma. Toxicity profiles for SAHA are well described and two clinical trials exploring the ability of SAHA to reactivate latent HIV *in vivo* are currently being carried out by David Margolis at the University of North Carolina and Sharon Lewin at the University of Melbourne. Preliminary studies from Margolis laboratory indicate that SAHA is able to reactivate latent HIV *in vivo*. Geleziunas described results with the HDACi, Romidepsin that is FDA approved for the treatment of cutaneous T cell lymphoma. Remarkably, Romidepsin is a thousand fold more potent then SAHA at inducing latent HIV and one thousand to twenty thousand more potent in inhibiting HDAC enzymatic activity. Romidepsin was able to activate HIV RNA production in twelve of thirteen HIV-1 infected subjects on suppressive c-ART. The average increase in viral RNA was approximately 8.6 fold. Therefore Romidepsin may be a better inducer of latent HIV *in vivo* and its favorable toxicity profiles would allow multiple dose studies. While this is an exciting development, an overarching question is whether the increases in viral RNA induced either by SAHA or Romidepsin will be sufficient to raise the amount of viral protein expression in reactivated cell to levels that lead to viral cytopathicity and/or elimination by cytotoxic T cells. Recent work from the Siliciano laboratory [25] indicates that after reversal of latency *in vitro*, reactivated resting T cells survived viral cytopathic effects even in the presence of autologous cytotoxic T lymphocytes from most patients on suppressive anti-retroviral therapy. Therefore, reactivation of viral latency may not be effective at eliminating the infected cell.

Susana Valente of the Scripts Research Institute in Jupiter, Florida described a novel compound that suppresses Tat-dependent HIV transcription [26]. Cortistatin A is a naturally occurring steroidal alkaloid isolated from marine sponges. Cortistatin A was originally shown to exert anti-proliferative activity against human umbilical vein endothelial cells and the laboratory of Valente became interested in Cortistatin A because it has also been described as a ligand of CDK11. Since the related CDK9 plays an essential role in activation of transcriptional elongation by HIV-1 Tat, Valente explored whether Cortistatin A may inhibit Tat activity.Cortistatin A was found to exert an inhibitory effect on acute HIV-1 infection at nanomolar concentrations and to repress transcription from the HIV promoter. Valente demonstrated that Cortistatin A binds to the basic domain of Tat and inhibits elongation from the HIV-1 promoter. Intriguingly, Cortistatin A was found to inhibit HIV reactivation from resting CD4 cells isolated from individuals on suppressive anti-retroviral therapy. Furthermore, Cortistatin A appeared to affect an irreversible effect on viral transcription since removal of Cortistatin A did not result in viral rebound. Therefore, Cortistatin A warrants serious consideration as an agent that can force HIV-1 into an irreversible state of latency. This approach would be fundamentally different from other approaches aimed at reactivating viral latency in order to purge infected cells.Cortistatin A may have the capacity to induce a permanent state of latency in cells of HIV-1 infected patients.

The laboratory of Tokameh Mahmoudi of Erasmus University Medical Center in Rotterdam provided evidence for the involvement of the Wnt signaling pathway in transcriptional regulation of the HIV-1 LTR [27]. A hallmark of Wnt signaling is stabilization of the transcriptional co-activator beta-catenin. Beta-catenin then regulates gene expression by binding members of the T-cell-specific transcription factor/lymphoid enhancer-binding factor 1 (TCF/LEF-1) family of transcription factors. Mahmoudi presented evidence that the HIV-1 LTR contains TCF/LEF binding sites and this prompted an investigation of the effect of Wnt activation on transcription of the latent HIV-1 LTR. LiCl, an inhibitor of Wnt signaling, was found to strongly synergize with valproic acid or SAHA in inducing reactivation of the latent HIV-1 LTR in a cell line model of HIV-1 latency. The level of activation of the latent LTR was found to correlate with the remodeling of NUC-1 by high resolution nucleosomal mapping. Regulators of the Wnt signaling pathway provide an additional strategy with which to promote reactivation of the latent LTR particularly in combination with HDACi.

Santiago Moreno summarized ongoing clinical trials aimed at reactivating viral latency *in vivo* [28].Disulfiram has been shown to activate HIV transcription in *in vitro* latency models of HIV. This prompted a pilot clinical trial involving 14 patients on c-ART with plasma viral loads below 50 copies/ml. Disulfiram was administrated for two weeks and the frequency of latently infected cells as well as residual viral viremia was measured during disulfiram administration. Overall, disulfiram was safe and well tolerated with few adverse events. Within two hours of initial administration of disulfiram, there was a significant increase in residual viremia from an average of 30 copies/ml to between 60 and 70 copies/ml. No significant changes in the size of the latent reservoir were observed at these intervals. Moreno then went on to summarize results from the SAHA trial being conducted by David Margolis at the University of North Carolina in Chapel Hill where SAHA administration resulted in a mean 4.8 fold increase in viral RNA expression in memory T cells. In contrast, there was no effect on residual viremia in this trial. Moreno also described a pilot clinical trial employing Bryostatin-1 in a Jurkat cell line model of HIV-1 latency. Bryostatin-1 has been show to reactivate HIV-1 through the PKC-dependent pathway and to down-regulate the expression of CD4 and CXCR4. Bryostatin-1 also synergizes with HDACi, VPA, and trichostatin A in reactivating HIV-1 latency. This has prompted a pilot clinical trial with a single dose of Bryostatin-1 followed by evaluation of latent cell reservoir size residual viremia and cell associated viral RNA. This pilot trial is ongoing.

In addition to the obstacles posed by reservoir of latently infected cells, a number of studies have raised the possibility that incomplete viral suppression may permit some degree of replenishment of the viral reservoir in patients on ART. In collaboration with Timothy Schacker and Ashley Haase at the University of Minnesota and Courtney Fletcher at the University of Nebraska, Mario Stevenson has been examining anti-retroviral therapy impacts on tissue reservoirs for HIV-1[29]. Gut associated lymphoid tissue (GALT) is the major site of viral replication in viremic patients since the majority of permissive lymphocytes are located within GALT. However, the impact of anti-retroviral therapy on this reservoir and viral activity in this reservoir in patients on suppressive therapy are not well understood.Stevenson and collaborators obtained lymphoid tissue for viremic individuals initiating c-ART. The virologic response was gauged by measuring unintegrated forms of viral DNA including linear forms and episomal forms (2-LTR circles). Within several weeks of initiating therapy plasma viremia fell to undetectable levels in all individuals. Despite this, unintegrated viral genomes were poorly resolved by one month and six months post initiation of anti-retroviral treatment and in some individuals levels of unintegrated DNA at 6 months exceed those at baseline or one-month intervals particularly in cells obtained from lymphoid tissue. Intracellular drug concentrations in cells from lymphoid tissue were found to be significantly lower than in cells from peripheral blood obtained at the same intervals. These preliminary data indicate discordance in the ability of anti-retrovirals to sequester within cells of lymphoid tissue and this raises the possibility that lymphoid tissue may provide conditions for *de novo* viral infection in the face of anti-retroviral suppression.

Clinical and therapeutic aspects

As Roy Gulick [30] pointed out in his presentation on new antiretroviral drugs, the number of agents currently pursued in phase 2 and 3 clinical trials is limited, and among those only the attachment inhibitor BMS-663068 represents a novel class with a new mode of action. This leaves little hope that novel compounds will overcome the problems of current drugs in the near future.

Jean-Michel Pawlotsky [31] gave an overview over recently available anti-HCV agents and compounds currently under development, as well as major clinical trials and very promising pilot studies investigating these agents and interferon-free regimens. As David Back [32] pointed out in his presentation on drug – drug interactions, the two recently licensed HCV protease inhibitors have opened a new arena of pharmacokinetic interactions with antiretroviral compounds, which are partly very challenging. He also described several important pharmacokinetic interactions between e.g. parenteral or topical corticosteroids and clarified that cobicistat, the novel pharmacokinetic booster contained in preparations of elvitegravir, will pose new questions regarding compatibility with concomitant medication. He made clear that the optimal use of these drugs requires an understanding of their interactions by physicians treating co-infected patients, and that more studies are needed to improve the strategies of dealing with those interactions.

In his presentation on salvage therapy in 2012, Stefano Vella [33] made the point that very few subjects in the developed world currently reach a level of treatment failure that would require their classification as true salvage patients. However, in developing countries patients reach the point beyond which no promising options are available much earlier due to economic constraints. He argued that this gap should be closed by making options for resistant viruses available in these settings and defining an optimal sequence of regimens.

Jürgen Rockstroh [34] presented on the issues regarding timing of anti-viral therapy, choice of regimen, complications, and HCV-treatment in HCV co-infected patients. He clarified that the beneficial effects of early ART clearly outweigh potential liver toxicities, but that physicians should stay alerted to the possibility of yet unexpected untoward effects, such as the association of portal hypertension with didanosine use. The treatment armamentarium for HIV now offers chances for regimens with less interaction with novel anti-HCV compounds, so that HCV coinfection may be managed actively.

In his presentation on pharmacogenomics, Amalio Telenti [35] outlined the wide-spread use of pharmacogenomics in other fields of medicine, the advances in the HIV field, especially with respect to management of toxicity (e.g. efavirenz, atazanavir, abacavir) or cardiovascular risk. He criticized the exceptionalism with respect to the application of genetic analyses to clinical medicine, especially in Europe and made a strong case for moving forward with the implementation of these diagnostic tools.

The question of when to initiate c-ART was also addressed in a presentation by Cécile Goujard [36] about the ANRS C06 Primo cohort, in which 1450 patients with primary HIV infection (PHI) have been included until 12/2011, 52% of whom initiated antiretroviral therapy at PHI. Of note, 77% of those included at a CD4 count of <500/μL showed progression to <350 CD4 cells/μL after two years, whereas none of the patients included at >750 CD4 cells/μL showed progression. In this cohort, the level of HIV DNA was an independent predictor of progression. When comparing patients with transient c-ART initiated at PHI with the SEROCO cohort, there was no obvious impact of c-ART on time off therapy. She also described the interesting observation of 14 cases in whom HIV RNA was persistently undetectable for more than 12 months following interruption of ART initiated at PHI. They did not find an overrepresentation of the HLA class one alleles classically associated with elite control. The virological and immunological arguments for starting ART as early as possible were elucidated by Jean-Pierre Routy [37] and Joseph Wong [38]. They talked about viral persistence as the principal obstacle to cure and made the point that clinical trials investigating functional or sterilizing cure will have to include analytical treatment interruptions.

For some of the hot topics in clinical HIV medicine, the organizers selected the format of a pro and con debate. Magnus Gisslén and Hans-Jürgen Stellbrink discussed the relevance of HIV-associated neurocognitive disorders, Mark Wainberg and Mark Nelson took the pro and con positions for PrEP, and Alain Lafeuillade and Jean-Pierre Routy discussed the prospects of HIV cure. The audience witnessed very lively discussions. Their votes reflected some changes in opinion after the discussions and provided a valuable feedback to the presenters regarding the perception of their argumentation.

In a review of HCV treatment outcome in the Hepatitis session, Stanislas Pol [39] clarified the clinically very important point that remodeling of fibrosis following

SVR is possible even in advanced liver disease, and that fibrosis reversal is associated with improvement of life expectancy. He clarified that ultrasound follow-up should be continued in patients with lack of fibrosis reversal following SVR, because progression to hepatocellular carcinoma may still occur in these subjects.

Viral hepatitis

The burden of viral hepatitis is enormous worldwide. Hepatitis B virus (HBV) and HCV are by far the most frequent agents of chronic viral hepatitis. Chronic HBV infection affects 350 million people, being the highest prevalence found in Asia. Of note, superinfection with the hepatitis delta virus (HDV) in chronic HBsAg + carriers leads to chronic hepatitis delta, which is the most aggressive form of viral hepatitis. A study from Taiwan that examined 1,186 HBsAg + patients found anti-HDV antibodies in up to 55% of 341 HIV-HBV coinfected individuals, stressing on the poor outcome of these patients. Delta superinfection was associated with intravenous drug use as well as with HCV coinfection [40]. Interestingly, HDV genotype IV predominated among injecting drug users whereas genotype II was the most frequent variant in other individuals with hepatitis delta in Taiwan.

Around 2% of the world population is infected by HCV, which represents 175 million people. The proportion of persons aware of their HCV infection is estimated to be below 40% in the United States and only rise up to 60% in France. Therefore, active HCV diagnosis remains crucial at a time that treatment for chronic hepatitis C has become much more successful following the arrival of directly acting antivirals (DAA). As in HIV, proper strategies pursuing *"test and treat"* should now be implemented for hepatitis C.

There are several reasons to explain why hepatitis C therapy in HIV-infected individuals attracted so much attention at ISHEID 2012. First, overall one third of HIV+ individuals are coinfected with HCV, being this rate disproportionately higher among IVDUs or persons who acquired the virus from contaminated blood products (i.e., hemophiliacs). Second, the way the new hepatitis C antiviral agents are used reminds much what we are already familiar in HIV therapeutics, considering variables such as viral load, drug resistance, geno/subtypes, viral kinetics, combination therapy, etc. [41]. Third, the pharmaceutical companies that are developing DAA are almost the same that already are marketing antiretroviral agents [31]. So, broad overlap exists between HCV and HIV at multiple areas. Ultimately, a shift in prescribers of the new HCV medications should be expected in many places moving from classical gastroenterologists to infectious diseases doctors.

Despite the previous considerations, significant biological features distinguish HIV from HCV, which translate into clinical and therapeutic differences [31]. First, in contrast with HIV there is no integration of the HCV genetic material into the chromosomes of infected cells during the virus replication cycle. This explains why HCV can be eradicated from the infected carrier whereas there is no elimination feasible for HIV even in long-term suppressed persons on antiretroviral therapy [42]. Second, the genetic variability in HCV is much greater than in HIV, accounting for significant differences in HCV susceptibility to antiviral agents across distinct HCV genotypes and subtypes. For instance, HCV subtype 1a responds less well to many DAA than HCV subtype 1b. Moreover, selection of drug resistance mutations to HCV protease inhibitors occurs at different positions in HCV subtypes 1a versus 1b [43].

The management of chronic hepatitis C in the setting of HIV infection is particularly challenging, being drug-drug interactions, overlapping toxicities and difficulties associated to polymedication amongst the most troublesome [41]. Both first-generation HCV protease inhibitors boceprevir and telaprevir reduce significantly exposure to HIV protease inhibitors but atazanavir for which this effect is lower. Likewise, significant drug interactions occur between telaprevir/boceprevir and HIV non-nucleoside polymerase inhibitors nevirapine and efavirenz (Additional file 1: Table S1). However, rilpivirine and etravirine do not interact significantly with DAA and therefore can be safely co-administered [32]. The same applies to raltegravir, which the most preferred third antiretroviral agent for HIV-HCV coinfected patients planned to be treated with DAA. Moreover, the good safety liver profile of this drug makes it particularly attractive for HIV-infected individuals with underlying liver disease [34].

The results so far available with boceprevir and telaprevir in HIV/HCV-coinfected patients were deeply discussed at ISHEID [41]. In the phase 2 boceprevir study, a total of 98 HCV genotype 1 patients were randomized to receive either triple therapy or standard of care (peginterferon-ribavirin) for one year. Two thirds of patients were infected with HCV subtype 1a. Seven patients experienced viral breakthrough during therapy, 3/64 in the boceprevir arm and 4/34 in the control arm. Severe anemia developed in 5% of patients assigned to boceprevir and in 3% of controls. Erythropoietin was prescribed in 38% of patients on triple therapy and in 21% of controls. The rate of sustained virological response 12 weeks after completion of therapy (SVR_{12}) was 61% versus 27%, respectively. Figure 2 records the proportion of patients with undetectable HCV-RNA in the two study arms at different time points. Although all patients were on antiretroviral therapy (mostly HIV protease inhibitors), a similar proportion of patients on boceprevir (3/64) and controls (4/34) experienced HIV-RNA rebounds during hepatitis C therapy.

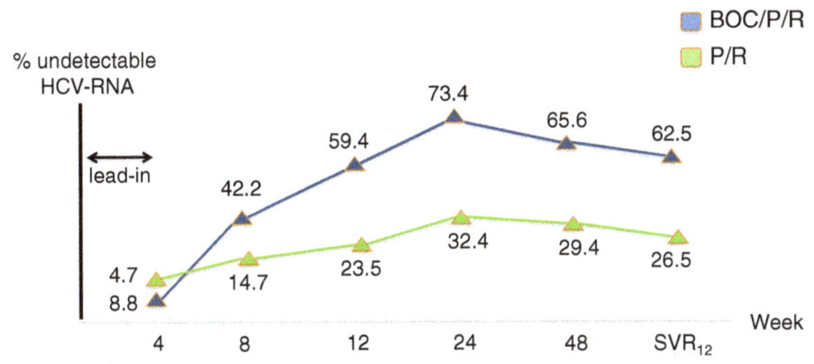

Figure 2 Treatment of chronic hepatitis C withBoceprevir in HIV/HCV coinfected patients. P: pegylated interferon, R: ribavirin, SVR_{12}: sustained virological response at 12 weeks.

In the phase 2 telaprevir trial (Study 110), 60 HIV-infected patients coinfected with HCV genotype 1 were randomized to receive either triple therapy or standard of care (peginterferon plus ribavirin). Of note, telaprevir only was given for the first 3 months of therapy, but all patients received peginterferon-ribavirin for one year. Thirteen patients did not receive antiretroviral therapy. Of the rest, 24 were on efavirenz and 23 on atazanavir/r. Early discontinuations due to side effects occurred in 3/38 patients on telaprevir and 0/22 in the control arm. Rash occurred in 13 (34%) patients on telaprevir and 5 (23%) controls. Anemia was recorded in 7 (18%) of patients on telaprevir and 4 (18%) of controls. SVR12 was 74% (28/38) on triple therapy versus 45% (10/22) on standard therapy. Relapses occurred in 1/32 (3%) of patients on telaprevir and 2/13 (15%) controls. Patients on atazanavir/r tended to respond better than those on efavirenz, although the numbers were too low to draw conclusions (Figure 3). All patients on antiretroviral therapy kept on undetectable plasma HIV-RNA. The unexplained high rate of response in controls might suggest that the population enrolled in the 110 trial was somewhat unique and particularly prone to respond. In fact, the variation between triple therapy and standard of care was more pronounced for boceprevir than telaprevir (35% versus 29%, respectively).

Successful treatment of hepatitis C translates into definitive elimination of the virus from the body, and regression of liver fibrosis occurs even in persons who already had developed cirrhosis [44]. Cure has allowed unveiling that chronic HCV infection results in other abnormalities than hepatic inflammation and fibrosis. This is the case for metabolic abnormalities, including dislipidemia and insulin resistance, which ameliorate once chronic hepatitis C is successfully treated. Likewise, most autoimmune phenomena associated with persistent HCV replication tend to resolve once the virus is cleared with treatment. Finally, the recent appreciation of a negative impact of persistent immune activation by continuous HCV replication on body systems and organs has encouraged to treat chronic hepatitis C even in patients with minimal liver damage [45]. Again, learning from the consequences of uncontrolled viral replication in the HIV field is pushing the management of hepatitis C.

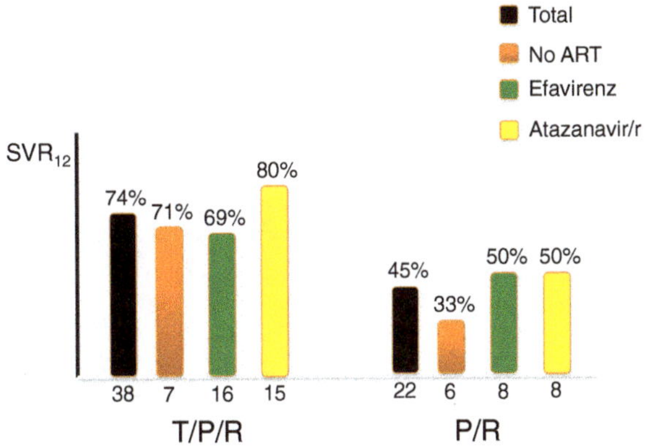

Figure 3 Treatment of chronic hepatitis C with Telaprevir in HIV/HCV coinfected patients. P: pegylated interferon, R: ribavirin.

Competing interests
The authors declare that they have no competing interests.

Authors' contributions
MSM wrote the epidemic, prevention and universal access section. AL, MS and JI wrote the HIV reservoirs & search for a cure section. HJS wrote the clinical and therapeutic section. VS wrote the hepatitis section. AL formatted the entire article. All authors read and approved the final manuscript.

Author details
[1]Department of Infectious Diseases, General Hospital, Toulon, France. [2]Department of Infectious Diseases Hospital Carlos III, Madrid, Spain. [3]INSERM, U912 (SESSTIM), Marseille, France. [4]Aix Marseille Université, IRD, UMR_S912, Marseille, France. [5]ORS PACA, Observatoire Régional de la Santé Provence Alpes Côte d'Azur, Marseille, France. [6]Miller MedicalSchool, University of Miami, Miami, FL, USA. [7]Laboratoire de Virologie, Institut

Fédératif de Biologie, Hôpital Purpan, Toulouse, France. [8]Infektions Medizinisches Centrum Hamburg Study Center, Hamburg, Germany.

References

1. Ekström A: **Update on HIV pandemic.** *Retrovirology* 2012, **9**(Suppl 1):I4.
2. Shamas S: **HIV epidemic in Bulgaria.** *Retrovirology* 2012, **9**(Suppl 1):P89.
3. WHO, UNAIDS, UNICEF: *Global HIV/AIDS response - Epidemic update and health sector progress towards universal access.* 2011. http://wwwunaidsorg/en/media/unaids/contentassets/documents/unaidspublication/2011/20111130_UA_Report_enpdf.
4. Souteyrand Y: **Universal access to anti-HIV therapy.** *Retrovirology* 2012, **9** (Suppl 1):I13.
5. Rosen S, Fox MP: **Retention in HIV care between testing and treatment in sub-Saharan Africa: a systematic review.** *PLoS Med* 2011, **8**(7):e1001056. Epub 2011 Jul 19.
6. Juárez-Figueroa L, González-Rodríguez A, Rodríguez-Nolasco E: **Integral HIV-STI diagnosis at the first VCT visit as strategy to prevent late ART initiation in the HIV-AIDS program of Mexico City (HIVPMC).** *Retrovirology* 2012, **9**(Suppl 1):P73.
7. WHO, UNAIDS: *The Treatment 2.0 Framework for Action: Catalysing the Next Phase of Treatment, Care and Support.* ; 2011. http://wwwunaidsorg/en/media/unaids/contentassets/documents/unaidspublication/2011/20110824_JC2208_outlook_treatment20_enpdf.
8. Fahim S, Shastri S, Washington R: **Scaling up HIV treatment-Karnataka, India experience.** *Retrovirology* 2012, **9**(Suppl 1):P71.
9. Fahim S, Shastri S, Rewari B: **Decentralizing treatment services with link ART centres- experience from Karnataka, South India.** *Retrovirology* 2012, **9**(Suppl 1):P82.
10. Grigoryan S, Mkrtchyan A: **Access to HIV treatment and care in Armenia.** *Retrovirology* 2012, **9**(Suppl 1):P75.
11. Granich R, Kahn JG, Bennett R, Holmes CB, Garg N, *et al*: **Expanding ART for treatment and prevention of HIV in South Africa: estimated cost and cost-effectiveness 2011–2050.** *PLoS One* 2012, **7**:e30216.
12. Sloan CE, Champenois K, Choisy P, Losina E, Walensky RP, *et al*: **Newer drugs and earlier treatment: impact on lifetime cost of care for HIV-infected adults.** *AIDS* 2012, **26**:45–56.
13. Yazdanpanah Y, Sloan CE, Charlois-Ou C, Le Vu S, Semaille C, *et al*: **Routine HIV screening in France: clinical impact and cost-effectiveness.** *PLoS One* 2010, **5**:e13132.
14. Paltiel AD, Freedberg KA, Scott CA, Schackman BR, Losina E, *et al*: **HIV preexposure prophylaxis in the United States: impact on lifetime infection risk, clinical outcomes, and cost-effectiveness.** *Clin Infect Dis* 2009, **48**:806–815.
15. Cohen J: **Breakthrough of the year. HIV treatment as prevention.** *Science* 2011, **334**:1628.
16. Lange JM: **"Test and treat": is it enough?** *Clin Infect Dis* 2011, **52**:801–802.
17. Gardner EM, McLees MP, Steiner JF, Del Rio C, Burman WJ: **The spectrum of engagement in HIV care and its relevance to test-and-treat strategies for prevention of HIV infection.** *Clin Infect Dis* 2011, **52**:793–800.
18. Wainberg MA: **Pre-exposure prophylaxis against HIV: pros and cons.** *Retrovirology* 2012, **9**(Suppl 1):I6.
19. Abdool-Karim SS, Abdool-Karim Q: **Antiretroviral prophylaxis: a defining moment in HIV control.** *Lancet* 2011, **378**:e23–e25.
20. ANRS: *ANRS IPERGAY - Intervention Préventive de l'Exposition aux Risques avec et pour les Gays.* 2012. http://wwwanrsfr/content/download/4097/21774/file/ANRS%20IPERGAYpdf.
21. Silvestri G: **Animal models of functional HIV cure.** *Retrovirology* 2012, **9** (suppl 1):I9.
22. Van Lint C: **Molecular control of HIV-1 postintegration latency: implications for therapeutic strategies.** *Retrovirology* 2012, **9**(suppl 1):I10.
23. Chun TW: **Towards a cure for HIV: a long road ahead.** *Retrovirology* 2012, **9** (suppl 1):I12.
24. Geleziunas R, Stepan G, Wei G, *et al*: **Search for small molecule activators of latent HIV.** *Retrovirology* 2012, **9**(Suppl 1):O2.
25. Shan L, Deng K, Shroff NS, *et al*: **Stimulation of HIV-1-specific cytolytic T lymphocytes facilitates elimination of latent viral reservoir after virus reactivation.** *Immunity* 2012, **36**(3):491 501. Epub 2012 Mar 8.
26. Mousseau G, Mark Clementz MA, Bakeman WN, *et al*: **Potent suppression of HIV viral replication by a novel inhibitor of Tat.** *Retrovirology* 2012, **9** (Suppl 1):O11.
27. Rafati H, Moshkin Y, Mahmoudi T, *et al*: **New transcription regulatory mechanisms of latent HIV LTR.** *Retrovirology* 2012, **9**(Suppl 1):O3.
28. Moreno S: **Anti-latency agents to purge HIV reservoirs.** *Retrovirology* 2012, **9**(Suppl 1):I16.
29. Stevenson M: **A roadmap to a cure.** *Retrovirology* 2012, **9**(Suppl 1):I11.
30. Gulick R: **New Antiretrovirals.** *Retrovirology* 2012, **9**(Suppl 1):I7.
31. Pawlotsky JM: **New antiviral agents for hepatitis C. F1000.** *Biol Rep* 2012, **4**:5. Epub 2012 Mar 1.
32. Back D: **New drug interactions in HIV and HCV.** *Retrovirology* 2012, **9**(Suppl 1):I8.
33. Vella S, Schwartländer B, Sow SP, Eholie SP, Murphy RL: **The history of antiretroviral therapy and of its implementation in resource-limited areas of the world.** *AIDS* 2012, **26**(10):1231–1241.
34. Rockstroh J: **Managing antiretrovirals in co-infected patients in 2012.** *Retrovirology* 2012, **9**(Suppl 1):I1.
35. Arab-Alameddine M, Décosterd LA, Buclin T, Telenti A, Csajka C: **Antiretroviral drug toxicity in relation to pharmacokinetics, metabolic profile and pharmacogenetics.** *Expert Opin Drug MetabToxicol* 2011, [Epub ahead of print].
36. Goujard C, Primary HIV: **infection: the French experience.** *Retrovirology* 2012, **9**(Suppl 1):I14.
37. Routy JP: **Treating since the beginning?** *Retrovirology* 2012, **9**(Suppl 1):I15.
38. Strain MC, Little SJ, Daar ES, *et al*: **Effect of treatment, during primary infection, on establishment and clearance of cellular reservoirs of HIV-1.** *J Infect Dis* 2005, **191**(9):1410–1418. Epub 2005 Mar 29.
39. Pol S: **What happens after hepatitis C eradication?** *Retrovirology* 2012, **9** (Suppl 1):I19.
40. Lin H, Lee S, Yu M, *et al*: **Epidemiology of hepatitis delta virus infection in HIV-infected individuals in Taiwan.** *Retrovirology* 2012, **9**(Suppl 1):P49.
41. Soriano V, Barreiro P, Vispo E, Labarga P, Soriano V: **Management and Treatment of Chronic Hepatitis C in HIV Patients.** *Semin Liver Dis* 2012, **32** (2):138–146. Epub 2012 Jul 3.
42. Soriano V, Zeuzem S, Zoulim F: **Why are there different dynamics in the selection of drug resistance in HIV and hepatitis B and C viruses?** *J AntimicrobChemother* 2008, **62**:1–4.
43. Halfon P: **HCV resistance.** *Retrovirology* 2012, **9**(Suppl 1):I18.
44. Cevik M, Singh G, Dickinson L, *et al*: **Raltegravir switch improves hepatitis C transaminitis in HIV-1 and hepatitis C (HCV) co-infected individuals.** *Retrovirology* 2012, **9**(Suppl 1):O7.
45. Andre P: **Hepatitis C as a metabolic disease.** *Retrovirology* 2012, **9**(Suppl 1):I17.

12

Influence of providers and nurses on completion of non-targeted HIV screening in an urgent care setting

Rachel A Bender Ignacio[1,9*†], Jacqueline Chu[2†], Melinda C Power[3], Jeffrey Douaiher[4], Jordan D Lane[5], Jeffrey P Collins[6,7] and Valerie E Stone[7,8]

Abstract

Introduction: Despite recommendations by the Centers for Disease Control (CDC) that all adults be offered non-targeted HIV screening in all care settings, screening in acute-care settings remains unacceptably low. We performed an observational study to evaluate an HIV screening pilot in an academic-community partnership health center urgent care clinic.

Methods: We collected visit data via encounter forms and demographic and laboratory data from electronic medical records. A post-pilot survey of perceptions of HIV screening was administered to providers and nurses. Multivariable analysis was used to identify factors associated with completion of testing.

Results: Visit provider and triage nurse were highly associated with both acceptance of screening and completion of testing, as were younger age, male gender, and race/ethnicity. 23.5% of patients completed tests, although 36.0% requested screening; time constraints as well as risk perceptions by both the provider and patient were cited as limiting completion of screening. Post-pilot surveys showed mixed support for ongoing HIV screening in this setting by providers and little support by nurses.

Conclusions: Visit provider and triage nurse were strongly associated with acceptance of testing, which may reflect variable opinions of HIV screening in this setting by clinical staff. Among patients accepting screening, visit provider remained strongly associated with completion of testing. Despite longstanding recommendations for non-targeted HIV screening, further changes to improve the testing and results process, as well as provider education and buy-in, are needed to improve screening rates.

Keywords: HIV, Screening, Patient care, Urgent care

Introduction

At the end of 2008, approximately 236,400 individuals were estimated to have undiagnosed HIV in the United States, representing 20% of the 1.1 million infected individuals [1]. In order to identify these individuals and initiate early treatment of HIV, in 2006 the Centers for Disease Control and Prevention (CDC) recommended that the United States adopt a voluntary, non-targeted opt-out HIV screening strategy for all individuals aged 13-64 years presenting to all health care settings where HIV prevalence is known to be $\geq 0.1\%$ [2]. Attempts at non-targeted screening, while logical in the primary care setting, are hindered by many constraints including stigma and lack of full access to primary care, especially among the most vulnerable populations [3,4]. In the more anonymous and accessible emergency department (ED) setting, adoption of non-targeted screening policies has been limited by time, concerns about follow up of test results, and competing priorities. Previous studies have demonstrated significant increases in detecting undiagnosed HIV

* Correspondence: rbi13@uw.edu
†Equal contributors
[1]Division of Allergy and Infectious Diseases, University of Washington, 1959 NE Pacific St, BB545, 98195 Seattle, WA, USA
[9]Fred Hutchinson Cancer Research Center, M1B-140 1100 Fairview Ave N, Seattle, WA 98109, USA

with non-targeted, rapid HIV tests in the ED setting [5,6], yet only about 25% of eligible patients complete testing in these studies [3,7-9]. In settings without explicit opt-out screening protocols, there were far lower rates of screening, such as the 1.5% overall screening rate observed within the 2009 National Hospital Ambulatory Medical Care Survey (NHAMCS) data [4]. A recent review of NHAMCS revealed that despite growing recommendations for non-targeted HIV screening in all clinical settings, no increase in screening in EDs had occurred between 1993 and 2010. However, HIV testing was significantly greater in outpatient ambulatory medical care departments (OPDs) than in EDs and physician offices, suggesting that non-targeted screening in urgent care (UC) settings may continue to be an important setting in which to expand HIV testing [4].

UCs may be an opportune setting for HIV screening because physicians may be less constrained by time or by acuity of the patient's condition compared to the ED setting [10]. At the same time, the UC setting maintains the function of a safety net for patients not linked to primary care who may have had fewer opportunities to be screened for HIV. While a logical and previously studied setting for implementing HIV screening, UCs in prior studies report lower rates of screening than expected. These studies cite the burden of pre- and post-test counseling, inconsistent practice patterns, and workflow as reasons for low screening rates [4,11].

Therefore, we undertook a study of non-targeted HIV screening at Massachusetts General Hospital-Chelsea Urgent Care (MGH-CUC), with the goal of creating infrastructure to streamline the screening process and increase screening rates. The MGH-CUC is a busy urban UC within a large academic-community health center, serving a racially and ethnically diverse underserved patient population. The health center serves a community with disproportionate rates of low health literacy, non-legal immigrant status, and poor social stability. Many of these patient characteristics not only increase the risk of acquiring HIV, but also decrease the likelihood that patients engage in routine primary care. Because no protocols existed for managing results or new HIV diagnoses, the baseline rate of HIV screening at this location was essentially zero. Our goal was to offer HIV screening to all patients by adding a triage questionnaire and testing protocol in the UC, as well as education sessions for all staff. The protocol employed an opt-in testing strategy since restrictions of Massachusetts legislation prior to 2012 required written informed consent for HIV testing (amended to verbal consent on April 27, 2012, which was after completion of this pilot) [12,13]. We examined factors predicting acceptance of HIV screening and completion of testing in this Urgent Care setting.

Methods

Study population and clinical pilot

We initiated a four-month pilot to demonstrate feasibility of non-targeted HIV screening in the UC. We performed an observational study augmented with electronic medical record (EMR) review and post-pilot provider and nurse surveys. We attempted enrollment of all patients age 18-65 presenting to the clinic between October 3, 2011 and January 30, 2012. We excluded minors aged 13-17 from the study, despite screening recommendations, because of the added complexity of written informed consent in the State of Massachusetts at the time of the study [12,14]. At triage, the nurses were requested to pair a study packet containing the data collection form (DCF), HIV consent/lab slip, and HIV testing explanatory material with the clinical encounter form for all patients aged 18-65 presenting with any complaint. Nursing staff documented self-report of HIV testing during the last 12 months and patient willingness to participate in HIV screening during that visit. Providers including physicians (MDs), nurse practitioners (NPs), and certified physician assistants (PA-Cs), were requested to offer each patient an HIV test, regardless of responses in triage, and obtain written consent for the test. Following state law, lab slips were not processed unless patient and provider signatures were obtained. Interpreters were used as necessary for the clinical visit. Patients who consented to testing had whole blood from peripheral venipuncture sent for 4th generation EIA/p24Ag HIV test (Abbott ARCHITECT Combo Assay), with positive tests confirmed with reflex Western Blot. Patients were then given additional printed information in multiple languages about HIV with an explanation of how to obtain their results.

For the first 2.5 months of the study, all patients received a provider phone call within 1-3 days of the visit; negative results were given during the call and patients with positive results were asked to return to clinic to receive their results. Interim feedback from providers suggested that calling all patients with their results was neither a successful method for reaching patients and conveying their results nor was it sustainable. For the remaining 1.5 months of the pilot, patients were instructed to obtain their printed results and explanatory information in envelopes held at the clinic's reception desk. As before, any patients with positive results were called personally and asked to return for a provider visit before the written result was released.

Provider and nurse surveys

All providers and nursing staff during the 4 months of the pilot were recruited to participate in our post-pilot survey via email. We asked staff to respond to the survey if they had worked a minimum of 1 shift during the pilot period. Staff who chose to participate followed a link to a secure, anonymous survey online. The survey used Likert scales to rate most negative to most positive responses to several statements regarding HIV testing in the Urgent Care Center and included free text for additional comments.

Data collection

The DCF accompanied the patient throughout the UC encounter. Nurses documented question responses during triage, and providers documented if patients were ultimately offered screening and then consented. If patients either were not offered or did not accept screening, providers documented the reason screening was not completed. Study data were collected and managed using REDCap electronic data capture tools hosted by Partners HealthCare Research Computing, Enterprise Research Infrastructure & Services (ERIS) group. REDCap (Research Electronic Data Capture) is a secure, web-based application designed to support data capture for research studies [15]. Medical record number (MRN) on the DCF was linked with the EMR, providing augmented demographic and clinical data for the patient encounter. HIV testing history back to 1998 was recorded when available from the EMR. The EMR was also used to obtain test results from the pilot and link entries from repeat encounters. DCFs without MRNs were excluded from analysis, as were patients who attended nurse-only visits. Patients with incomplete data due to acuity of visit or provider omission were included in the study and documented as "not completed, lack of documentation/other reason" if a DCF was initiated.

Data analysis

Data tabulated included self-report of HIV testing within 12 months, age category by 5-year increment, gender, race/ethnicity, Primary Care Physician (PCP) location, area of residence (same city, within clinic catchment, outside catchment area), month of UC visit, prior HIV tests during last 12 months, documentation of HIV test ever in the EMR, triaging RN, and provider seen. We evaluated the univariate relationship between each of these characteristics and completion of screening using Chi-Square tests. We used logistic regression to identify independent predictors of completing screening from the above variables among all participants. We created a second multivariable model restricted to only those patients indicating they desired screening in triage. Repeat visits during the study period were excluded from the primary analysis but included in a repeater analysis. We evaluated the rate of repeat visits in which testing took place both when testing was initially performed and when testing was not initially performed. We report 95% confidence intervals and consider a p-value of <0.05 statistically significant throughout. We performed a qualitative analysis of post-pilot surveys given the small number of surveys. Data was analyzed with SAS, Version 9.3 (Cary, NC, USA).

Human subjects

Institutional review board (IRB) approval was obtained from the Partners Healthcare System Human Subjects Research Committee for the medical records review and evaluation of the pilot. The pilot itself was considered IRB exempt since it was an innovation of national clinical guidelines. Informed consent was waived for the observational study as consent was obtained routinely for the HIV test. A separate IRB application was submitted and received approval for the provider/nurse survey. Informed consent was implied by response to the survey invitation. The survey recruitment email stated clearly that participation in the survey was optional and responses were free from personal or professional repercussions.

Results

HIV screening uptake

Figure 1 illustrates the data collection and HIV screening process. Over the four-month pilot period, 5,164 vistis were made by patients aged 18-65 at the Urgent Care Center out of 8,114 total visits. There were 3,996 unique eligible patients during the pilot period, 8 of whom had previously diagnosed HIV (0.2%). We observed 2,465 eligible visits (47.7%) at which DCFs were initiated. The first visit from each of 2,188 unique patients with eligible visits was included in the primary analysis (after excluding 157 repeat visits and 120 visits where the MRN was missing or the patient was not seen by a provider). The 157 repeat visits made by 141 patients were evaluated in a separate analysis. Of enrolled unique patients, 514 (23.5%) completed HIV screening at their first visit, accounting for only 12.9% of total eligible patients. 788 (36.0%) patients indicated in triage that they were agreeable to screening at their initial enrolled visit. Of 141 patients with 157 repeat visits to the UC during the study period, 17.3% of those not initially screened completed screening on a subsequent visit, while only 5.4% tested more than once during the study period.

One new diagnosis of HIV was made during the screening pilot, with one additional diagnosis made by targeted testing of the partner. There were no indeterminate or false positive tests. Of 514 patients screened, the rate of previously undiagnosed HIV was 0.19%. The newly diagnosed patients were linked to care with an HIV provider within one week at the same health center.

Patient characteristics

The 2,188 unique patients included in our primary analysis reflected the demographic makeup of the local population [Table 1], with Hispanics predominating (55.7%,

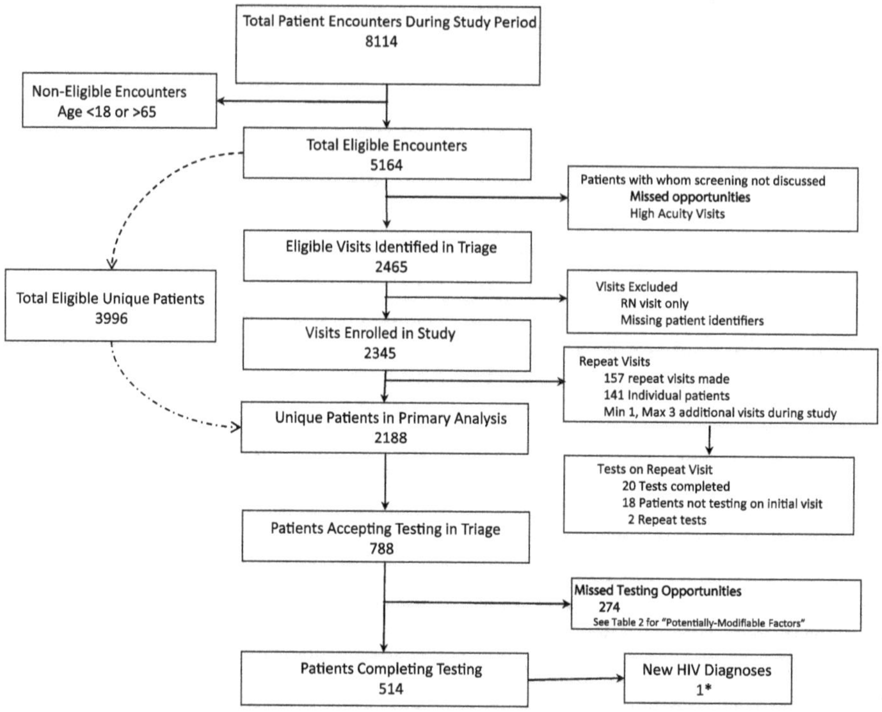

Figure 1 Patient flow through urgent care clinic during the four month study period. One new diagnoses resulted from screening. One additional diagnosis resulted from targeted partner testing of the study patient.

mainly of Central American background). The average age was 37 years (SD 12.6 years); 61.6% were male. 1439 patients (65.5%) identified a PCP within the hospital's primary care network. 49.0% lived within the same city, 40.0% within the adjoining catchment zone of the clinic, and only 11.1% from outside the local area.

Of patients with a listed in-network PCP, 55.4% had no HIV test documented in our EMR dating back to 1998. 10.8% had tests documented within the last 12 months. There was a large disparity with respect to prior testing by gender, with 53.0% of women and only 30.6% of men having documented prior tests; self-report of HIV screening was more gender-balanced (26.3% of women and 25.1% of men).

Patient factors associated with completion of screening

Several patient demographic factors were considered in multivariable analysis predicting completion of HIV screening. Younger age was strongly associated with screening acceptance, with screening declining significantly with older age (Odds ratio (OR) 5.2, 95% Confidence Interval (CI) 2.2, 12.2 for patients 18-25 compared against age 60-65, $p < 0.0001$ for trend) [Table 2]. Men screened more frequently than women (OR 1.4, 95% CI 1.1, 1.8). Race/ethnicity also was a significant factor, with Hispanic ethnicity (OR 3.7, 95% CI 2.7, 5.2) or black race (OR 4.1 95% CI 2.5, 6.9) associated with increased rates of screening compared to non-Hispanic white patients ($p < 0.0001$). There was no statistically significant screening difference between those with a PCP at the health center, those with an in-system PCP, or no listed PCP ($p = 0.24$). In the study population, 565 (25.8%) reported that they had previously been tested for HIV in the past year; this strongly predicted against screening in this study with an OR 0.3 (95% CI 0.2, 0.3, $p < 0.0001$).

In the separate multivariable model restricted to those 788 patients accepting screening, only male gender continued to be a significant patient factor associated with completing the screening test (OR 1.6, 95% CI 1.1, 2.2, $p = 0.01$).

Association of provider and nurse on completion of screening

During the four-month pilot period, a staff of 19 clinicians, including Internal Medicine and Medicine-Pediatrics physicians (MDs), NPs, and PA-Cs, provided care, and 11 RNs triaged patients at the UC. In multivariable analysis, the visit provider and the triaging RN were each independent factors associated with completion of screening, contributing more highly in both effect size and level of significance of association ($p = 0.0005$ for RN, <0.0001 for provider) than many individual patient demographic factors [Table 2 for individual ORs]. There was a 2.6-fold difference in screening rates between those seeing the RNs with the lowest and highest odds of screening completion

Table 1 Baseline demographic characteristics of patients presenting to the urgent care during the HIV screening pilot

Variable	Total sample N=2188	Accepting HIV screening N=788 (36.0)	Tested for HIV N=514 (23.5)	Not tested for HIV N=1674 (76.5)
Age	37.1 +/- 12.6	34.5+/-11.7	33.8 +/- 11.233.8 +/- 11.2	38.1 +/- 12.8
Male	1342 (61.3)	471 (59.8)	291 (56.6)	1051 (62.8)
Male Gender	1342 (61.3)	471 (59.8)	471 (59.8)	1051 (62.8)
Female Gender	846 (38.7)	317 (40.2)	223 (43.4)	623 (37.2)
Race/Ethnicity				
Non-Hispanic White	610 (28.0)	112 (14.2)	61 (11.9)	549 (32.8)
Hispanic	1219 (55.7)	556 (70.6)	373 (72.6)	846 (50.5)
African/Black	127 (5.8)	54 (6.9)	40 (7.8)	87 (5.2)
Asian/Pacific Islander	49 (2.2)	11 (1.4)	6 (1.2)	43 (2.6)
Other/Not Listed	183 (8.4)	55 (7.0)	34 (6.6)	149 (8.9)
Area of Residence†				
Same Zip Code	1072 (49.0)	444 (56.4)	307 (59.7)	765 (45.7)
Clinic Catchment	874 (40.0)	281 (35.7)	169 (32.9)	705 (42.1)
Outside Catchment	242 (11.1)	63 (8.0)	38 (7.4)	204 (12.2)
Pilot Month of Visit Date				
1	789 (36.1)	323 (41.0)	202 (39.3)	587 (35.1)
2	583 (26.7)	184 (23.4)	131 (25.5)	452 (27.0)
3	397 (18.1)	128 (16.2)	77 (15.0)	320 (19.1)
4	419 (19.5)	153 (19.4)	104 (20.2)	315 (18.8)
PCP Location				
At Same Location	989 (45.0)	360 (45.7)	234 (45.5)	750 (44.8)
In System‡	442 (20.5)	134 (17.0)	93 (18.1)	355 (21.1)
No In System PCP	756 (34.6)	294 (37.3)	187 (36.4)	569 (34.0)
Prior HIV Test by EMR				
Ever	966 (44.6)		722 (43.1)	248 (48.3)
> 1 year ago	737 (33.4)		541 (32.3)	192 (37.4)
Within 1 year	239 (10.8)		181 (10.8)	56 (10.9)
Prior HIV Test by Self-Report				
Within 1 year	565 (25.8)		261 (71.7)	103 (28.3)
Total Patients	2188	788 (36.0)	514 (23.5)	1674 (76.5)

Data are No. (percentage) +/- Standard Deviation.
Abbreviations: HIV, Human Immunodeficiency Virus; PCP, Primary Care Physician; EMR, Electronic Medical Record.
†Local: same city and zip code as clinic, Clinic Catchment Area: The 5 towns/cities encompassing the 6 zip codes from which >85% of UC population is drawn, Outside Clinic Catchment: a zip code not other than above.
‡In system PCP defined as affiliation with any primary MD or NP affiliated with Partners Healthcare System.

in the multivariable analysis. There was an 8.7-fold difference in testing rates among providers. In the subset of patients "accepting screening", the odds of completing screening varied more than 90-fold between providers ($p < 0.0001$). Point estimates suggest that NPs and PA-Cs tested at lower rates than MDs.

Acceptance of screening vs completion of HIV test

Starting with all patients age 18-65 eligible for screening, we witnessed a "screening cascade" with drop-offs measured at each phase from entry in the clinic to completion of screening and retrieval of results [Figure 2]. In the flow through the clinic visit, there were clear points where screening opportunities were lost. As described above, 52.3% of eligible visits did initiate a screening questionnaire (DCF) at triage. While 36.0% of patients in those observed visits did accept screening at triage, only 23.5% actually completed the test. 1294 (77.3%) of the 1674 persons not screened had reasons documented that we categorized as visit-based or potentially modifiable factors, such that under different circumstances (less acute visit, different provider) the patient may have accepted and

Table 2 Adjusted odds ratios (ORs) and 95% confidence intervals (CIs) for predictors of completing HIV testing from multivariate analysis

	Full sample (n=2188)	Persons accepting HIV screening at triage (n=788)		
Characteristic	**OR (95%CI)**	**p-value**	**OR (95%CI)**	**p-value**
		<0.0001		0.2
18 to 24	5.2 (2.2, 12.2)		5.5 (1.7,17.3)	
25 to 29	3.8 (1.6, 9.1)		4.2 (1.3, 13.6)	
30 to 34	4.9 (2.0, 11.6)		4.8 (1.5, 15.3)	
35 to 39	3.0 (1.2, 7.3)		4.1 (1.2, 13.6)	
40 to 44	2.8 (1.2, 6.9)		4.4 (1.3, 14.8)	
45 to 49	2.6 (1.1, 6.4)		4.3 (1.2, 14.9)	
50 to 54	1.9 (0.8, 4.8)		3.4 (0.9, 12.2)	
55 to 59	1.0 (0.7, 5.0)		2.5 (0.7, 9.7)	
60 to 65	ref		ref	
Gender				
		0.004		0.01
Male	1.4 (1.1, 1.8)		1.6 (1.1, 2.2)	
Female	ref		ref	
Month				
		0.56		0.94
1	ref		ref	
2	0.8 (0.6, 1.1)		1.1 (0.7, 1.8)	
3	0.8 (0.6, 1.2)		0.9 (0.6, 1.6)	
4	0.9 (0.7, 1.3)		1.0 (0.6, 1.7)	
Area of Residence				
		0.08		0.08
Outside Clinic Catchment	0.8 (0.6, 1.0)		0.7 (0.5, 1.0)	
Within Catchment	0.7 (0.4, 1.0)		0.7 (0.4, 1.4)	
Same Zip Code	ref		ref	
Race				
		<0.0001		0.23
Black/African	4.1 (2.5, 6.9)		2.0 (0.9, 4.4)	
Asian/Pacific Islander	1.3 (0.5, 3.2)		0.5 (0.1, 2.1)	
Hispanic	3.7 (2.7, 5.2)		1.5 (0.9, 2.4)	
Other/Unknown	2.0 (1.2, 3.2)		1.2 (0.6, 1.5)	
Non-Hispanic White	ref		ref	
PCP Location				
		0.24		0.44
No In System PCP	1.3 (1.0, 1.7)		1.0 (0.6, 1.5)	
In System PCP	1.1 (0.8, 1.5)		1.3 (0.8, 2.2)	
At Same Location	ref		ref	
Self-Report of HIV Test Within 1 Year				
		<0.0001		0.32
Yes	0.3 (0.2, 0.3)		0.7 (0.4, 1.1)	
Not Reported	0.4, (0.1, 1.2)		1.2 (0.2, 7.3)	

Table 2 Adjusted odds ratios (ORs) and 95% confidence intervals (CIs) for predictors of completing HIV testing from multivariate analysis *(Continued)*

No	ref		ref	
HIV Test in EMR		0.008		
Within 1 year	1.6 (1.1, 2.5)		1.1 (0.6, 2.0)	
1 year ago	1.5 (1.1, 1.9)		1.3 (0.8, 1.9)	
Never	ref		ref	
Triage RN		0.0005		0.19
A	1.0 (0.5, 2.1)		1.0 (0.4, 2.9)	
B	1.5 (0.5, 4.2)		5.2 (0.5, 49.8)	
C	1.8 (1.0, 3.3)		1.7 (0.7, 4.2)	
D	1.2 (0.6, 2.5)		1.3 (0.4, 3.8)	
E	1.6 (0.9, 2.8)		2.6 (1.1, 5.1)	
F	1.1 (0.8, 1.5)		1.4 (0.9, 2.2)	
G	1.3 (0.6, 2.9)		1.6 (0.5, 5.0)	
H	2.3 (1.4, 3.9)		2.4 (1.2, 5.1)	
I	2.6 (1.7, 4.0)		1.9 (1.0, 3.4)	
J	1.2 (0.2, 6.7)		0.4 (0.1, 2.9)	
K	ref		ref	
Provider		<0.0001		<0.0001
A	2.9 (1.6, 5.3)		3.4 (1.6, 7.0)	
B	3.3 (1.8, 6.0)		4.9 (2.1, 11.3)	
C	6.9 (3.3, 14.4)		46.1 (5.5, 390.7)	
D	2.4 (1.2, 4.6)		3.0 (1.2, 7.4)	
E	2.4 (1.0, 5.8)		4.3 (1.1, 16.8)	
F	4.6 (1.9, 11.0)		11.1 (2.1, 60.3)	
G	2.7 (1.3, 5.8)		3.8 (1.2, 12.4)	
H	2.2 (1.2, 4.0)		2.6 (1.3, 5.5)	
I	2.1 (0.6, 7.5)		2.2 (0.4, 11.8)	
J	2.2 (0.9, 5.4)		4.9 (1.1, 21.1)	
K	1.6 (0.6, 4.5)		2.2 (0.5, 9.3)	
L	7.6 (3.4, 17.0)		14.1 (3.4, 58.2)	
M	1.0 (0.2, 5.4)		2.5 (0.2, 32.5)	
N*	1.7 (0.8, 3.4)		1.7 (0.7, 4.3)	
O*	1.6 (0.9, 2.9)		1.5 (0.7, 4.3)	
P*	1.0 (0.5, 2.2)		0.5 (0.2, 1.3)	
Q*	1.6 (0.8, 3.2)		1.6 (0.7, 4.0)	
R*	2.5 (1.2, 5.2)		1.8 (0.7, 4.4)	
S*	3.6 (1.3, 10.4)		10.1 (1.1, 91.2)	
T	ref		ref	

Abbreviations: PCP, Primary Care Physician; HIV, Human Immunodeficiency Virus; EMR, Electronic Medical Record.
*Denotes mid-level providers, either certified physicians assistants (PA-C) or nurse practitioners (NP).

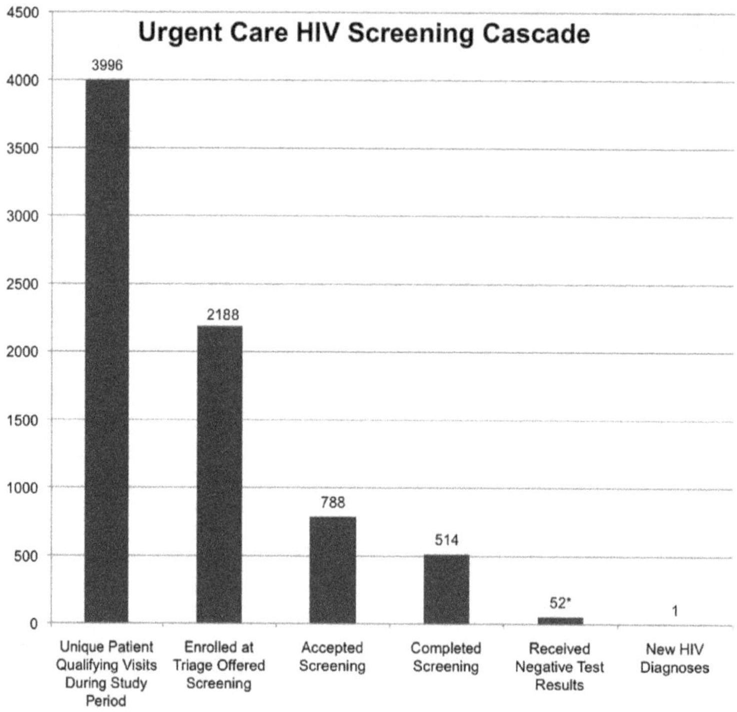

Figure 2 Cascade of Lost Testing Opportunities. This cascade shows lost opportunities for screening at each phase in the visit. The largest decrements were in identifying appropriate patients to screen at triage (54.8% of eligible patients identified and enrolled) and obtaining patient acceptance of screening (36.0% of those identified to screen). Of the 788 patients amenable to screening, 34.8% did not complete the consent and blood work. *Approximately 10% returned to receive negative test results. 0.19% of screened patients were found to have HIV.

completed screening. Frequently reported modifiable reasons for not completing tested included visit acuity/ lack of time (8.1%) or provider not offering testing (8.4%) [See Table 3 for full data]. A small proportion of patients desired HIV screening but provider deferred testing to an upcoming PCP visit (1.2%) or prenatal appointment (1.1%). We included in the "potentially modifiable" list the 552 visits (33%) for which no reason was documented. The majority of these visits had a time-sensitive chief complaint such as chest pain or foreign body in the eye listed in the medical record. An additional 28.1% of visits where screening was not completed were associated with a "patient-based factor", which we define as a feature of that patient unlikely to change if other visit-based variables were different. Such patient-based reasons included patient report of recent testing in last year (19.8%) or greater than 1 year ago without recent perceived risk (3.5%) or fear of needles (0.24%) [Table 3]. For several encounters, greater than 1 reason was recorded.

Provider and nurse post-pilot surveys

Seven of 11 eligible RNs (63.6%) completed a post-pilot survey. Only one RN felt it was acceptable to continue HIV screening after the pilot, 3 had a neutral/no opinion, and 3 were slightly opposed to continue screening. There were less strong patterns with response to other questions and willingness to formalize the screening process; the majority of responses were neutral to slightly negative across the board, especially with respect to logistical difficulties caused by adding screening to the visit and negative impact of work-flow [Figure 3a]. Several open-ended responses from RNs included concerns that it was not appropriate to involve RNs in HIV screening or that RNs did not feel well equipped to discuss patients' risk of HIV or answer patient questions on this topic.

Twelve of 19 eligible providers (63.1%) completed post-pilot surveys with questions that differed slightly from those in the RN survey as appropriate for roll in HIV screening. Of these, 58.3% were in favor of continuing uniform non-targeted screening after completion of the pilot. 25% preferred to screen only a subset of patients, for example, targeted screening based on patient factors and when sufficient visit time allowed. One provider each wished to screen only if the patient requested screening or not at all. Overall, there was a trend in willingness to continue HIV screening following the pilot with positive responses to the following: provider comfort with discussing screening, perceptions of responsibility of UC providers to participate in screening, appropriateness of time use, burden of results management, and value added to patients by offering screening as a service [Figure 3b].

Table 3 Reported reasons HIV screening not performed during urgent care visit

Reason screening not performed Sums to > 100% with multiple responses	Number (%)
Visit-Based or Potentially Modifiable Factors	1294 (77.3)
Provider felt patient to not be at risk	60 (3.6)
Patient felt themselves to be at low risk	367 (21.9)
Provider did not offer	141 (8.4)
Visit Acuity or Lack of Time†	135 (8.1)
Patient desired testing, deferred to future PCP visit	20 (1.2)
Pregnancy diagnosed: testing deferred to PNV	8 (1.1)
Patient or provider perceived cost of testing‡	7 (0.42)
Patient felt too ill to test	4 (0.24)
Other reason not listed/lack of documentation†	552 (33.0)
Patient-Based Factors	471 (28.1)
Patient reported testing in the last 12 months	332 (19.8)
Patient declined, no reason given	68 (4.1)
Patient reported testing > 12 mos prior	59 (3.5)
Previously known HIV+ status	8 (0.48)
Fear of needles	4 (0.24)
Total Patients Not Screened/Enrolled Patients	1674 (100%)

Abbreviations: PNV, Pre-Natal Visit.
†135 visits documented high-acuity of visit on the study form as reason testing not performed, however EMR review showed that the vast majority of the 552 visits with "Other Reason Not Listed" were also visits of high acuity, but without provider documentation on the study form. Examples of "High-acuity visits" determined by EMR review included presentation with probable cardiac chest pain, asthma exacerbation, foreign body in the eye, or other visit requiring emergent medical interventions and/or ambulance transfer to Emergency Department. Most visits fitting the above description of "High-acuity" also had incomplete HIV screening documentation, presumably because of the urgency of the patient encounter.
‡The Commonwealth of Massachusetts offers "universal" health care coverage. For those not already enrolled in the hospital-based safety net system, the vast majority of patients are enrolled following first contact with CHC and covered retroactively, including all lab testing associated with the visit. Despite education regarding this, a small number of providers and/or patients remained concerned about cost of testing.

Discussion

We evaluated predictors of completing non-targeted HIV screening in an Urgent Care center at an academic-community partnership health center serving a racially and ethnically diverse and socioeconomically disadvantaged community. We attempted to enhance the nil HIV screening rate at baseline by establishing a protocol at the UC to offer routine screening. The overall rate of testing at the end of the study was 23.5%, within the range reported by prior studies performed in ED and UC settings [3,7-9]. In the process, we identified a previously unrecognized, independent predictor for completing HIV screening: the health care professional who treated the patient in the UC. Of the responders to the survey, about half of providers were neutral or opposed to the UC setting being the appropriate setting for a screening test, but as illustrated by the heat map of survey responses [Figure 3b], a majority of respondents favored continuing screening. Altogether, provider opinion, whether in favor or opposition to screening, likely contributes to broad range of screening completion rates by provider. This suggests that successful implementation of non-targeted screening is unlikely to occur until there is buy-in by providers in UCs and EDs, despite strong national-level guidelines.

Providers may have offered, completed or deferred screening based on perceived time constraints or because they felt screening was of low value to the patient encounter because of lack of perceived risk, among other factors. While the latter runs counter to the principle of implementing non-targeted testing in acute-care settings, the finding is consistent with previous studies [17,18]. Other studies have demonstrated that physicians have variable knowledge about the CDC recommendations, and when they are informed, often have doubts about guidelines, fear of mistrust from their patients, or fear of what to do with a positive result [17-19].

RN responders to the survey were largely neutral about their role as it related to the screening pilot and were relatively negative with respect to whether they would support non-targeted HIV screening moving forward. In this model of HIV screening, the particular nurse screening a patient could strongly influence the patient's response as to whether or not he/she was amenable to screening. Since willingness to be screened was evaluated by the triage RN, the group accepting screening was likely selected based on a combination of RN opinion on screening in general, and how the RN did or did not resolve their own perceptions and patient perceptions about who is at risk for HIV.

Based on our results and a recently published study reporting that RN-initiated screening has lower uptake than provider-initiated screening [7], we do not recommend that future non-targeted screening programs use RN-initiated screening protocols in the ED or UC setting. However, because HIV screening inherently involves RNs for other steps in the screening process, it is important to include nursing staff in education and design of HIV screening programs.

In this pilot we identified several points during the encounter where improvements could be made to increase both screening uptake and test completion. As depicted in Figure 2, in the flow through the clinic visit, there were clear points where testing opportunities were lost; while there may be several patient factors impacting uptake of screening, our pilot suggests that the person offering the screening is extremely influential in the patient's testing decision. Not all patients were enrolled in the pilot and offered HIV screening in triage. A lower number of patients than expected were agreeable to screening, possibly reflecting initiation of screening by triage RNs.

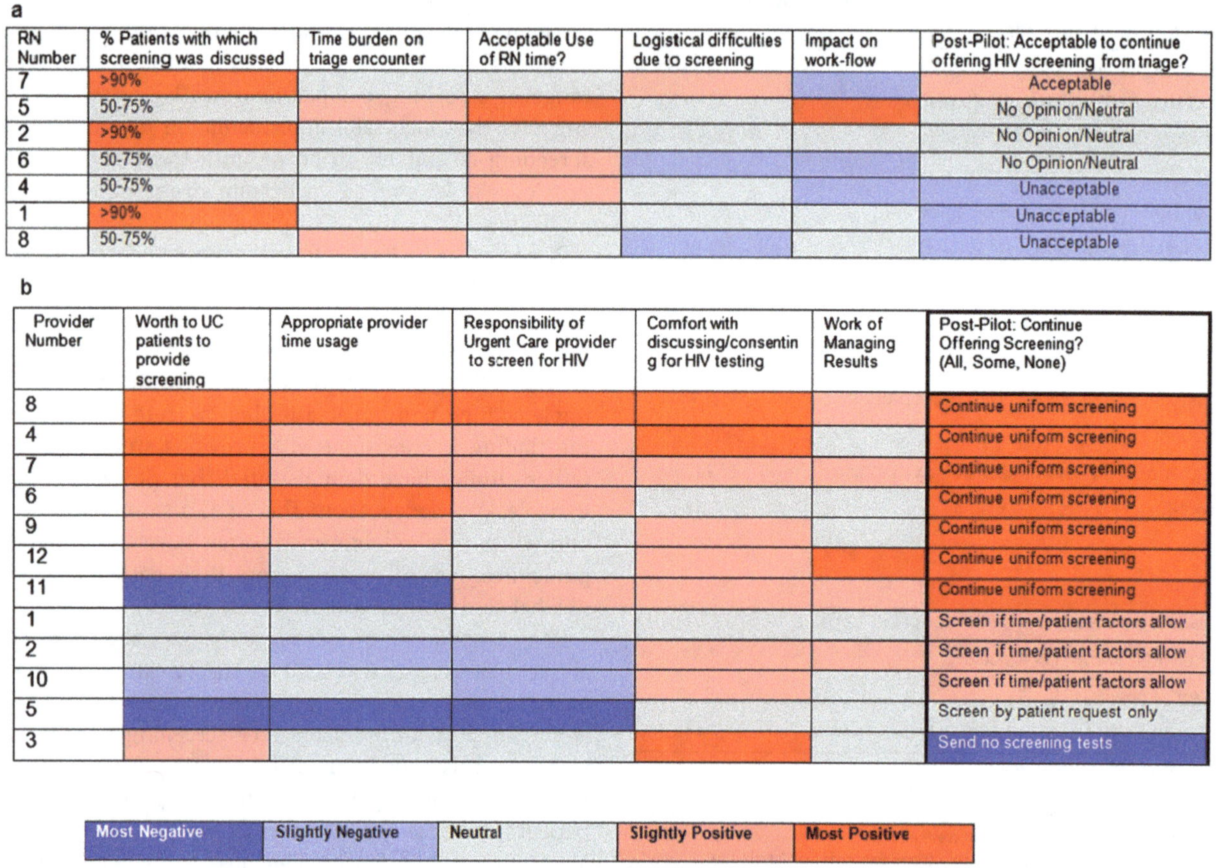

Figure 3 Heat map representation of post-pilot survey responses a) nursing survey responses. 7 of 11 eligible RNs responded via secure online anonymous survey. Response scale converted to color coding from "Most Positive" to "Most Negative" response based responses to questions given in the form of Likert Scales as per key. **b)** Provider survey responses. 12 of 19 eligible providers responded via secure online anonymous survey. Response scale converted to color coding from "Most Positive" to "Most Negative" response based responses to questions given in the form of Likert Scales as per key. The final column demonstrates provider self-prediction of their future testing practices after completion of the screening pilot (Screen all patients, only screen some patients depending on patient request/other factors, not perform HIV screening).

Our study also affirmed the previously documented findings that younger age groups, Hispanics, and Blacks were more likely to complete HIV screening [11,16].

Limitations

Our study has limitations. We performed a single center study, with the intent to evaluate predictors for screening at our site only; patients may have had previous tests performed with outside providers and we relied on their self-report of these tests. Furthermore, a large proportion of visits meeting criteria for enrollment in the study were not enrolled at triage. As the pilot was performed in Massachusetts prior to April 2012, the legal obligation to use written informed consent forced an opt-in strategy. This created an additional barrier to screening that is no longer required by most states. Settings where point-of-care testing is used and where written consent is no longer required may have greater screening uptake.

Conclusions

The wide variability in completion of screening associated with interacting with different care providers has not previously been reported in the literature. In this single-center observational study we found that the provider and the nurse serving each study participant were each independently associated with acceptance of testing. Based upon our qualitative data, time and comfort level with HIV testing may have contributed to low rates of testing.

While the pilot aimed to educate providers and streamline the screening process, screening drop-off still occurred at points of contact between patients and clinical staff. Survey data suggested that providers maintain bias against uniform non-targeted screening. We can use this knowledge as an opportunity to educate providers on the CDC guidelines and its rationale in order to increase screening in acute care settings. This issue warrants future operational research and clinical innovation projects to enhance the implementation of non-targeted HIV screening across all care settings.

Abbreviations

HIV: Human immunodeficiency virus; CDC: Centers for disease control and prevention; ED: Emergency department; NHAMCS: National hospital ambulatory medical care survey; OPD: Outpatient ambulatory medical care departments; UC: Urgent care; EMR: Electronic medical record; DCF: Data collection form; MD: Medical doctor, physician; NP: Nurse practitioner; PA: Physicians' assistant; RN: Registered nurse; IRB: Institutional review board; PCP: Primary care physician; SD: Standard deviation; OR: Odds Ratio; CI: Confidence Interval.

Competing interests

The authors declare they have no competing interests.

Authors' contributions

RBI and JTC designed and conducted the study, interpreted the data and prepared and edited the manuscript. MC provided statistical expertise, interpreted the data and edited the manuscript. JD and JDL assisted with study implementation and preparing the manuscript. JPC assisted with study design. VES provided oversight of study design and manuscript preparation, and edited the manuscript. All authors have read and approve the manuscript.

Acknowledgements

RBI and this study were funded in part by the Winickoff Fellowship Program in Primary Care of the General Medicine Division, Massachusetts General Hospital.
REDCaps is hosted by Harvard Catalyst | The Harvard Clinical and Translational Science Center (NIH Award #UL1 RR 025758 and financial contributions from Harvard University and its affiliated academic health care centers).

Author details

[1]Division of Allergy and Infectious Diseases, University of Washington, 1959 NE Pacific St, BB545, 98195 Seattle, WA, USA. [2]Department of Medicine, Massachusetts General Hospital, Grey/Bigelow 740, 55 Fruit St, 02114 Boston, MA, USA. [3]Johns Hopkins Bloomberg School of Public Health, Department of Epidemiology, 615 North Wolfe Street, W6508, 21205 Baltimore, MD, USA. [4]Department of Surgery, Johns Hopkins Hospital, 600 N Wolfe St, 21287 Baltimore, MD, USA. [5]Harvard Medical School, Tosteson Medical Education Center, 260 Longwood Ave, 02115 Boston, MA, USA. [6]Department of Medicine, CHC Urgent Care, Massachusetts General Hospital Chelsea Healthcare Center, 151 Everett Ave, 02150 Chelsea, MA, USA. [7]Department of Medicine, Harvard Medical School, 25 Shattuck St, 02115 Boston, MA, USA. [8]Department of Medicine, Mount Auburn Hospital, 330 Mount Auburn Street, 02138 Cambridge, MA, USA. [9]Fred Hutchinson Cancer Research Center, M1B-140 1100 Fairview Ave N, Seattle, WA 98109, USA.

References

1. Centers for Disease Control and Prevention: **HIV surveillance–United States, 1981-2008.** *MMWR Morb Mortal Wkly Rep* 2011, **60**(21):689.
2. Branson BM, Handsfield HH, Lampe MA, Janssen RS, Taylor AW, Lyss SB, Clark JE: **Revised recommendations for HIV testing of adults, adolescents, and pregnant women in health-care settings.** *MMWR Morbidity and mortality weekly Report.* **55**(RR-14):1–17. CDC 2006 Sep 22.
3. Walensky RP, Losina E, Malatesta L, Barton GE, O'Connor CA, Skolnik PR, Hall JM, McGuire JF, Freedberg KA: **Effective HIV case identification through routine HIV screening at urgent care centers in Massachusetts.** *Am J Public Health* 2005, **95**(1):71.
4. Tai M, Merchant RC: **HIV testing in US emergency departments, outpatient ambulatory medical departments, and physician offices, 1992–2010.** *AIDS Care* 2014, **26**(9):1105–1108. Epub 2014 Jan 2.
5. Haukoos JS, Hopkins E, Conroy AA, Silverman M, Byyny RL, Eisert S, Thurn MW, Wilson ML, Hutchinson AB, Forsyth J: **Routine opt-out rapid HIV screening and detection of HIV infection in emergency department patients.** *JAMA* 2010, **304**(3):284–292.
6. Hoover JB, Tao G, Heffelfinger JD: **Monitoring HIV testing at visits to emergency departments in the United States: very-low rate of HIV testing.** *J AIDS* 2013, **62**(1):90–94.
7. Haukoos JS, Hopkins E, Byyny RL, Conroy AA, Silverman M, Eisert S, Thurn M, Wilson M, Boyett B, Heffelfinger JD: ***Design and Implementation of a Controlled Clinical Trial to Evaluate the Effectiveness and Efficiency of Routine Opt out Rapid Human Immunodeficiency Virus Screening in the Emergency* Department.** *Acad Emerg Med* 2009, **16**(8):800–808.
8. Liddicoat RV, Losina E, Kang M, Freedberg KA, Walensky RP: **Refusing HIV testing in an urgent care setting: results from the" Think HIV" program.** *AIDS Pat Care STDs* 2006, **20**(2):84–92.
9. Kinsler JJ, Sayles JN, Cunningham WE, Mahajan: **Preference for physician vs nurse-initiated opt-out screening on HIV test acceptance.** *AIDS Care* 2013, **25**(11):1442–1445.
10. White DA, Scribner AN, Schulden JD, Branson BM, Heffelfinger JD: **Results of a rapid HIV screening and diagnostic testing program in an urban emergency department.** *Ann Emerg Med* 2009, **54**(1):56–64.
11. Murphy K, Grusky O, Roberts KJ, Swanson AN: **HIV testing in an urgent-care clinic.** *Sex Health* 2005, **2**(4):245–250.
12. **Massachusetts General Law, Part I, Title XVI, Chapter 111, § 70F. "Public Health" Commonwealth of Massachusetts.** [https://malegislature.gov/Laws/GeneralLaws/PartI/TitleXVI/Chapter111]
13. **Massachusetts General Law Part I, Title XVI, Chapter 111, Session 2012: Chapter 84, "An Act Increasing Screening for HIV", Approved 27 April 2012. "Public Health" Commonwealth of Massachusetts.** [https://malegislature.gov/Laws/GeneralLaws/PartI/TitleXVI/Chapter111]
14. **Massachusetts General Law, Part I, Title XVI, Chapter 112 § 12 F. "Registration of Certain Professions and Occupations" Commonwealth of Massachusetts.** [https://malegislature.gov/Laws/GeneralLaws/PartI/TitleXVI/Chapter112/Section12F]
15. Harris PA, Taylor R, Thielke R, Payne J, Gonzalez N, Conde JG: **Research electronic data capture (REDCap)—a metadata-driven methodology and workflow process for providing translational research informatics support.** *J Biomed Inform* 2009, **42**(2):377–381.
16. Haukoos JS, Hopkins E, Bender B, Sasson C, Al-Tayyib AA, Thrun MW: **Comparison of enhanced targeted rapid HIV screening using the Denver HIV risk score to nontargeted rapid HIV screening in the emergency department.** *Ann Emerg Med* 2013, **61**(3):353–361.
17. Burke RC, Sepkowitz KA, Bernstein KT, Karpati AM, Myers JE, Tsoi BW, Begier EM: **Why don't physicians test for HIV? A review of the US literature.** *AIDS* 2007, **21**(12):1617–1624.
18. Hudson AL, Heilemann MV, Rodriguez M: **Missed Opportunities for universal HIV screening in primary care clinics.** *J Clin Med Res* 2012, **4**(4):242.
19. Sison N, Yolken A, Poceta J, Mena L, Chan PA, Barnes A, Smith E, Nunn A: **Healthcare provider attitudes, practices, and recommendations for enhancing routine HIV testing and linkage to care in the Mississippi Delta region.** *AIDS Pat Care STDs* 2013, **27**(9):511–517.

13

The utility of self-emulsifying oil formulation to improve the poor solubility of the anti HIV drug CSIC

Nicholas C Obitte[1*], Lisa C Rohan[2], Christianah M Adeyeye[3], Michael A Parniak[4] and Charles O Esimone[5]

Abstract

Background: CSIC (5-chloro-3-phenylsulfonylindole-2-carboxamide), a non-nucleoside reverse transcriptase inhibitor (NNRTI) has not been advanced as a therapeutic anti-HIV candidate drug due to its low aqueous solubility and poor bioavailability.

Objective: The objective of this work was to formulate CSIC into self-emulsifying oil formulations for the purpose of improving its aqueous solubility and evaluating *in vitro* antiretroviral activity.

Methods: CSIC self-emulsifying oil formulations (SEFs) were formulated and evaluated for droplet size, zeta potential, polydispersity index (PDI), viscosity, emulsification time, stability and bioactivity.

Results: Results showed significantly improved solubility of CSIC in the SEFs.The concentration of co-surfactant affected the droplet size, zeta potential and polydispersity index. *In vitro* bioactivity studies showed that the CSIC SEFs retained full anti-HIV activity.

Conclusion: The *in vitro* data from this first attempt to formulate CSIC SEFs suggest that improvement on the aqueous solubility of CSIC through this delivery system may accentuate its antiretroviral effectiveness *in vivo* via bioavailability enhancement. The formulation is therefore intended as an oral anti-HIV agent for prophylactic and therapeutic uses.

Keywords: Anti-HIV, Poorly soluble, Self-emulsification, CSIC, Bioactivity, Anhydrous emulsion

Introduction

Approximately 40% of all new drug entities have poor aqueous solubility characteristics [1]. Specific to the HIV field a number of newly developed drug candidates including several non nucleoside reverse transcriptase are extremely hydrophobic. Poorly soluble drugs tend to exhibit low bioavailability, high intra- and inter-subject variability, and a lack of dose proportionality, which pose a significant challenge when administered per orally [2,3]. Drugs that belong to the Class II Biopharmaceutic classification system are frequently caught up in this web of poor solubility [4]. Enhancement of solubility has been achieved by some drug manufacturers through use of special excipients or formulation carriers that enhance drug dissolution and hence, bioavailability. Several approaches including, solid dispersions, inclusion complexes, nanoparticles or lipid vehicles [4-6] are available as potential formulation options for hydrophobic drug candidates. An additional option is self-emulsifying oil formulation.

Self-emulsifying oil formulation (SEF) is a lipid composition with inherent capability of improving drug solubility and bioavailability. SEF is a thermodynamically stable isotropic mixture of oil, surfactant and co-surfactant, which on gentle agitation in aqueous medium self-emulsifies to yield micro or nano-emulsion [7,8]. SEF, in its native form comes as anhydrous emulsion (emulsion pre-concentrate), but upon dispersion in aqueous medium it transforms into oil-in-water (O/W) or water-in-oil (W/O) micro-emulsion or nano-emulsion which constitutes micro-domains of oil droplets stabilized by the interfacial film created by the surfactant and co-surfactant mixture [9,10].

The advantages of SEF over ordinary oil or surfactant dispersions of drugs include the combination of permeability and/or absorption enhancement, thermodynamic stability

* Correspondence: obittenick@yahoo.com
[1]Department of Pharmaceutical Technology and Industrial Pharmacy, Faculty of Pharmaceutical Sciences, University of Nigeria, Nsukka, Nigeria

(long shelf life), ease of preparation (zero interfacial tension and formation spontaneity), optical isotropy, ease of sterilization via filtration, high surface area, very small particle size (that promotes adherence to membranes) [11] and the lipoid characteristic which promotes drug intactness in the droplet prior to absorption. Long shelf life, ease of scale-up and manufacturing, improvement on dissolution and lymphatic transport of poorly soluble or lipophilic drugs rate them better than other novel colloidal drug delivery systems [7]. In the SEF front there are commercially available SEF-based antiretroviral drugs which, demonstrate the contribution of SEFs in bioavailability enhancement. Norvir® (ritonavir), Fortavase® (saquinavir) and Aptivus® (tipranavir) are antiretroviral drugs in the market which have been formulated based on this approach [12,13]. The dose-limiting side effects associated with hydrophobic antiretroviral drugs may be mitigated if formulated in a SEF. This is because erratic drug release common with poorly soluble drugs [2,3] may sometimes lead to the utilization of excessively high drug dose in traditional formulations. SEF ranks well as a reliable carrier that promotes consistent absorption and bioavailability of hydrophobic drugs [2,14].

NNRTIs such as efavirenz, UC781, dapivirine and 5-chloro-3-phenylsulfonylindole-2-carboxamide (CSIC) are potent tight-binding inhibitors of HIV RT, a property that may enhance their utility in both therapeutic and prophylactic use [15]. Efavirenz is poorly soluble, with a bioavailability of 40-45% and belongs to class II Biopharmaceutic classification system (BCS) [16-18]. Similarly CSIC is poorly soluble and has a limited bioavailability which precludes its further development despite superior *in vitro* cell-protective ability [15,19].

CSIC pretreatment of uninfected cells to protect them from subsequent HIV infection in the absence of exogenous drug, resulted to sequestration of CSIC in the cell plasma membrane [15]. This may be suggestive of possible high *in vivo* membrane permeability [20-22]. Nonetheless, the poor aqueous solubility of CSIC may restrict access to absorption through GIT membrane. In this work SEF was explored as a formulation strategy to overcome the limited aqueous solubility and associated bioavailability limitations of CSIC. This is because it offers a nano-sized non-ionic molecular form of the soluble drug which enhances permeability and absorption. Therefore, the objective of this work was to formulate CSIC into SEFs for the purpose of improving its aqueous solubility and evaluating *in vitro* cell-based antiretroviral bioactivity.

Materials and methods

Materials

The excipients used included triacetin (Acros Organics of Fisher Scientific, U.S.A), lauroglycol 90® (propylene glycol monolaurate, Gattefosse, France), and Labrasol® (caprylocaproyl macrogol-8-glycerides, Gattefosse, France). CSIC was obtained from Dr. Michael Parniak at the University of Pittsburgh.

Pseudo ternary phase diagram construction

Labrasol® (surfactant) and lauroglycol 90® (co-surfactant) ratios were varied at five fixed triacetin (oil) ratios (0.5, 1.0, 1.5, 2.0 and 2.5) to generate 30 different oil/surfactant/co-surfactant homogenous isotropic preconcentrate formulations. Oil (triacetin) concentration was evaluated at levels of 10, 20, 30, 40, and 50%. The remainder of the formulations studied consisted of a combination of surfactant and co-surfactant. Labrasol® (surfactant) and lauroglycol 90® (co-surfactant) were evaluated at levels of 10 to 80%. The titration method was adopted for the determination of self-emulsifying region. A 0.1 mL quantity of the SEF was pipetted into a 10 mL beaker. Drop-wise quantities of Milli-Q water (Millipore, USA) filtered through a 0.22 micrometer filter were introduced into the beaker until a stable transparent system was formed. SEF formulations resulting in phase separation or non-transparent emulsions were discarded. The different amounts of the ingredients that contributed to transparent SEFs were determined and a phase diagram plotted using JMP version 4.0.4 software (SAS Institute Inc).

Assay of CSIC

A liquid chromatography method was used to assay CSIC. A Waters Acquity UPLC was employed. A 1 mg quantity of CSIC was dissolved in 5 mL of Acetonitrile. From the stock solution serial dilutions were made to attain the concentration range of 10, 20, 50, 100 and 150 μg/mL respectively. The corresponding Area under the curve values and the resultant calibration curve were determined using the UPLC machine (Acquity UPLC,Waters USA). CSIC was separated with a C18 (2.1 × 50 mm, 1.7 micrometer) column using a mobile phase of 0.05 v/v% trifluoroacetic acid (TFA) in acetonitrile and 0.08 v/v% of TFA in water at a flow rate of 0.4 ml/min. UV detection was at 302 nm. CSIC eluted at 6 min under these conditions.

Solubility of CSIC in triacetin

An excess quantity of CSIC was introduced into a vial containing triacetin (oil). The suspension was first vortexed for 10 min and subsequently mixed intermittently for 5 h using a mechanical shaker, prior to storage for 24 h. Using a 0.1 micrometer filter (Fisher Scientific, USA) 20 μL of the suspension was double-filtered, diluted to 1 mL with acetonitrile and assayed for CSIC content using the UPLC method described above. A total of seven replicate samples were analyzed.

Differential scanning calorimetry

A 2–10 mg quantity of CSIC powder was sealed in a small aluminum pan using a mechanical punch (Perkin Elmer, USA). A sealed empty pan served as control over the temperature range 30 - 400°C. The samples were analyzed using the software, Pyris Series- DSC 7. DSC enabled the determination of melting point of CSIC.

Formulation of CSIC SEFs

From the experiment described under pseudo ternary phase diagram section the optimal SEF formulations were identified as those which did not result in phase separation and maintained transparency. These formulations are detailed in Table 1. CSIC was combined with each of these formulations at the ratio 0.5 mg CSIC/0.3 ml SEF. Briefly, 0.5 mg CSIC was mixed with triacetin, and then the appropriate amounts of surfactant and co-surfactant were added sequentially with stirring until a homogenous mix was achieved.

Characterization of CSIC SEFs

The content of CSIC in each formulation was determined. In these studies a 0.3 mL quantity of SEF was sampled from each of the five formulations described in Table 1 and diluted to 1 mL with acetonitrile. After shaking to ensure complete mixing, the mixtures were assayed for CSIC content using the described UPLC method. Each experiment was carried out in triplicates. Additionally viscosity, droplet size, polydispersity index and zeta potential were also determined for each formulation. Viscosity was measured using 0.5 ml samples with a DV-111 ultra programmable Rheometer (Brookfield Engineering Labs, USA) equipped with a CPE 51 Spindle. Data were calculated with Rheocalc V3.1-2 software. Triplicate determinations were made. A Malvern Zeta Sizer (Malvern Instruments Ltd., UK) was used to determine droplet size, polydispersity index and zeta potential. In these studies transparent emulsions were prepared by gentle agitation of the anhydrous SEF with an appropriate quantity of water. Droplet size was evaluated using cuvette containing 2.5 ml of the nano/microemulsion, and zeta potential was measured using 1 ml in capillary cuvettes. All measurements were performed in triplicates.

Table 1 The % concentrations (w/w) of the different components in stable and transparent emulsions

Formulation	Oil:surfactant: cosurfactant	Oil (% w/w)	Surfactant/ cosurfactant mix (%w/w)	Water (%w/w)
A	10:80:10	1.2	8.6	90.2
B	10:70:20	1.8	12.5	85.7
C	20:70:10	2.7	8.5	88.8
D	20:60:20	2.7	8.4	88.9
E	30:60:10	5.4	9.8	84.8

Stability studies for CSIC SEFs

Stability testing for each of the CSIC formulations was evaluated. In these studies each of the CSIC formulations was introduced into vials and stored under three different conditions: (1) 25°C and 60% relative humidity (RH) using a Caron 6010 Humidity Chamber, (2) 40°C and 86% RH using a Caron 6010 Humidity Chamber, and (3) 50°C (Former Scientific Inc., U.S.A). Drug content was determined weekly over a four week period. Additionally stability under stressed conditions was evaluated. Firstly, the effect of centrifugation was studied to evaluate potential metastable conditions, including phase separation and/or drug precipitation. This was done by centrifuging each CSIC formulation at 2000 rpm for 30 min and visually observing for phase separation and drug precipitation. Secondly, the formulations were also stressed by temperature cycling. In brief, the formulations were subjected to a cycle of 12 h refrigeration (4°C) and 12 h storage at room temperature (25°C) for a period of one week. Formulations were then evaluated visually for phase separation or drug precipitation.

Emulsification time

An adaptation of the method of Koo et al. [23] was used. A 0.3 mL quantity of the SEF was introduced into a beaker containing 200 mL milli-Q water at 37°C. The sample was stirred and visually monitored to determine the time for complete emulsification.

Drug release/dispersion studies

Drug release/dispersion was measured using a Sotax dissolution apparatus (Sotax CP 7, USA). The dissolution chambers were filled with 100 mL 0.1 N HCl. Analyses were carried out at 37°C and drug content evaluated at 3 min intervals over 40 min.

Bioactivity testing

Two types of bioactivity tests were carried out, (i) standard antiviral assessments in which cells were simultaneously exposed to varying concentrations of drug and HIV, with drug being present throughout the infection process, and (ii) protective or memory effect assessments in which cells were pretreated with varying concentrations of drug for 16 h, then exogenous drug was removed by extensive washing and the cells exposed to HIV in the absence of exogenous drug. HIV replication was evaluated in single replication cycle HIV assays, using P4R5 HIV infection indicator cells (from Dr. John Mellors, University of Pittsburgh). Cells were maintained in DMEM/10% FBS supplemented with puromycin (0.5 g/mL). P4R5 cells express CD4, CXCR4 and CCR5 as well as a β-galactosidase reporter gene under the control of an HIV LTR promoter [24]. Viral infectivity was assessed in 96-well micro-plate assays using P4R5 cells (5x10^{3}cells/well). Cells were inoculated with 25 ng HIV-1 p24/well and the extent of infection was evaluated 48 h post-infection using fluorescence-based β-galactosidase detection assay. Briefly, infected cells were washed, then incubated with 100 L lysis buffer (60 mM Na_2HPO_4, 40 mM NaH_2PO_4 (pH 7.2), 1 mM $MgSO_4$, 100 mM -mercaptoethanol, 2% [v/v] Triton X-100) for 1 h at 37°C. β-Galactosidase activity was assessed by addition of 50 L 4-MUG to a final concentration of 0.5 mM, incubation for 1 h at 37°C, and then quenched with 150 L 0.2 M Na_2CO_3, pH 11.2. Fluorescence intensity was assessed with a SPECTRA max GEMINI XS dual-scanning micro-plate spectrofluorometer (Molecular Devices, Sunnyvale, CA) using an excitation wavelength of 355 nm and an emission wavelength of 480 nm, with cutoff filter set to 475 nm.

Statistics

Results were presented as the mean ± standard deviation. One-way analysis of variance (ANOVA) was employed in the determination of statistical significance using Graph Pad Instat Demo (Graph pad software, Inc., USA). $P < 0.05$ was considered statistically significant.

Results

Pseudo ternary phase diagram

Of the 30 formulations tested, only five (A-E) (Table 1) formed transparent micro/nano-emulsions without phase separation. These were evaluated as potential SEFs for CSIC. The pseudo ternary phase diagram is an important preliminary strategy adopted in SEFs to delineate self-emulsifying regions [11]. Preparation of SEFs without a preliminary phase diagram construction may result in loss of formulation stability after a period of storage. The pseudo ternary phase diagram is shown in Figure 1.

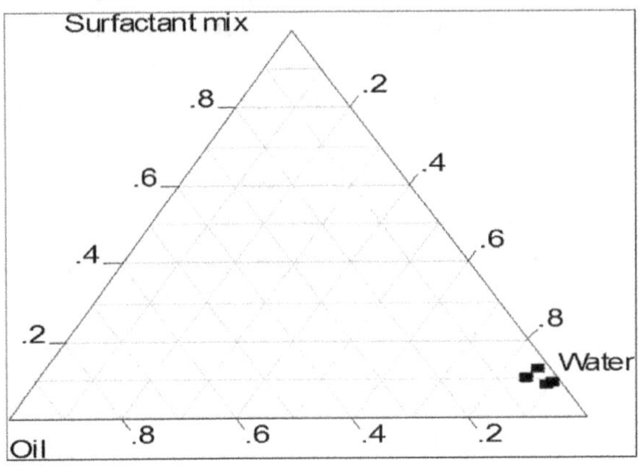

Figure 1 Pseudo-ternary phase diagram for oil, surfactant mix and water.

Solubility, stability and drug content

The mean solubility of CSIC in triacetin was 0.75 ± 0.04 mg/mL. This limited the unit dose of the formulation to 0.5 mg CSIC. Solubility assessments in the surfactants were not done, since the triacetin oil component was the primary determinant for the drug to remain intact in the droplet post-emulsification. The drug content of the SEFs was between 0.42-0.48 mg (83-93%) (Table 2). Studies to evaluate the effect of temperature and relative humidity on the stability of CSIC in the SEFs showed no substantial changes in CSIC content over the 4 week duration of the experiment (Table 3). Differential scanning calorimetry of CSIC showed a melting peak of 243.67°C.

Droplet size, polydispersity index, zeta potential, viscosity and emulsification time

One-Way Analysis of Variance (ANOVA)-based Tukey-Kramer multiple comparisons Test showed that the droplet sizes of placebo and drug-loaded formulations A, C and E respectively were significantly ($p < 0.05$) smaller than those of formulations B and D (Table 4). Furthermore ANOVA-based Student-Newman-Keuls Multiple Comparisons Test revealed that drug-loading did not significantly ($p < 0.05$) affect the droplet sizes of the formulations in comparison with placebo batches (Table 4). Placebo formulation D showed significantly ($p < 0.05$) higher PDI values (Table 4) than those of A, C and E, while B was only significantly ($p < 0.05$) higher than C and E. Drug-loaded formulations A, C and E recorded significantly ($p < 0.05$) lower PDI than B and D. On the contrary, drug-loading did not significantly ($p < 0.05$) contribute to increased PDI. Low polydispersity indices are preferable as emulsions with higher values may be prone to instability. Negative zeta potential often associated with oil-in-water emulsions was generally the case, with minor variations amongst the batches. The viscosity values of the SEFs were 51mpa.s, 48.8mpa.s, 44.3mpa.s, 37.8mpa.s, and 35.7mpa.s for formulations A through E respectively. All formulations displayed a Newtonian flow pattern. The rate of emulsification was too fast (within a few seconds) to be accurately measured. The high rate of emulsification precluded determination of a dissolution profile, as the formulations showed 100% drug release within the earliest time point measured (3 minutes).

Table 2 Drug content (% CSIC recovery) in various SEFs

Formulation	Oil:surfactant: cosurfactant	Drug assay content	
		(mg)	% recovery
A	10:80:10	0.468 ± 0.0006	93.62
B	10:70:20	0.436 ± 0.0028	87.12
C	20:70:10	0.453 ± 0.002	90.58
D	20:60:20	0.449 ± 0.0002	89.88
E	30:60:10	0.420 ± 0.001	83.98

Table 3 Thermal stability of CSIC in CSIC SEF

FC[1]	Week 0	Amount of CSIC remaining (mg)								
		Week 2			Week 3			Week 4		
		25°C	40°C	50°C	25°C	40°C	50°C	25°C	40°C	50°C
A	0.47	0.40 ± 0.01	0.45 ± 0.002	0.48 ± 0.02	0.36 ± 0.001	0.37 ± 0.01	0.39 ± 0.03	0.39 ± 0.04	0.47 ± 0.01	0.49 ± 0.03
B	0.44	0.40 ± 0.008	0.45 ± 0	0.50 ± 0.1	0.35 ± 0.01	0.37 ± 0.02	0.40 ± 0.01	0.39 ± 0.02	0.47 ± 0.02	0.47 ± 0.02
C	0.45	0.414 ± 0.001	0.50 ± 0.01	0.50 ± 0.1	0.36 ± 0	0.39 ± 0.01	0.38 ± 0.02	0.40 ± 0.003	0.48 ± 0.003	0.46 ± 0.02
D	0.45	0.42 ± 0.004	0.45 ± 0.01	0.46 ± 0.01	0.34 ± 0.02	0.39 ± 0.02	0.4 ± 0.01	0.42 ± 0.004	0.46 ± 0.01	0.50 ± 0.001
E	0.42	0.39 ± 0.001	0.44 ± 0.04	0.43 ± 0.01	0.34 ± 0.01	0.36 ± 0.01	0.38 ± 0.01	0.39 ± 0.001	0.44 ± 0.002	0.47 ± 0.005

1 = Formulation code.

Bioactivity studies

In order to establish that the formulation did not result in loss of bioactivity, *in vitro* anti HIV testing was conducted using the five formulations (A-E). Figure 2 illustrates the antiviral activity for each of the formulations tested. This data showed that the formulations did not result in any loss of antiretroviral bioactivity when compared to unformulated drug substance. Furthermore, the highest concentration tested in these experiments was 0.5 μM. No toxicity was seen at this level indicating that the SEFs did not result in increased toxicity at the 0.5 μM level of dosing. The "memory effect" of the SEFs at 0.1, 1.0, and 10 μM was also tested. Cells were incubated with these concentrations for 16 h, then washed and exposed to HIV. All SEFs were very toxic at 10 μM, and partially toxic at 1 μM. CSIC alone was not toxic at any of these concentrations. All CSIC samples either tested unformulated or in SEFs gave complete protection without discernible toxicity at 0.1 μM. The potent protective or memory effect exerted by the SEFs at 0.1 μM showed that the cells maintained ready access to the formulated drug, essentially similar to that of the free unformulated CSIC. On the contrary when the placebo SEFs, were tested there was no anti-HIV activity.

Discussion

In this study it was found that higher oil and lower surfactant ratios (eg, formulation D) provided a narrow transition window from anhydrous to transparent nano-emulsion than did lower oil and higher surfactant ratios (eg, formulation A). Figure 1 clearly portrays a narrow self-emulsifying region, since only a few formulations formed stable micro/nano-emulsions upon titration with water. Out of the 30 batches evaluated only 5 formed transparent emulsions upon aqueous dilution. The rest either witnessed phase separation or formed nontransparent emulsions with outrageous droplet sizes. Thus they were excluded. Our choice of the five stable batches was for comparative purposes.

The determination of the amount of drug that could be dissolved in the anhydrous emulsion is crucial to avoid post-formulation drug precipitation either during storage or following *in vivo* dispersion in the aqueous GIT environment [21,25]. CSIC was found to dissolve very slowly, but once dissolved in the anhydrous emulsion it did not precipitate out. Dissolution in SEF involves molecular interaction with the excipients that renders the crystalline drug amorphous [26]. The 0.75 mg solubility in triacetin motivated the choice of 0.5 mg per dose of SEF. Our bioactivity studies results have confirmed 0.5 mg as pharmacologically effective. However, establishment of minimum effective concentration and unit dose is anticipated in our next investigation.

Experimental evaluations of the thermodynamic stability of SEFs are important to assess the possibility of drug precipitation or phase separation after centrifugation or repeated refrigeration/warming cycles. With conventional emulsions, the index of stability is the absence of phase separation after centrifugation [27], but in SEFs an additional organoleptic index includes the presence/

Table 4 Droplet size, zeta potential and polydispersity index values for the nano/micro-emulsions

[1]FC	Placebo nano/micro-emulsion			Drug-loaded nano/micro-emulsion		
	Droplet size (nm)	Polydispersity index	Zeta potential (-)(mV)	Droplet size (nm)	Polydispersity index	Zeta potential (-)(mV)
A	40.36 ± 0.69	0.159 ± 0.001	0.635 ± 0.03	67.84 ± 1.6	0.283 ± 0.001	0.635 ± 0.01
B	296.5 ± 54	0.432 ±0.16	0.979 ± 0.002	269 ± 6.1	0.533 ± 0.003	1.58 ± 0.07
C	41.1 ± 0.23	0.134 ± 0.01	1.32 ± 0.02	58.6 ± 0.3	0.283 ± 0.004	1.72 ± 0.04
D	288.5 ± 13	0.559 ± 0.02	1.51 ± 0.01	286 ± 11	0.587 ± 0.001	2.18 ± 0.08
E	52.8 ± 1.4	0.136 ± 0.005	0.970 ± 0.002	65.39 ± 0.9	0.251 ± 0.003	2.25 ± 0.02

1 = Formulation code.

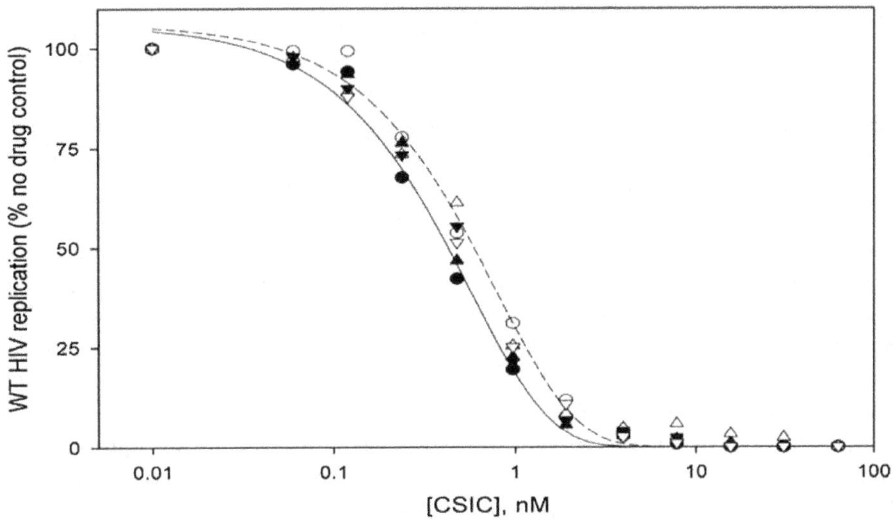

Figure 2 Antiviral activity of CSIC powder and CSIC SEF.

absence of drug precipitate. All the SEFs maintained thermodynamic stability both in the centrifugation and refrigeration/warming cycle protocols. This may be a clue that this formulation strategy is superior to macro-emulsions or colloidal formulations [5,11]. Furthermore at different temperature and humidity conditions CSIC demonstrated stability in the SEFs. The high melting point of CSIC (Figure 3) was an indication of thermal stability or non-heat sensitivity. This may be why stability studies lacked evidence of thermal drug degradation.

In all the formulations, as the concentrations of oil and surfactant were simultaneously increased and decreased respectively, co-surfactant was held at a fixed concentration of either 10% (formulations A, C, E) or 20% (formulations B, D) (Table 1). It thus appears that droplet size may be related to the co-surfactant concentration used in the formulation; larger droplet sizes resulted from 20% co-surfactant concentration. The contribution of co-surfactant to droplet size may be connected to its supportive functionality during emulsification, where it

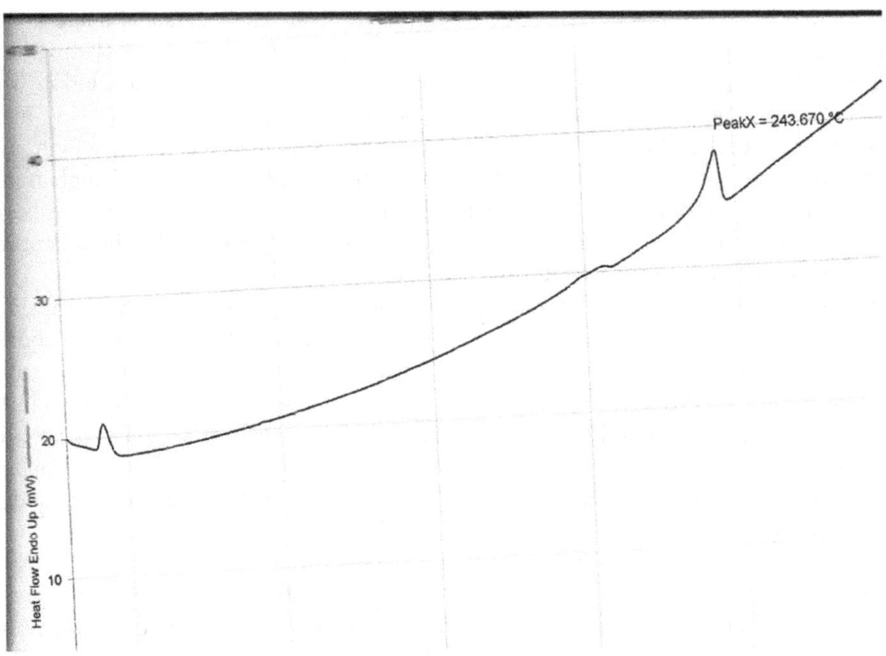

Figure 3 DSC thermogram for CSIC.

stabilizes the interfacial role of the surfactant. In micro-emulsions, the interfacial tension is so low that the interfacial energy assumes a similar or lower value than the entropy of dispersion. This renders the free energy zero or negative [28,29]. The use of only one surfactant may hardly achieve transient negative interfacial tension and fluid interfacial film; hence the need for incorporation of a co-surfactant [30]. Generally, co-surfactants lower the interfacial bending stress and consequently predispose the interfacial film to possess enough flexibility to assume various curvatures required for nano/micro-emulsion formation over a wide range of compositions [11,31]. In addition, lauroglycol 90® has a potential dual role of co-surfactant and oil. Higher co-surfactant concentration may have simultaneously increased the interfacial thickness and curvature flexibility of the emulsion droplets with consequent size enlargement. Although the three constituents were miscible, upon emulsification in aqueous phase the cosurfactant with low HLB as the oil may have had better interaction with the oil than the surfactant (with high HLB) and the oil. The polar head of the surfactant may have protruded towards and interacted more with the aqueous medium.

During emulsification more work and energy may be required for droplet formation in high drug-loaded than placebo formulations. Apparently the placebo formulations may ultimately offer lower resistance in aqueous medium during the emulsification process and form smaller droplets than the drug-loaded ones. However in this present investigation the low drug loading (0.5 mg/dose) did not impel significant droplet size or PDI increase [32] probably because little resistance may have been posed.

The oil constituent of the SEFs may be responsible for the negative zeta potential of the nano/micro-emulsions [33]. The viscosity of SEFs is critical during dispersion in aqueous phase. Higher viscosities tend to slow down the emulsification rate which may be detrimental when faster *in vivo* drug release and smooth post-absorption bioavailability profiles are crucial. The low values recorded by the SEF formulations in the present study were low enough to preclude the possibility of erratic or slow self-emulsification.

Self-emulsification occurs when the entropy change favoring dispersion is more than the energy needed to increase the surface area of the dispersion [34,35]. Two minutes has been suggested as an upper acceptable limit for emulsification time [23]; thus the SEFs of the present work were well within this limit. High emulsification rate was responsible for 100% drug release within three minutes.

For an orally administered drug, gastrointestinal and pharmaceutical barriers must be overcome before absorption can take place. Aqueous solubility of the drug in question is a crucial factor because only drug in solution is destined for possible absorption [26]. Since the dissolution rate is the rate-determining step to absorption of poorly soluble drugs, improvement on aqueous solubility will promote absorption and bioavailability [4,36]. Consequently, only the relative quantity of drug that emerges after systemic absorption may be available at the receptor site for pharmacological activity. The bioactivity investigation conducted within this study attempted to predict the absorption status of CSIC. It did not account for the *in vivo* gastrointestinal interactions between drug, food and aqueous GIT fluid. The unformulated CSIC had similar antiviral activity as the CSIC SEF formulations. However the CSIC powder was first dissolved in an aqueous solution of dimethyl sulphoxide (DMSO) since it is poorly water soluble. Otherwise, unaided dispersion in water would be unsolubilised and difficult to acces the cells. This may be the predictable *in vivo* fate when administered orally in that form. The stock solution of the CSIC in DMSO was diluted with excess water and vigorously shaken otherwise drug crystallization would take place. Obviously our SEF formulation offers a less tedious and more commercially viable approach. Two important observations made in our study indicated CSIC SEFs' therapeutic and prophylactic potentials. Bioactivity established at 0.5 μM and cell protection at, 0.1 μM essentially corroborate drug permeability and activity within the cells. Consequently in the GIT the formulation may witness smooth absorption via the villi of the small intestine. Suffice it to say that of utmost significance was the established improvement on CSIC aqueous solubility which may overcome barrier to its further development as an HIV therapeutic agent [15,19]. Poor water solubility of some antiretroviral drugs may predispose to impaired and inconsistent dissolution within the GIT and consequent erratic absorption. This may cause delay in reaching peak plasma concentration and predispose to sublethal drug concentration. Subpharmacological concentrations may induce resistance. The burden of resistance associated with some hydrophobic antiretrovirals may be due to the above reason.

These studies suggest that this formulation approach could address pharmaceutical product development limitations for the anti-HIV drug candidate CSIC such as poor aqueous solubility and cellular permeability. Furthermore this formulation strategy provides a platform which can be extended to other hydrophobic anti-retroviral agents facilitating their advancement in development.

Conclusion

Further development of CSIC had been stalled due to poor aqueous solubility and low bioavailability. However, in these studies a self-emulsifying oil formulation has been shown to be a reliable formulation approach for the improvement of CSIC aqueous solubility. The *in vitro* antiretroviral bioactivity of the CSIC SEF formulations developed was also established. We therefore conclude that self-emulsifying oil formulation may provide improved bioavailability for this poorly soluble drug making it a viable drug candidate for evaluation in HIV therapy. Further research works are ongoing in our laboratory. Areas of further investigative concern include use of wider spectrum of surfactants, cosurfactants and oils. Extensive stability and bioavailability studies are also contemplated.

Competing interests

The authors declare that they have no conflict of interest to declare.

Authors' contributions

ONC, RLC, ACM and ECO were involved in the conception, design and preparation of self-emulsifying oil formulations. All the authors were involved in the preparation and editing of the manuscript. PMA designed and carried out the bioactivity studies. All authors read and approved the final manuscript.

Acknowledgements

This work was funded in part by the STEP-B project, University of Nigeria, Nsukka, Nigeria and by NIH NIAID grants AI079801 and AI082623. Labrasol® and lauroglycol 90® were free samples from Gattefosse, USA. The work was arranged by Dr. Adeyeye to be carried out in Dr. Rohan's lab at the Magee Women's Research Institute at the University of Pittsburgh.

Author details

[1]Department of Pharmaceutical Technology and Industrial Pharmacy, Faculty of Pharmaceutical Sciences, University of Nigeria, Nsukka, Nigeria. [2]Department of Pharmaceutical Sciences, School of Pharmacy, Magee Womens Research Institute, University of Pittsburgh, Pittsburgh, PA, USA. [3]Department of Biopharmaceutical Sciences, College of Pharmacy, Roosevelt University Schaumburg, Shaumburgh, IL, USA. [4]Department of Microbiology and Molecular Genetics, School of Medicine, University of Pittsburgh, Pittsburgh, PA, USA. [5]Department of Pharmaceutical Microbiology and Biotechnology, Faculty of Pharmaceutical Sciences, Nnamdi Azikiwe university, Awka, Anambra, Nigeria.

References

1. Tang B, Cheng G, Gu J, Xu C: **Development of solid self-emulsifying drug delivery systems: preparation techniques and dosage forms.** *Drg Disc Tod* 2008, **13**:13–14.
2. Kommuru TR, Gurley B, Khan MA, Reddy IK: **Self-emulsifyingdrug delivery systems (SEDDS) of coenzyme Q10: formulationdevelopment and bioavailability assessment.** *Int J Pharm* 2001, **212**:233–246.
3. Tang J, Sun J, He Z: **Self-emulsifying drug delivery systems: Strategy for improving oral delivery of poorly soluble drugs.** *Curr Drg Ther* 2007, **2**:85–93.
4. Valizadeh H, Zakeri-Milani P, Barzegar-Jalali M, Mohammadi G, Danesh-Bahreini M, Adibkia K, Nokhodchi A: **Preparation and characterization of solid dispersions of piroxicam with hydrophilic carriers.** *Drug Dev Ind Pharm* 2007, **33**(1):45–56.
5. Patel HM, Suhagia BN, Shah SA, Rathod IS, Parmar VK: **Preparation and characterization of etoricoxib-b-cyclodextrin complexes prepared by the kneading method.** *Acta Pharm* 2007, **57**:351–359.
6. Che E, Zheng X, Sun C, Chang D, Jiang T, Wang S: **Drug nanocrystals: a state of the art formulation strategy for preparing the poorly water-soluble drugs.** *Asian Journ Pharm Scs* 2012, **7**(2):85–95.
7. Joshi M, Pathak S, Sharma S, Patravale V: **Solid microemulsion preconcentrate (NanOsorb) of artemether for effective treatment of malaria.** *Int J Pharm* 2008, **362**:172–178.
8. Watnasirichaikul S, Davies NM, Rades T, Tucker IG: **Preparation of Biodegradable insulin nanocapsules from biocompatible microemulsions.** *Pharm Res* 2000, **17**:6.
9. Lawrence MJ, Rees GD: **Microemulsion-based media as novel drug delivery systems.** *Adv Drug Deliv Rev* 2000, **45**:89–121.
10. Shafiq S, Faiyaz S, Sushma T, Farhan JA, Khar RK, Ali M: **Development and bioavailability assessment of ramipril nanoemulsion formulation.** *Eur J Pharm Biopharm* 2007, **66**:227–243.
11. Talegaonkar S, Azeem A, Ahmad FJ, Khar RK, Pathan SA, Khan ZI: **Microemulsions: a novel approach to enhanced drug delivery.** *Recent Pat Drug Deliv Formul* 2008, **2**:238–257.
12. Pouton CW, Porter JH: **Formulation of lipid-based delivery systems for oral administration: materials, methods and strategies.** *Adv Drug Deliv Rev* 2008, **60**:625–637.
13. Sha X, Wu J, Chen Y, Fang X: **Self-microemulsifying drug-delivery system for improved oral bioavailability of probucol: preparation and evaluation.** *Int Journ Nanomed* 2012, **7**:705–712.
14. Stegemanna S, Leveillerb F: **When poor solubility becomes an issue: from early stage to proof of concept.** *Eur Journ Pharm Sci* 2007, **31**:249–261.
15. Motakis D, Parniak MA: **A tight-binding mode of inhibition is essential for anti-human immunodeficiency virus type 1 virucidal activity of nonnucleoside reverse transcriptase inhibitors.** *Antim Agent Chem* 2002, **6**(46):1851–1856.
16. Hari BV, Dhevendaran K, Narayanan N: **Development of Efavirenz nanoparticle for enhanced efficiency of anti-retroviral therapy against HIV and AIDS.** *BMC Infect Dis* 2012, **12**(Suppl 1):7.
17. Kasim NA, Whitehouse M, Ramachandran C, Bermejo M, Lennernaes H, Hussain AS, Junginger HE, Stavchansky SA, Midha KK, Shah VP, *et al*: **Molecular properties of WHO essential drugs and provisional biopharmaceutical classification.** *Mol Pharm* 2004, **1**:85–96.
18. Williams TM, Ciccaro TM, MacTough SC, Rooney CS, Balani SC, Condra JH, Emini EA, Goldman ME, Greenlee WJ, Kaufman LR, *et al*: **5-Chloro-3-(phenylsulfonyl)indole-2-carboxamide: a novel, non-nucleoside inhibitor of HIV-1 reverse transcriptase.** *J Med Chem* 1993, **36**:1291–1294.
19. Roehr B: **Fashioning new tools to deter HIV transmission.** *J Int Assoc Phys AIDS Care* 2000:157–168.
20. Araya H, Tomita M, Hayashi M: **The novel formulation design of self-emulsifying drug delivery systems (SEDDS) type o/w microemulsion 11: stable gastrointestinal absorption of a poorly water soluble new compound, ER-1258 in bile-fistula rats.** *Drug Metab Pharmacokinet* 2005, **20**(4):257–267.
21. Pouton CW: **Formulation of poorly water-soluble drugs for oral administration: physicochemical and physiological issues and the lipid formulation classification system.** *Europ J Pharm Sci* 2006, **29**:278–287.
22. Yu LX, Amidon GL, Polli JE, Zhao H, Mehta MU, Conner DP, Shah VP, Lesko LJ, Chen ML, Lee VH, *et al*: **Biopharmaceutics classification system: the scientific basis for biowaiver extensions.** *Pharm Res* 2002, **19**:921–925.
23. Khoo SM, Humberstone AJ, Porter CJ, Edwards GA, Charman WN: **Formulation design and bioavailability assessment of lipidicselfemulsifying formulations of halofantrine.** *Int J Pharm* 1998, **167**:155–164.
24. Munk C, Brandt SM, Lucero G, Landau NR: **A dominant block to HIV-1 replication at reverse transcription in simian cells.** *Proc Natl Acad Sci USA* 2002, **99**(21):13843–13848.
25. Patel AR, Vavia PR: **Preparation and *in vivo* evaluation of SMEDDS (Self-microemulsifying drug delivery system) containing fenofibrate.** *AAPS J* 2007, **3**:41.
26. Sinha S, Ali M, Baboota S, Ahuja A, Kumar A, Ali J: **Solid dispersion as an approach for bioavailability enhancement of poorly water-soluble drug ritonavir.** *AAPS PharmSciTech* 2010, **11**(2):518–527.
27. Wilkinson JB, Moore RJ: *Emulsions. In Harry's cosmeticology.* 7th edn, Burnt Mill Essex UK: George Godwin publishers, Longman House; 1982.
28. Hoar TP, Schulman JH: **Transparent water-in-oil dispersions: the oleopathic hydro-micelle.** *Nature* 1943, **152**:102–103.
29. Patel MR, Patel RB, Parikh JR, Bhatt KK, Kundawala AJ: **Microemulsions: as novel drug delivery vehicle.** *Latest Reviews* 2007, **5**:6.
30. Baboota S, Shakeel F, Ahuja A, Ali J, Shafiq S: **Design, development and evaluation of novel nanoemulsion formulations for transdermal potential of celecoxib.** *Acta Pharm* 2007, **57**:315–332.
31. Kawakami K, Yoshikawa T, Moroto Y, Kanaoka E, Takahashi K, Nishihara Y, Masuda K: **Microemulsion formulation for enhanced absorption of poorly soluble drugs, I. Prescription design.** *J Control Release* 2002, **81**:65–74.
32. Dixit AR, Rajput SJ, Patel SG: **Preparation and bioavailability assessment of SMEDDS containing valsartan.** *AAPS Pharm Sci Tech* 2010, **11**(1):314–321.

33. Gershanik T, Benita S: **Positively-charged self-emulsifying oil formulation for improving oral bioavailability of progesterone.** *Pharm Dev Technol* 1996, **1**:147–157.
34. Reiss H: **Entropy-induced dispersion of bulk liquids.** *J Colloids Interface Sci* 1975, **53**:61–70.
35. Lam AC, Schechter RS: **The theory of diffusion in microemulsions.** *J Colloid Interface Sci* 1987, **120**:56–63.
36. Hecqa J, Deleers M, Fanara D, Vranckx H, Amighi K: **Preparation and characterization of nanocrystals for solubility and dissolution rate enhancement of nifedipine.** *Int J Pharm* 2005, **299**:167–177.

Utility of the point of care CD4 analyzer, PIMA, to enumerate CD4 counts in the field settings

Madhuri Thakar[1*], Bharati Mahajan[1], Nawaj Shaikh[1], Salman Bagwan[1], Suvarna Sane[1], Sandhya Kabra[2], Bharat Rewari[2], Mohamad Shaukat[2], Namita Singh[3], Peter Trevor[3] and Ramesh Paranjape[1]

Abstract

Background: In resource limited settings non-availability of CD4 count facility at the site could adversely affect the ART roll out programme. Point of care CD4 enumerating equipments can make the CD4 count available at the site of care and improve the patients' management considerably. This study is aimed at determining the utility of a Point of Care PIMA CD4 analyzer (Alere, Germany) in the field settings in India.

Method: The blood samples were collected from 1790 participants at 21 ART centers from different parts of the country and tested using PIMA and the reference methods (FACSCalibur, FACSCount and CyFlow SL3). The paired finger prick and venous blood samples from 175 participants were tested by the PIMA CD4 Analyzer and then by FACSCalibur.

Result: The CD4 counts obtained by PIMA CD4 analyzer showed excellent correlation with the counts obtained by the reference methods; for venous blood the Pearson's r was 0.921, $p < 0.001$ and the relative bias was 0.2% (range: -42 to 42%) and for finger prick samples, the Pearson's r was 0.856 and the relative bias was −9.1% (range: -46% to 27%). For CD4 ranges; <250, 251–350, 351–500 and >500 cells/mm3, the differences in the median CD4 counts obtained by the reference method and the PIMA analyzer were not significant ($P > 0.05$) and the relative bias were low (−7 to 5.1%). The Intermachine comparison showed variation within the acceptable limit of%CV of 10%.

Conclusion: In the field settings, the POC PIMA CD4 analyzer gave CD4 counts comparable to the reference methods for all CD4 ranges. The POC equipment could identify the patients eligible for ART in 91% cases. Adequate training is necessary for finger prick sample collection for optimum results. Decentralization of CD4 testing by making the CD4 counts available at primary health centers, especially in remote areas with minimum or no infrastructure would reduce the missed visits and improve adherence of the patients.

Keywords: CD4+ T-cell count, HIV, Point-of-care, PIMA CD4 analyzer

Introduction

CD4 count estimation is a mainstay of monitoring the HIV disease progression and initiation and monitoring of anti-retroviral treatment (ART) [1-4]. The World Health Organization (WHO) has recommended using CD4 counts for initiation and monitoring of ART in HIV infected individuals in recourse limited settings [1]. The scaling up of the public ART programmes increased the demand for CD4 counts globally [5]. In a resource limited setting CD4 count facility is not available in peripheral areas and often the patients need to travel long distances or the samples need to be transported to the centres where the facility for CD4 count estimation is available. This could be a barrier for expansion and decentralization of the ART programme and adherence to treatment.

A point of care CD4 assay may be able to fill this gap and help in expanding the ART services and increase adherence. The Point-Of-Care (POC) CD4 equipments will be able to give the results in a very short time on the

* Correspondence: mthakar@nariindia.org
[1]Department of Immunology, National AIDS Research Institute, G-73, MIDC, Bhosari, Pune 411 026, India

same day of collection and thus would avoid need for another visit for collecting results. PIMA CD4 analyzer (Alere) is one of the POC equipment. The closed disposable cartridge used in the analyzer contains the reagents required for the CD4+ T cell count estimation. It can also work on finger prick sample and give results within 20 minutes of the sample collection. The validation studies showed that the PIMA analyzer could give CD4 counts comparable to those obtained with the standard flow cytometers such as FACSCount and FACSCalibur [6-8]. For efficient working of the POC machines it is important to know the accuracy of the PIMA analyzer at different CD4 levels.

In the present study we assessed the feasibility of use of PIMA POC CD4 analyzer in the field setting in Indian ART programme. The PIMA CD4 analyzers were placed at 21 different ART centers in different parts of the country with maximum load of 25 patients per day. The Intermachine comparisons and repeatability of the CD4 counts were assessed using venous blood samples. The finger prick samples collected at the field settings were also tested for the accuracy of CD4 counts in comparison with the paired venous samples.

Methods

Study centres

The study was conducted at 21 ART centres having minimum (5-10/day) to moderate (25-30/day) patient load. Of these 21 centres, 2 had FACSCalibur, 13 had FACSCount (both from Becton Dickinson, USA) and 6 had CyFlow® SL3 counter from Partec, Germany. All these equipments are under the external proficiency assessment conducted with Quality Assessment and Standardization for Immunological measures relevant to HIV/AIDS, Public Health Agency, Canada (QASI) for the last three years and performing satisfactorily. Also the inter machine comparison between these equipments using fresh blood samples has been published earlier [9,10]. These equipments were considered as reference method in the study. The technologists from these centers were trained for two days for finger prick sample collection and the CD4 count estimation using PIMA analyzer including the use of calibrators. The equipments were handed over to the technologists during training.

Study participants

During June to August 2011, each centre consecutively enrolled 5 to 10 HIV positive patients for CD4 count estimation every day after obtaining written informed consent for CD4 count estimation. Approximately 100 patients were enrolled by each centre. The inclusion criteria included age between 18 to 60 years and willingness to give blood sample for CD4 count estimation.

The paired finger prick and the venous blood samples were collected at NARI, Pune from 175 HIV infected individuals who gave written informed consent for collection of finger prick samples.

Blood collection and processing

Three ml of venous blood sample was collected in K3 EDTA vacutainers. The capillary blood sample was collected from the finger tip using lancet finger stick. A puncture depth of 1.8 mm with a blade-type lancet (Sarstedt) was used to achieve sufficient capillary blood flow. The venous or the finger prick samples were first tested in the ART centre using PIMA CD4 analyzer and the results were stored in the centre. The samples were then sent to the attached laboratory for processing by the respective reference methodologies. The technicians estimating CD4 count by reference method were blinded for PIMA results. The CD4 counts obtained by the reference method were provided to the patients.

CD4 count estimation

Test method- pima™ CD4

The samples were run in the PIMA CD4 analyzer only after the normal and Low value control cartridges gave acceptable value. After collection of venous sample, 25 μl of blood was immediately added to the PIMA CD4 cartridge. In case of finger prick sample, the sample was directly collected on the cartridge. The cartridge was capped and inserted immediately into the PIMA analyzer. The PIMA analyzer works on volumetric principle. Hence every time 5 μl of blood was drawn into the detection channel of the PIMA cartridge from the blood added in the receptacle.

During the incubation, freeze-dried fluorescently labeled antibodies (anti-CD3 and anti-CD4) get mixed with the blood and the images of the CD3+ and CD4+ cells are captured by the camera and the results are then expressed as cells/μl within 20 minutes. In the study, the print out of the CD4 count obtained from the PIMA analyzer was checked by the supervisor and stored in the clinic itself.

Reference method-flow cytometry

In the laboratory, the blood samples were tested by respective reference methodology on the day of collection. The daily calibration and internal quality controls were included in every run. The samples were acquired and analyzed only when the quality control indicators were passed.

FACSCalibur (Becton Dickinson, USA)

Twenty μL of liquid antibody reagent (MultiTEST CD3 FITC, CD4 PE, CD45 PerCP, Becton Dickinson, USA) and 50 μL of whole blood was added to the TruCOUNT tube (Becton Dickinson, USA) containing the reference beads. After incubation, the RBCs were lysed using 450 µl of 1:10 diluted lysing solution for 15 minutes in the dark at ambient temperature. The stained sample was acquired on FACSCalibur (Becton Dickinson, USA) and analyzed automatically using the MultiSET software (BD Biosciences) by gating CD45+ T cells in first place and these cells were further gated in CD3 + CD4+ versus CD3 + CD4- T cells.

FACSCount (Becton Dickinson, USA)

Fifty µL of whole blood was added to FACSCount tube containing CD3 PE /CD4 PE.Cychrome (PE.Cy5) monoclonal antibodies and a known number of reference beads in a liquid format (Becton Dickinson, USA). After incubation, 50 µL of fixative (5% formaldehyde in PBS) was added. The stained sample was acquired and analyzed on the FACSCount using the automated analyzing software by gating on CD3 + CD4+ T cells.

CyFlow® SL3 (partec, Germany)

Twenty µL of whole blood and 20 µL of CD4-PE (Partec, Germany) monoclonal antibody were added to the sample tube (Partec, Germany). After incubation, 800 µl of no lyse buffer (Partec, Germany) was added into the sample tube. The stained sample was then acquired on the CyFlow SL_3. The acquired data was analyzed using the inbuilt CyView software by gating on the histogram of CD4+ T cells. The histogram and absolute counts are displayed and printed automatically.. The results were printed and stored after review.

Assessment of inter machine variation for PIMA CD4 analyzer

Before distribution of the machines to respective centers, the inter-machine variation was assessed by running the commercially available stabilized blood samples with Normal and low level CD4 count (Immuno Trol controls, Beckman Coulter, USA) and 2 freshly collected blood samples with low and high CD4 counts.

Additionally the onsite inter machine variation was assessed using the low (CD4 count range: 129 to 201 cells/mm^3) and normal (CD4 count range: 857 to 1075 cells/mm^3) level PIMA Bead standards which were used by these centers daily.

Statistical analysis

For assessing the precision as well as inter-machine variability amongst all 21 machines, the percent CV value less than 10% was considered to be an acceptable value.

The Pearson's correlation coefficient was used to estimate the strength of the correlation between the CD4 counts obtained by the PIMA CD4 analyzer and the respective reference methods. The data was analyzed using Bland-Altman analysis to find out whether the methods agree sufficiently well [11]. Since the data was collected on a wide range of CD4 counts the relative bias was calculated which is expected to normalize wide range of absolute count data and thus would allow direct comparison between PIMA and various reference methods. The relative bias was calculated by converting the ratio of the difference between the CD4 counts obtained from two machines and the average of both readings into percentages.

Similar analyses were performed for comparison of the finger prick sample with the venous sample. To determine the accuracy of the PIMA analyzer at different CD4 levels, the median values obtained for different CD4 ranges (<250, 251–350, 351–500 and >500 cells/mm^3) by both, the reference method and the PIMA analyzer were compared. The relative bias was also calculated for these CD4 ranges. To determine the clinical significance of the variations in the CD4 estimations in the decision on treatment initiation, the sensitivity and specificity of PIMA CD4 analyzer to identify patients requiring ART (CD4 count < 350 cells/µL) was determined.

Results

Before distribution, the inter machine variation for all 21 machines was assessed using fresh as well as stabilized blood samples with high and low CD4 counts. Using the stabilized blood samples, the% CV was found to be 4% and 3% for low (130 cells/mm^3) and high (649 cells/mm^3) Immuno Trol controls respectively. Whereas for the freshly collected samples, the%CV was 10% for low count (180 cells/ mm^3) and 8% for the normal count (749 cells/mm^3). When the machines were installed on site, the onsite variation was assessed by the values of low and normal level PIMA Bead standards which were used by all centers daily before processing the samples. The mean% CV of all the centers for low control was 2.3 (range 0.67 -7.59) where as the mean%CV for high control was 1.6 (range: 0.39- 7.19). The data collected for the inter machine comparison between the three reference analyzers at a single center at two different out-patient clinics showed that the% CV between these analyzers was 8% with a range of 2.4% to 9% (N = 25, range of CD4 count: 114–965).

A total of 1790 participants were enrolled in the study (958 Male and 832 Female). The median age of the participants was 36 years (range: 19 to 55 years). The data showed excellent correlation between the CD4 counts obtained by PIMA CD4 analyzer and the respective reference methods (N = 1790, r = 0.921, p < 0.001, Figure 1A) at all centers. The Bland Altman plot analysis for the agreement between the values obtained with PIMA CD4 analyzer and the respective reference methods showed low relative bias of 0.2% (Mean ± SD: -42 to 42) (Figure 1B). The CD4 counts obtained using individual reference

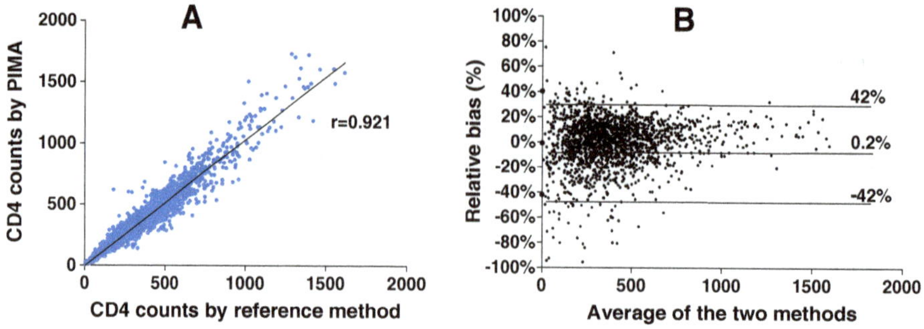

Figure 1 Comparison of the CD4 counts obtained by PIMA analyzer and reference methods using venous blood from 1790 samples. Figure 1**A**: Linear regression analysis: The CD4 counts obtained by PIMA CD4 analyzer at 21 centers are plotted on Y axis and the counts obtained by the respective reference methods are plotted on X axis. Figure 1**B**: The agreement analysis using the Bland Altman plots. The percent relative bias for PIMA analyzer and the respective reference method is plotted on the Y axis and the average of the CD4 count by both the methods is plotted on X axis. The black line represents the mean% relative bias where as the blue lines represent the range of Mean ± SD.

methods also showed good correlation with the counts obtained using PIMA CD4 analyzer FACSCount ($r = 0.983$, $P < 0.01$), FACSCalibur ($r = 0.988$, $P < 0.01$) and Cyflow SL3 ($r = 0.977$, $P < 0.01$). The CD4 counts obtained using PIMA analyzer were compared with those obtained using either of the three reference methods at different clinically relevant CD4 levels such as <250, 251–350, 351–500 and >500 cells/mm^3 (Table 1). The differences in the median CD4 counts obtained by the reference method and the PIMA analyzer were not significant ($P > 0.05$) for all CD4 ranges. The relative bias was also ranged between −7 to 5.1%.

WHO recommends to initiate ART at CD4 count < 350 cells/mm^3(1). Hence, the sensitivity and specificity of the PIMA CD4 analyzer to identify patients with CD4 count <350 cells/mm^3 was found to be 91% indicating that the chances of 9% wrong counts. When the data within the CD4 range of 251–500 cells/mm3 was assessed it was observed that 50% of the mismatched values were within the 320 to 380 cells/mm^3. The data was analyzed for individual reference analyzer (Table 2) which also showed the sensitivity and specificity of the PIMA analyzer ranged between 91 to 96% and the mean relative bias between −5 to 8%.

In 175 patients, the finger prick sample was obtained in addition to venous blood. The CD4 counts obtained from the finger prick samples using PIMA CD4 analyzer correlated well with the CD4 counts obtained by reference method, FACSCalibur using the venous blood ($r = 0.856$, $P < 0.01$, Figure 2A) with a relative bias of -9.1%(range: -46% to 27%, Figure 2B). The CD4 counts obtained using PIMA analyzer on both, finger prick and venous blood were also comparable with $r = 0.854$ and slightly better relative bias on 2.8% (range: -37% to 43%) (Figure 2C and D).

The users of the equipment at various centers expressed that the analyzer was compact and hence could fit in the small space available at the centers. The equipment is battery operated, showed a battery backup of 3–4 hours eliminating the requirement of continuous electricity. The rate of invalid cartridges was 1 to 2 percent at these centers and thus repeat testing needed to be done in such cases.

Discussion

The present field based study showed that the PIMA analyzer gave comparable results with the reference methodologies for different CD4 ranges; one of the

Table 1 Comparison of CD4 counts obtained by PIMA analyzer and the reference methods within different CD4 ranges

CD4 Range (Cells/mm^3)	N	Median CD4 Count (Range)* Cells/mm^3		Mean relative bias (±2SD)
		Reference Method	PIMA Analyzer	
All	1790	356 (2–1726)	354 (6–1615)	−1% (−43, 42)
<250	508	165 (2–250)	168 (6–348)	−7% (−65, 51)
<350	877	228 (2–350)	225(6–542)	5% (−45,55)
251-350	369	298 (251–350)	299 (153–542)	−2% (−40, 36)
351-500	423	417 (351–500)	415 (213–676)	0% (−30, 30)
>500	490	648 (502–1726)	637 (179–1615)	5.1% (−23, 33)

*: The differences between the median CD4 counts obtained by the one of the reference methods and the PIMA analyzer was statistically insignificant for all CD4 ranges ($P > 0.05$).

Table 2 Sensitivity of PIMA analyzer to identify patients with CD4 count <350; a cut off used for ART initiation

Reference method	PIMA analyzer			
	N	Sensitivity	Specificity	Mean Relative bias (±2SD)
FACSCalibur	121	96%	91%	4(−48, 56)
FACSCount	206	92%	91%	−5(−49, 59)
Partec	550	91%	96%	8(−8.4, -7.6)

important characteristics for the validation of a new technology. The study could analyze more than 300 samples (range 369 to 508) samples at each CD4 range; <250, 251–350, 351–500 and >500 cells/mm^3 and the analysis showed very low relative bias within the PIMA and reference methodologies. Before distribution of the machines to various centers the inter machine comparison showed less than 10 percent%CV for both high and low CD4 counts for either the stabilized blood samples or fresh blood samples indicating good precision. The onsite inter-instrument variation was also within the 10% limit indicating the efficient use of PIMA analyzer as POC machine. The sensitivity and specificity of the PIMA analyzer to identify the patients with CD4 count less than 350, was found to be 91%. This indicated that the use of PIMA would put additional burden on the treatment providers as the treatment would be given to the patients who still have CD4 counts above 350. However the analysis showed that more than 50% mismatched results were between CD4 counts of 320 to 380; indicating that most of the patients would need ART in short time. The previously reported study has showed higher sensitivity but lower specificity to identify patients with CD4 counts lower than 350 cells (8). Previous studies have also shown less precision for the finger prick samples and also indicated that the finger prick sample collection required adequate training for correct use of the samples (7,8,12). Our study confirmed that

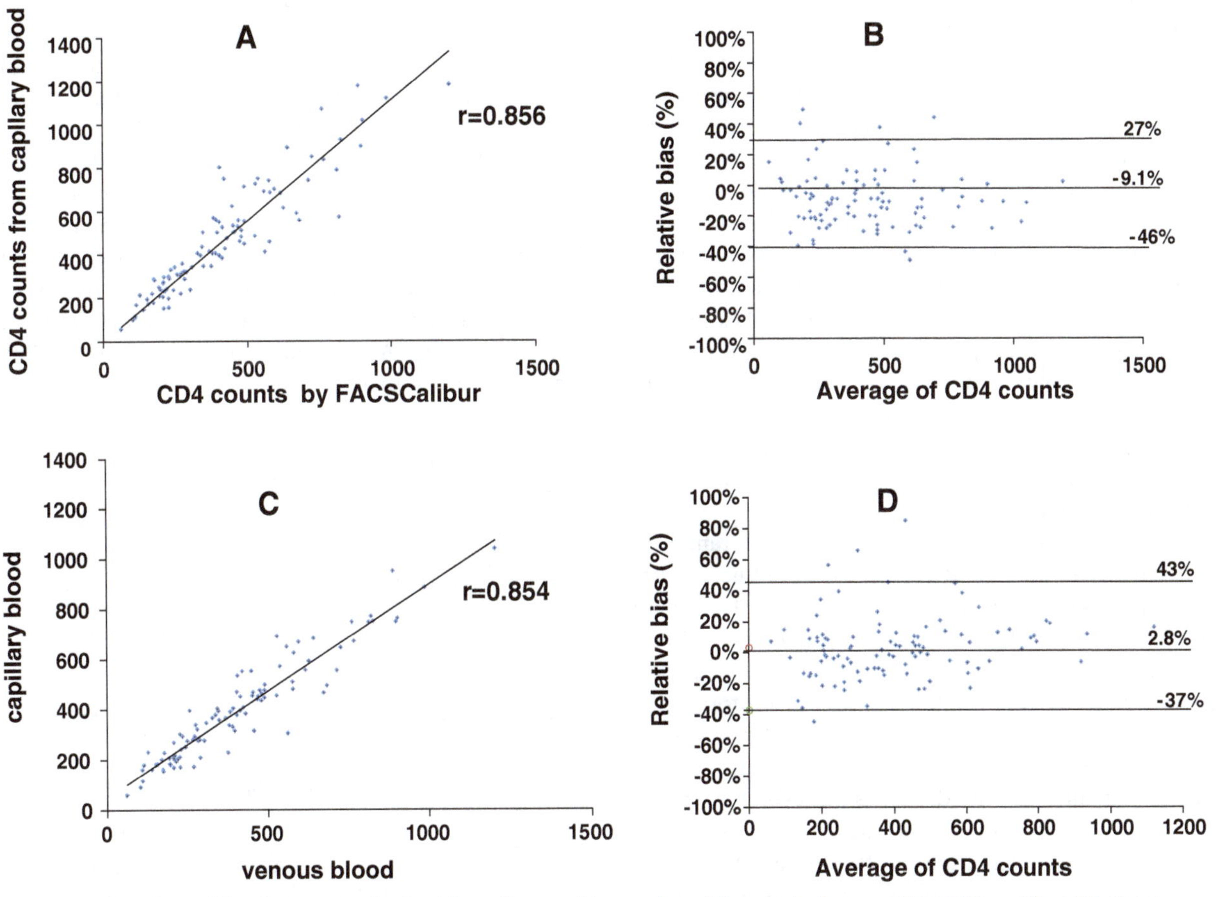

Figure 2 Comparison of the CD4 counts obtained from finger prick sample and from paired venous blood. Figure 2**A** and **C**: Linear regression analysis: The correlation between the CD4 counts obtained from finger prick sample using PIMA CD4 analyzer (Y axis) and from venous blood using FACSCalibur (2A) and PIMA (2C) (X axis) is assessed. Figure 2**B** and **D**: The agreement analysis using the Bland Altman plots. The percent relative bias for CD4 counts from finger prick sample and the paired venous blood using FACSCalibur (Figure 2B) and PIMA (Figure 2D) is plotted on the Y axis and the average of the CD4 count by both the samples is plotted on X axis. The black line represents the mean% relative bias of where as the blue lines represent the range of Mean ± SD.

the finger prick samples could be tested on PIMA analyzer with slightly less efficiency and also confirmed the requirement of the operator training for proper collection of finger prick sample to avoid multiple pricks. It was observed that in case of insufficient and improper finger-prick sample collection, the reliability of the CD4 counts by PIMA analyzer was questionable. Also our study participants preferred to give venous blood sample. The primary reasons were requirement of blood collection for other investigations using venous blood and a fear of being subjected to multiple pricks if sufficient volume of blood is not obtained in a single prick. Hence the finger prick blood sample could be the method of choice when only CD4 testing has to be carried out. The PIMA CD4 analyzer is battery operated and the reagents are stable at room temperature making it suitable for use in the areas where the reliable electric supply is not available and the ambient temperatures are often high. The cartridges have shelf life of six months making it suitable for remote areas where the shipment, delivery and storage, would be difficult. The testing does not require any additional equipment. The analyzer can be used after a minimum training and can be run by the clinical staff such as nurses where multi-tasking may be necessary due to shortage of trained staff or lack of sufficient workload [12].

The stabilized blood samples could be tested reliably by PIMA analyzer indicating amenability of the system for participation in the External Quality Assurance Scheme.

Unlike other CD4 enumerating equipments, in PIMA analyzer, the complete process of staining takes place in the equipment itself. Hence the sample throughput would be relatively low and the analyzer would be useful at the centres with 10–20 patients load/day. However, it is not expected that peripheral centres will have higher patient load and more than one machine could be installed in the centres if required.

The countrywide national ART roll out programme in India comprises of 300 ART centers and 550 linked centers with 3,64,000 adult populations on ART by January 2011 [13].The availability of CD4 counts in selected centers required either long distance travel for the patient or transport of the sample to the laboratory. This resulted in missed visits of the patients and problems in patient management. The loss to follow up of HIV infected patients after the diagnosis has been reported to be in the range of 16 to 25% in India [14, personal communication]. Although multiple factors are responsible for loss to follow up, availability of CD4 testing at point of care will help in reducing the number of clinic visits, thus helping in reducing loss to follow up. A recent report from Africa showed that POC CD4 testing could successfully reduce the pretreatment loss to follow-up [15]. Also the implementation of 350 CD4 count as a cut off for ART initiation instead of earlier cutoff of 250 would increase the burden on CD4 testing facility. Hence the decentralization of CD4 testing by providing CD4 count at primary health centers in combination with HIV diagnosis could enable proper monitoring of disease progression and ART initiation at the primary health centers only and would maximize the public health benefit of POC technology.

The PIMA analyzer does not provide percentage of CD4+ cells; hence, it would not be useful for monitoring the paediatric population younger than 5 years. As the movement of the paediatric patients/samples is difficult in the periphery, unavailability of CD4 percentage at the peripheral centre could be one of the limitations of this POC machine. In such cases the dual platform technology can be used by using absolute lymphocyte counts from hematology analyzer or from peripheral blood smear and the absolute CD4 counts from PIMA analyzer to calculate CD4 percentages. However the disadvantages would be of influence of the variation due to another system.

The cost of the PIMA analyzer is lesser than the available single platform CD4 machines and the cost of the cartridge is around 10 US$ which is slightly higher which might pose problem if not procured in bulk amount where the cost benefit could be obtained.

In conclusion, the study showed that the POC PIMA CD4 analyzer would be suitable for use in remote areas with minimum or no infrastructure. The availability of the CD4 counts on the same day of sample collection would reduce the number of repeat visits and improve patient management. Hence the integration of POC CD4 testing into the national AIDS control program would facilitate the better patient management in HIV infection.

Competing interests

The authors have declared that no competing interests exist.

Authors' contributions

MT: Planning, execution, analysis of the data and manuscript writing. BM, NS, SB: Execution of the study, data collection and training. SS: statistical analysis. SK, BR, MS, NS, PT: Execution and manuscript writing. RP: Planning and manuscript writing. All authors read and approved the final manuscript.

Acknowledgements

The authors would like to thank the clinical and laboratory staff of the 21 ART centers from India for conducting the CD4 count estimations by PIMA analyzer and the reference methods and also to the study volunteers for their participation. The study was funded by UNITAID.

Author details

[1]Department of Immunology, National AIDS Research Institute, G-73, MIDC, Bhosari, Pune 411 026, India. [2]National AIDS Control Organization, New Delhi, India. [3]Clinton Health Access Initiative, New Delhi, India.

References

1. World Health Organization: *Antiretroviral therapy for HIV infection in adults and adolescents: Recommendations for a public health approach.* 2010. http://whqlibdoc.who.int/publications/2010/9789241599764_eng.pdf.

2. Phillips AN, Pillay D, Miners AH, Bennett DE, Gilks CF, Lundgren JD: **Outcomes from monitoring of patients on antiretroviral therapy in resource limited settings with viral load, CD4 cell count, or clinical observation alone: a computer simulation model.** *Lancet* 2008, **371**:1443–1451.
3. Lawn SD, Little F, Bekker LG, Kaplan R, Campbel E, Orrell C, Wood R: **Changing mortality risk associated with CD4 cell response to antiretroviral therapy in South Africa.** *AIDS* 2009, **23**:335–342.
4. Sterne JA, May M, Costagliola D, de Wolf F, Phillips AN, Harris R, Funk MJ, Geskus RB, Gill J, Dabis F, Miró JM, Justice AC, Ledergerber B, Fätkenheuer G, Hogg RS, Monforte AD, Saag M, Smith C, Staszewski S, Egger M, Cole SR: **When To Start Consortium: Timing of initiation of antiretroviral therapy in AIDS-free HIV-1-infected patients: a collaborative analysis of 18 HIV cohort studies.** *Lancet* 2009, **373**:1352–1363.
5. UNAIDS: *Report on the global AIDS epidemic.* 2010. http://www.unaids.org/globalreport/Global_report.htm.
6. Sukapirom K, Onlamoon N, Thepthai C, Polsrila K, Tassaneetrithep B, Pattanapanyasat K: **Performance Evaluation of the Alere PIMA CD4 Test for Monitoring HIV-Infected Individuals in Resource-Constrained Settings.** *J Acquir Immune Defic Syndr* 2011, **58**(2):141–147.
7. Mtapuri-Zinyowera S, Chideme M, Mangwanya D, Mugurungi O, Gudukeya S, Hatzold K, Mangwiro A, Bhattacharya G, Lehe J, Peter T: **Evaluation of the PIMA point-of-care CD4 analyzer in VCT clinics in Zimbabwe.** *J Acquir Immune Defic Syndr* 2010, **55**(1):1–7.
8. Papa Alassane D, Géraldine D, Abdoul Aziz C, Birahim Pierre N, Djibril W, Makhtar CamaraSouleymane M, Luc K, Tandakha Ndiaye D: **Multisite Evaluation of a Point-of-Care Instrument for CD4+ T-Cell Enumeration Using Venous and Finger-Prick Blood: The PIMA CD4.** *J Acquir Immune Defic Syndr* 2011, **58**:103–111.
9. Pattanapanyasat K, Phuang-Ngern Y, Sukapirom K, Lerdwana S, Thepthai C, Tassaneetrithep B: **Comparison of 5 flow cytometric immunophenotyping systems for absolute CD4+ T-lymphocyte counts in HIV-1-infected patients living in resource-limited settings.** *J Acquir Immune Defic Syndr* 2008, **49**(4):339–347.
10. Zijenah LS, Kadzirange G, Madzime S, Borok M, Mudiwa C, Tobaiwa O, Mucheche M, Rusakaniko S, Katzenstein DA: **Affordable flow cytometry for enumeration of absolute CD4+ T-lymphocytes to identify subtype C HIV-1 infected adults requiring antiretroviral therapy (ART) and monitoring response to ART in a resource-limited setting.** *J Transl Med.* 2006, **4**:33.
11. Bland JM, Altman DG: **Statistical methods for assessing agreement between two methods of clinical measurement.** *Lancet* 1986, **1**:307–310.
12. Jani IV, Sitoe NE, Chongo PL, Alfai ER, Quevedo JI, Tobaiwa O, Lehe JD, Peter TF: **Accurate CD4 T-cell enumeration and antiretroviral drug toxicity monitoring in primary healthcare clinics using point-of-care testing.** *AIDS* 2011, **25**:807–812.
13. Annual Report, 2010-11. National AIDS Control Organization: *Department of AIDS Control, Ministry of Health & Family Welfare Government of India.* http://www.nacoonline.org/upload/REPORTS/NACO%20Annual%20Report%202010-11.pdf.
14. Bachani D, Garg R, Rewari B, Hegg L, Rajasekaran S, Deshpande A, Emmanuel K, Polin C, Rao S: **Two-year treatment outcomes of patients enrolled in India's national first-line antiretroviral therapy programme.** *Natl Med J India* 2010, **23**(1):7–12.
15. Jani IV, Sitoe NE, Alfai ER, Chongo PL, Quevedo JI, Rocha BM, Lehe JD, Peter TF: **Effect of point-of-care CD4 cell count tests on retention of patients and rates of antiretroviral therapy initiation in primary health clinics: an observational cohort study.** *Lancet.* doi:10.1016/S0140-6736(11)61052-0. Published online September 26, 2011.

15

Antiretroviral regimens sparing agents from the nucleoside(tide) reverse transcriptase inhibitor class

Amit C Achhra* and Mark A Boyd

Abstract

The nucleoside(tide) reverse transcriptase inhibitors (NRTIs) have traditionally been an important 'back-bone' of an antiretroviral therapy (ART) regimen. However all agents have been associated with both short- and long-term toxicity. There have also been concerns regarding the efficacy and safety of a treatment sequencing strategy in which those with past exposure and/or resistance to one or more NRTIs are re-exposed to 'recycled' NRTIs in subsequent ART regimens. Newer, potent and possible safer, agents from various ART classes continue to become available. There has therefore been growing interest in evaluating NRTI-sparing regimens. In this review, we examined studies of NRTI-sparing regimens in adult HIV-positive patients with varying degrees of ART experience. We found that in treatment experienced patients currently on a failing regimen with detectable viral load, there now exists a robust evidence for the use of NRTI-sparing regimens including raltegravir with a boosted-protease inhibitor with or without a third agent. In those on a virologically suppressive regimen switching to a NRTI-sparing regimen or in those ART-naïve patients initiating an NRTI-sparing regimen, evidence is sparse and largely comes from small exploratory trials or observational studies. Overall, these studies suggest that caution needs to be exercised in carefully selecting the right candidate and agents, especially in the context of a dual-therapy regimen, to minimise the risks of virological failure. There is residual toxicity conferred by the ritonavir boost in protease-inhibitor containing NRTI-sparing regimens. Fully-powered studies are needed to explore the place of N (t)RTI-sparing regimens in the sequencing of ART. Additionally research is required to explore how to minimise the adverse effects associated with ritonavir-based pharmacoenhancement.

Keywords: HAART, Toxicity, NRTI, NNRTI, NRTI-sparing, Class-sparing, HIV, Dual therapy, Raltegravir, Maraviroc

Introduction

The nucleoside(tide) reverse transcriptase inhibitor (NRTI) class has formed the 'back-bone' of antiretroviral therapy (ART) regimens since the early ART era. All major treatment guidelines currently recommend the selection of 2 NRTIs and a third agent from a separate class in the initial management of ART naïve HIV-positive patients; some guidelines suggest recycling NRTI agents as far as possible in ART-experienced HIV-positive patients experiencing virological failure [1-4]. However, concerns about long-term toxicities and cross–resistance within the NRTI class combined with the continuing development of newer, seemingly safer agents in several independent classes of drugs has led to a growing interest in the potential use of feasible, innovative and appealing NRTI-sparing options.

The main purpose of this review is to explore the current state of our knowledge on the efficacy and safety of NRTI class-sparing antiretroviral regimens used in the management of adult HIV-positive patients. The review is restricted to studies conducted on adult HIV-1 mono-infected individuals published in the English language. The review has a greater focus on studies published since 2006 (so as to ensure relevance to contemporary practice). We included clinical trials as well as non-randomised small clinical studies, both published and unpublished (conference presentations).

* Correspondence: aachhra@kirby.unsw.edu.au
The Kirby Institute, University of New South Wales, Sydney, Australia

Rationale for NRTI-sparing regimens

The thymidine analogue NRTIs, such as zidovudine and in particular stavudine (d4T) have been associated with serious mitochondrial toxicity which has been linked to lipoatrophy. In addition, zidovudine has been associated with anaemia and didanosine with peripheral neuropathy. As a consequence these agents are no longer recommended as preferred components of therapy; in the case of stavudine it has been recommended that it's use be phased out, even in low- and middle-income countries [2]. However, one of the most important push factors for the assessment of NRTI-sparing regimens has been a growing understanding of the long-term toxicity profile of even the newer, relatively safe NRTIs in common use such as tenofovir and abacavir. Tenofovir has been associated with nephrotoxicity, including acute and chronic renal failure, proximal tubular dysfunction, nephrogenic diabetes insipidus and nephrotic syndrome [1,4,5]. In a large EuroSIDA cohort study, tenofovir use was associated with a 20% increased risk of chronic kidney disease [6]. Further, clinical trials and observational studies have consistently demonstrated decline in bone-mineral density (BMD) of about 2-10% in the short-term attributable to the use of tenofovir [7,8]. Cumulative use of tenofovir has been associated with a higher risk of osteoporotic fracture [9]. Finally, one observational study attributed increased risk of heart failure to the tenofovir use, although this observation has not been replicated [10]. Abacavir, another commonly used NRTI has been implicated in the risk of myocardial infarction by some large cohort studies and a clinical trial [10-12]. However, the evidence is not definitive as this association has not been seen in other studies [13]. Nevertheless, it has generated considerable anxiety in the provider community, especially for its use in patients with a high cardiovascular risk. Further, abacavir is associated with the risk of severe hypersensitivity reactions which can only be eliminated by screening out those carrying the HLA-B57*01 allele [1,14].

One of the main concerns prompting studies on NRTI-sparing regimens in failing patients has been that of possible reduced potency of NRTI agents due to current or archived nucleoside mutations such as thymidine analogue associated mutations (TAMs). As a result, if NRTIs are being recycled in such patients, they could potentially be exposed to a regimen with <2 or 3 fully-active agents. This is especially of concern in resource limited settings where NRTIs are recommended for recycling following treatment failure identified through immunological or virological failure. This surrogate means of identifying virological failure is associated with substantial degrees of resistance which may significantly compromise the action of recycled NRTIs in future ART regimens [15]. Moreover, access to agents beyond NRTIs and the ritonavir-boosted protease inhibitors atazanavir, lopinavir and darunavir is limited [2]. Switching a specific anchor agent to one with a lower genetic barrier (e.g. LPV/r replaced by raltegravir [16] or PI replaced with another NRTI [17]) with a compromised NRTI backbone could result in higher rates of treatment failure. Finally, recycling NRTIs might mean exposing patients to long term NRTI agents which may result in unanticipated, cumulative adverse effects.

Several newer agents from various classes with a good safety profile to date continue to become available. These include new integrase inhibitors, newer non-nucleoside reverse transcriptase inhibotors (NNRTIs, e.g. etravirine and rilpivirine), the CCR5 attachment inhibitor maraviroc and the PIs lopinavir, darunavir and atazanavir. It is therefore possible to construct regimens containing 2-3 fully-active agents which are NRTI-sparing.

We next discuss NRTI-sparing regimens that have been evaluated in each of the three main types of patient populations: treatment-experienced failing patients where most of the evidence is concentrated; virologically suppressed patients; and ART-naïve patients.

NRTI-sparing regimens in treatment-experienced failing patients

Recent large clinical trials have evaluated NRTI-sparing regimens in treatment experienced patients experiencing virological failure (key studies summarised in Table 1 [18-25]). The regimen most of interest has been that of a boosted-PI with raltegravir, and/or maraviroc and/or etravirine.

The SECOND-LINE study (n=541) [18] evaluated ritonavir-boosted lopinavir (LPV/r) with raltegravir vs. LPV/r + NRTIs (the WHO standard of care of recycling NRTIs in HIV-positive patients with demonstrable virological failure of first-line NNRTI-based ART), with no previous PI or integrase inhibitor exposure. The use of resistance testing at randomization was optional. Of the 492 patients with resistance tests available, 89% had ≥1 NRTI mutations and 60% had M184V with ≥ NRTI mutations at baseline. Patients were randomised (stratified by baseline HIV RNA ≤ or > 100,000 copies/mL) to receive LPV/r with raltegravir or LPV/r with physician-chosen NRTIs. At 48 weeks, the NRTI-sparing raltegravir arm was non-inferior to the NRTI-containing control arm for the primary endpoint of virological control <200 copies/mL with an overall 81.7% virological response rate. The NRTI control-arm resulted in a 2-4% greater decline in BMD compared to the NRTI-sparing arm (likely due to patients switching to tenofovir) [25]. On the other hand the raltegravir arm was associated with a greater degree of hypercholesterolaemia. Despite this there was no difference in the resultant total: HDL cholesterol ratio. Finally, emergence of PI mutations was negligible in those experiencing virological failure, attesting to the high genetic

Table 1 Key recent studies of NRTI-sparing regimens in treatment experienced patients

Author, name of the trial, if any/year/published?	Design	Comparison	N	Follow-up (weeks)	Results
Boyd et al. [18], SECOND-LINE/2013/Yes	Phase-3/4 RCT, non-inferiority	(i) LPV/r + RAL vs. (ii) LPV/r + recycled NRTIs in those failing 1st line NNRTI-based ART	541 (271 vs. 270)	48	-Arm (i) non-inferior to arm (ii) for virological outcome -No major differences in serious adverse events -Greater decline in BMD in arm (ii) [25]
Paton et al. [19], EARNEST/2013/No	Phase-3/4 RCT, non-inferiority	(i) LPV/r + RAL (ii) LPV/r monotherapy after induction with LPV/r + RAL (iii) LPV/r + recycled NRTIs (control) in those failing 1st line NNRTI-based ART	(i) 433; (ii) 418; (iii) 426	96	-Arm (i) non-inferior to arm (iii) for a composite of virological and clinical endpoint -Arm (ii) inferior to other arms for virological outcome and higher LPV/r resistance -No differences in grade 3/4 events
Tashima et al. [20], OPTIONS/2013/No	Phase-3/4 RCT, non-inferiority	(i) NRTI-omitting optimised regimen (ii) NRTI-including optimised regimen in triple-class experienced failing patients	(i) 179; (ii) 181	48	-Similar virlogical outcomes in both arms -No differences in grade 3/4 events -Higher mortality in arm (ii).
Ruane et al. [24], INROADS/2013/No	Single-arm exploratory phase-2b trial	DRV/r + ETV in failing patients (78%) or ART naïve patients with transmitted resistance (22%)	54 (75% completed the study)	48	-100% of ART naïve and 87% of failing patients achieved virological success. -2 patients developed ETV mutations and none had DRV mutations.
Imaz et al. [21]/2011/Yes	Observational	Salvage regimen of at least three active agents from DRV, ETV, RAL and MVC, with or without NRTIs	122	48	-78% virologically suppressed (equal in both arms) -Higher baseline viral load associated with worse outcomes.
Nozza et al. [22]/2011/Yes	Observational	Salvage regimen of RAL + MVC + ETV	28	96	-96% virologically suppressed (<50 copies/ml)
Florence et al. [23]/2010/Yes	Observational	Salvage regimen of ETV + optimised regimen, 40% without NRTIs	941	24	-70% and 90% had viral load <50 and 400 copies/mL respectively.

barrier of LPV/r under conditions of frequent (3 monthly) virological monitoring.

The EARNEST study [19] was similarly designed to SECOND-LINE and performed in an identical patient population (with an additional arm of LPV/r monotherapy after a 12 week induction combined with raltegravir). After 96 weeks of follow-up the investigators found no difference between the raltegravir and NRTI-arms in the study's primary composite endpoint of "good disease control" (i.e. alive with no WHO stage 4 disease, CD4 >250/mm^3 and viral load <10,000 or >10,000 copies/mL with no PI mutations), as well as virological outcome (viral load <200 or <50 copies/mL). The investigators also found no difference in grade 3/4 events at 96-weeks follow-up. Of note, the monotherapy arm was found to be virologically inferior to the control and LPV/r plus raltegravir arms.

The OPTIONS study [20] was conducted on a set of treatment experienced patients failing a PI-based regimen and with past exposure to NRTIs and NNRTIs (n=360). Patients were randomised to either NRTI-including or NRTI-excluding optimised regimen arms containing >2 fully active agents (not including NRTIs). In the NRTI-sparing arm, the most common regimens were raltegravir with boosted-darunavir (DRV/r) and either etravirine (56%), maraviroc (14%) or both (9%). At 1 year of follow-up, virological suppression rates were similar in both arms. Of note, the study only had the power to find a non-inferiority margin of 15%. Finally, though there were no major differences in the grade 3/4 safety outcomes the NRTI-arm experienced greater mortality. It is unclear if causes of deaths were NRTI-related.

A few smaller observational studies confirm these findings in routine clinic settings (Table 1). In one study of 122 patients with prior triple-class failure, the regimen of raltegravir with DRV/r and maraviroc or etravirine demonstrated similar virological efficacy (>75%) compared to those using NRTI agents at 48 weeks [21].

Collectively, these studies confirm that in virologically failing patients, the strategy of selecting 2 or 3 fully-active pharmacologically compatible agents is a feasible strategy. Of note, all of these studies have included a boosted-PI, and because of their high genetic barrier to resistance, the data should not be extrapolated to other 2-class regimens. Also, recycled NRTI agents seem to retain efficacy (i.e. non-inferior to the comparator arms), which is reassuring in settings where newer agents are not yet widely available.

NRTI-sparing regimens in patients receiving suppressive ART

Switching to a NRTI-sparing regimen in a virologically suppressed patient needs consideration of several factors. These include the treatment history, archived mutations, duration of viral suppression, expected level of adherence, the choice of agents as well as the patient motivation to switch from a stable regimen. Large, well powered trials in such patients are few and difficult to recruit, although several smaller studies have identified promising regimens. Key studies on this patient population are summarised in Table 2 [26-36].

In the ACTG 5116 trial [34], virologically suppressed patients receiving a standard PI- or NNRTI-based ART regimen were randomised to efavirenz with LPV/r or efavirenz with NRTIs (standard ART arm). Though not a fully powered trial, the NRTI-sparing arm performed poorly due largely to higher rates of discontinuation and toxicity as well as dyslipidemia. This study suggests that the choice of agents will be important in constructing such regimens as they will need to provide clear evidence of greater safety before convincing ART providers and/or patients to consider a switch.

In a more recent small exploratory study (the KITE trial [31]), virologically suppressed patients with no history of failure to PI-based regimens were randomised to standard ART (n=20) or LPV/r with raltegravir (n=40). At 42 weeks, there were no differences in virological suppression rates (90-92%) and no treatment limiting side effects, although there was a trend for higher triglycerides in the NRTI-sparing arm. Another similar exploratory single-arm trial [33] (n=29) reported similar results with raltegravir plus a boosted-PI (mainly darunavir) regimen with no serious dyslipidaemia at 24 weeks.

Since most studies on NRTI-sparing regimens have included a boosted-PI regimen, residual toxicity concerns with ritonavir as the booster (such as gastrointestinal upset and dyslipidemia) have been seen as a relative disadvantage. With several new agents now available, it is now possible to conceive regimens which exclude not only NRTIs but also ritonavir, as well as first-generation NNRTIs such as efavirenz (also associated with dyslipidaemia and neurotoxicity) or nevirapine. This strategy is especially attractive in virologically suppressed patients with minimal treatment experience, where good adherence can be presumed and the possible adverse impact of high viral load on regimen efficacy is less of a concern.

In one recent cohort study on treatment experienced, virologically suppressed patients switching to dual therapy of etravirine with raltegravir, 91% maintained virological suppression at 48 weeks [36]. In another exploratory observational study of 62 patients (the majority with HIV RNA <400 copies/mL) switching to NRTI-sparing regimens, 92% had undetectable viral loads at 42 months [26]. The most common regimens used were: raltegravir, unboosted atazanavir, and maraviroc (33%); raltegravir and unboosted atazanavir (22%); raltegravir, maraviroc, and etravirine (13%). Of note, 3 out of 15 people receiving a two drug regimen demonstrated low-level viremia (i.e. >50 but <200 copies/mL), the clinical meaning of which is debated. In another study, called No Nuc No Boost [29], ART-naïve R5 tropic patients with high CD4 counts and baseline viral load $<10^3$ log copies/mL were first treated with tenofovir/emtricitabine, raltegravir and maraviroc for six months after which those with plasma viral load <50 copies/mL at 24 weeks were continued on a two-drug combination of raltegravir and maraviroc for a further 24 weeks. All patients retained viral load <50 copies/mL on dual therapy. However, in another similar study (RocNRaL) on more treatment experienced patients, this dual regimen demonstrated lower efficacy [28]. Collectively, these studies suggest that while such unconventional regimens are promising in carefully selected patients, caution must be exercised when using dual therapy regimens without the support of a high genetic barrier to the selection of resistance like LPV/r or DRV/r.

Boosted-PI monotherapy

Given the high genetic barrier of boosted PIs, several large studies have evaluated this simplification strategy. Boosted-PI monotherapy trials have been extensively reviewed previously [37,38] and are therefore not covered in detail here. In the 96-week trial of LPV/r monotherapy in virologically suppressed patients receiving a boosted-PI + NRTI regimen with no history of failure (OK trial), although the virological success rate was similar, the monotherapy arm had a significantly higher rate of low-level viremia (12%) necessitating reinduction with NRTIs [39]. A similar trial with DRV/r monotherapy (MONET) [40] also demonstrated a high virological success rate with DRV/r however the monotherapy arm had a higher rate of low-level viremia. Overall, although the virological response rates in LPV/r or DRV/r monotherapy arms are high and PI mutations are rare in the setting of regular virological monitoring, there appears to be a greater risk of consistent low-level viremia which may herald virological failure in the monotherapy arms. In the fully powered EARNEST study [19] described above, the PI monotherapy arm (combined for the first

Table 2 Key recent studies of switch to NRTI-sparing regimens in virologically suppressed patients on standard ART

Author, name of the trial, if any/year/published?	Design	Comparison	N	Follow-up (weeks)	Results
Monteiro et al. [36]/2013/Yes	Observational	RAL + ETV	25	48	-91% virologically suppressed in per-protocol analysis -Lipids improved
Ward et al. [26]/2013/No	Observational	Switching for toxicity concerns to a RAL + 1 or 2 agents, most commonly on RAL + ATV/r with or without ETV or MVC	62	168	-92% virologically suppressed; -3 of 15 on dual therapy had to add third agent for low-level viremia
Calin et al. [27]/2013/No	Observational	Switching to RAL + ETV regimen	91	48	-93% had viral load <50 copies/mL -4/5 with virological failures had past NNRTI mutations -3 patients had RAL mutations
Katlama et al. [28], ROCnRAL/2013/No	Single-arm exploratory trial	R5-trophic suppressed patients switched to MVC + RAL	41	48	-Failure in 11.4% -RAL mutations in 3/5 patients who failed -1/5 had R5 to ×4 virus switch
Cotte et al. [29], No Nuc No Boost/2013/No	Single-arm exploratory trial	MVC + RAL	10	48	-No virological failures (>50 copies/mL) -No serious adverse event
Burgos et al. [30]/2012/No	Observational	Switching for toxicity concerns to a PI/r + 2nd agent, many with no NRTI	131	56	- > 90% virologically suppressed.
Ofotokun et al. [31], KITE/2012/No	Exploratory pilot trial	(i) LPV/r + RAL; (ii) standard ART	60	48	-92% in arm (i) and 88% in arm (ii) with viral load <50 copies/mL; -Higher triglycerides in arm (i) -No difference in BMD or body composition.
Carey et al. [32], SPARTA/2012/Yes	Pilot cross-over RCT	Patients receiving ATV/r randomized to: (i) ATV/r (300/100 mg respectively once daily) + RAL (800 mg once daily) (ii) ATV (300 mg twice daily) + RAL (400 mg twice daily)	25	76% in follow-up for 48 weeks	-Both agents pharmacologically compatible. -All patients remained virologically suppressed
Cordery et al. [35]/2010/Yes	Observational	RAL + ATV (unboosted)	20	72	-Only 1 (5%) failure
Allavena et al. [33]/2009/Yes	Observational	Switching for toxicity concerns to a PI/r + RAL.	29	48	-100% virologically suppressed
Fischl et al. [34]/2007/Yes	RCT, not fully powered	(i) LPV/r + EFV; (ii) EFV + NRTIs	236	96	-Arm (i): shorter time to failure or discontinuation; -Arm (i): greater increase in triglycerides

12 weeks of treatment with RAL 400 mg bid) was found to be significantly inferior to the standard ART arm. The authors concluded that such a strategy is unsuitable for a public health approach. Presently, none of the major treatment guidelines recommend PI monotherapy because of concerns regarding efficacy [1-4].

NRTI-sparing regimens in ART naïve patients

Large, fully powered trials evaluating NRTI sparing regimens in ART naïve patients are few and most smaller studies have suggested that care must be exercised in selecting both suitable agents and candidates for such regimens. Key studies are summarised in Table 3 [41-48].

The ACTG 5142 trial randomised ART-naïve patients to standard ART arms with LPV/r or efavirenz, both given with investigator selected 2NRTIs and a NRTI-sparing arm of LPV/r and efavirenz [46]. Though the NRTI-sparing arm showed comparable virological efficacy overall at 96 weeks, it performed poorly in those with baseline viral load >100,000 copies/mL and the rate of discontinuation due to adverse events was significantly higher than other two arms. Of note, the dose of LPV/r was increased due to its interaction with efavirenz, which may have contributed to the additional toxicity in this arm.

More recent pilot studies have explored a dual therapy regimen of raltegravir with a boosted-PI. These studies

Table 3 Key recent studies of switch to NRTI-sparing first-line ART regimens in ART naïve patients

Author, name of the trial, if any/year/published?	Design	Comparison	N	Follow-up (weeks)	Results
Mills et al. [41], A4001078/2013/Yes	RCT, phase-2b pilot	(i) MVC + ATV/r (ii) TDF + FTC + ATV/r	121	48	-75% in arm (i) and 84% in arm (ii) had viral load <50 copies/mL. -More hyperbilirubenmia in arm (i) -Nine in arm (i) and 3 in arm (ii) had low-level viremia after virological suppression
Reynes et al. [42], PROGRESS/2013/Yes	RCT pilot study	(i) LPV/r + RAL (ii) LPV/r + TDF + FTC	(i) 101; (ii) 105	96	-66.3% in arm (i) and 68.6% in arm (ii) responded by FDA-TLOVR -Better body comp in arm (i) -Greater decline in eGFR in arm (ii)
Kozal et al. [47], SPARTAN/2012/Yes	RCT pilot study	(i) ATV + RAL (ii) ATV/r + TDF + FTC	(i) 63; (ii) 31	24	-74.6% in arm (i) and 63.3% in arm (ii) had viral load <50 copies/mL -4/6 failures in arm (i) had RAL mutations. -20% incidence of grade-4 hyperbilirubenimia in arm (i).
Taiwo et al. [43,48], MIDAS/2013/Yes	Single-arm pilot	MVC + DRV/r	25	96	-Viral load < 50 copies/mL: 8.3% and 10% at week 48 and 96, respectively. -Virological failures mainly explained be high baseline viral load >100000 copies/mL
Bedimo R et al. [44], RADAR/2011/No	RCT pilot	(i) RAL + DRV/r (ii) DRV/r + TDF + FTC	80	24	-86% in arm (i) and 87% in arm (ii) had viral load <50 copies/mL
Taiwo et al. [45], ACTG5262/2011/Yes	Single-arm pilot	DRV/r + RAL	112	48	-26% with viral load > 50 copies/mL, majority with low-level viremia (<200 copies/mL) -Baseline viral load >100000 copies/mL strongly associated with failure
Riddler et al. [46], ACTG5142/2008/Yes	RCT	(i) EFV + NRTIs (ii) LPV/r + NRTIs (iii) LPV/r + EFV	(i) 250 (ii) 253 (iii) 250	96	-89%, 77% and 83% had viral load <50 copies/mL in arms (i), (ii) and (iii) respectively -No difference in time to toxic effects -At failure, resistance mutations more common in arm (iii)

NOTE for Tables 1, 2, 3: ATV/r = ritonavir boosted atazanavir, DRV/r = ritonavir boosted darunavir, LPV/r = ritonavir boosted lopinavir, RAL = raltegravir, ETV = etravirine, MVC = maraviroc, EFV = efavirenz, TDF = tenofovir, FTC = emtricitabine, NRTI = Nucleoside(tide) reverse transcriptase inhibitors, PI = protease inhibitors.

suggest that a high baseline plasma viral load could adversely impact the success of the regimen in such patients. In a single arm study of 112 patients receiving raltegravir and DRV/r, virological failure (>50 copies/mL) was 26% at 48 weeks [45]. Most (21/28) of the patients with virological failure and all of those with integrase mutations had a baseline plasma viral load >100,000 copies/mL . Almost 50% of failures were that of low level viremia (>50 but <200 or <400 copies/mL). No PI mutations were detected. However, the similar fully-powered trial of DRV/r + RAL (NEAT protocol 001, see below) is ongoing and has not been stopped by Data Safety Monitoring Board. In the RADAR study (small randomised study of DRV/r with either raltegravir or NRTIs), response rates were poorer in the raltegravir arm which also experienced higher rates of dyslipidemia [44]. In the SPARTAN pilot study evaluating experimental unboosted atazanavir (300 mg) with raltegravir (vs. NRTI with boosted-atazanavir), most raltegravir resistance mutations occurred in those with baseline viral load >100,000 copies/mL [47]. Also, the rate of hyperbilirubinemia in the raltegravir arm was higher (possibly due to the higher dose of atazanavir used in that arm (300 mg bid) and the known pharmacoenhancement effect of RAL on ATV) [47]. In a randomised study of LPV/r with raltegravir or with NRTIs (PROGRESS trial), virological response did not differ by baseline viral load although there were only a few patients with high viral load at baseline [42]. Of note, in this study, surrogate renal and bone outcomes were significantly more favourable in the NRTI-sparing arm.

Overall, these studies suggest that while NRTI-sparing regimens are promising, caution needs to be exercised in the selection of patients. In particular, the impact of the baseline plasma viral load on regimen efficacy and the risk of baseline or archived resistance mutations for failure need further study. Dual-therapy regimens in general have resulted in mixed results. Well designed, appropriately powered randomised controlled trials are required to reach definitive conclusions. In a recent well-powered trial of LPV/r with lamivudine (a relatively safe NtRTI) vs. LPV/r+2 NRTIs, the dual therapy arm demonstrated non-inferior efficacy of >85% at 48 weeks regardless of baseline viral load, with fewer toxicity-related discontinuations [49]. This study indicates that carefully selected dual therapy could be a reasonable option even in ART-naïve patients. Of note, however, dyslipidemia tended to be more pronounced in the dual therapy arm, which may be due to the absence of tenofovir which is known to be associated with a favourable lipid profile [50,51]. On the other hand, the MODERN study – a well powered study of maraviroc + DRV/r vs. standard ART (n=791) was prematurely stopped at 48 weeks due to inferior performance of the dual-therapy arm (unpublished data) [52]. Ongoing studies such as A4001095 (DRV/r with maraviroc or NRTIs) (Trial Identifier: NCT01345630)and the NEAT protocol 001/ ANRS 143 (DRV/r with raltegravir or NRTIs) (Trial Identifier: NCT01066962) should provide a clearer understanding of the use of such regimens in ART-naïve patients.

Limitations, conclusions and future directions

NRTI-sparing regimens appear to be promising and if established, will be an important step towards optimising ART to maximise patient safety. However, there are a few important points to consider. First, trials evaluating such regimens will need to show a clear benefit in terms of long-term safety so as to convince clinicians to move away from much more familiar NRTI-based regimens. Promising regimens such as the use of a boosted-PI with raltegravir have shown a higher risk of dyslipidemia in some studies likely attributable to ritonavir and possibly the absence of tenofovir. Future studies considering regimens without NRTIs, ritonavir and efavirenz (due to neuro-psychaitric adverse events) will be important in identifying safer, better tolerated ART regimens. A recent study by our group suggested that most HIV-positive patients will have such regimen options available to them regardless of their treatment experience [53].

In addition, most clinical trials follow participants up for 48 to 96 weeks, which, along with their enrolment number, is not of sufficient duration to demonstrate differences in hard clinical endpoints such as renal failure or fractures. Cohort studies will be instrumental in this regard. Also, most of the studies are small and unpublished. Better quality evidence is therefore clearly needed in this area.

Second, many of the studies on NRTI-sparing two drug regimens suggest that in selected patients (e.g. those with high baseline viral loads), the risk of virological failure and selection of resistance mutations to the non-PI component are a risk. This suggests that such regimens, especially ones without a boosted-PI support, should ideally be first evaluated in virologically suppressed patients.

Finally, many NRTI-sparing regimens are may require twice daily dosing frequency and ≥1-2 pills/day. This may impact the adherence (example selective lower adherence to the 2nd dose of raltegravir in DRV/r + raltegravir regimen). However, both etravirine and maraviroc have pharmacokinetic and clinical data supporting once-daily dosing [41,54], and RAL is being studied in a 1200-mg once-daily formulation. Therefore, NRTI-sparing once-daily regimens could be possible in future.

In conclusion, there has now accumulated a sizeable evidence base that supports the use of NRTI-sparing regimens of 2–3 fully-active agents for HIV-positive patients currently on a failing ART regimen. For virologically suppressed patients, an NRTI-sparing regimen may be an option is some patients although further, more definitive studies are needed. Finally, the evidence is sparse for such regimens in the ART naïve patient population and more research is required to generate robust evidence. Future studies such as A4001095 and NEAT protocol 001/ ANRS 143 will be instrumental in informing the evidence base for such regimens.

Competing interests

ACA has received Gilead Australia Fellowship for the year 2013. MB has received research grant support and honoraria for serving on advisory boards and educational presentations from AbbVie, Boehringer Ingelheim, Bristol Myers Squibb, Gilead Sciences, Janssen Pharmaceuticals, and Merck.

Authors' contributions

MAB conceived the idea. ACA and MAB both performed the literature search and planned the structure of the review. ACA conducted the review and wrote the first draft and subsequent changes to the manuscript. MAB provided key input to the contents and provided overall supervision of the project. All authors read and approved the final manuscript.

References

1. Thompson MA, Aberg JA, Hoy JF, Telenti A, Benson C, Cahn P, Eron JJ, Gunthard HF, Hammer SM, Reiss P, *et al*: **Antiretroviral treatment of adult HIV infection: 2012 recommendations of the International Antiviral Society-USA panel.** *JAMA* 2012, **308**:387–402.
2. World Health Organisation: *Consolidated guidelines on the use of antiretroviral drugs for treating and preventing HIV infection.* 2013. http://www.who.int/hiv/pub/guidelines/arv2013/en/. Accessed on October 2013.
3. European AIDS Clinical Society: *European Guidelines for treatment of HIV-infected adults in Europe.* Available at http://www.eacsociety.org/Guidelines.aspx. Accessed on October 2013.
4. Panel on Antiretroviral Guidelines for Adults and Adolescents: *Guidelines for the use of antiretroviral agents in HIV-1-infected adults and adolescents.* http://aidsinfo.nih.gov/contentfiles/lvguidelines/AdultandAdolescentGL.pdf. Assesed on October 2013.
5. Calza L: **Renal toxicity associated with antiretroviral therapy.** *HIV Clin Trials* 2012, **13**:189–211.

6. Mocroft A, Kirk O, Reiss P, De Wit S, Sedlacek D, Beniowski M, Gatell J, Phillips AN, Ledergerber B, Lundgren JD, Group ftES: **Estimated glomerular filtration rate, chronic kidney disease and antiretroviral drug use in HIV-positive patients.** *AIDS* 2010, **24**:1667–1678.
7. Brown TT, McComsey GA, King MS, Qaqish RB, Bernstein BM, da Silva BA: **Loss of bone mineral density after antiretroviral therapy initiation, independent of antiretroviral regimen.** *J Acquir Immune Defic Syndr* 2009, **51**:554–561.
8. McComsey GA, Kitch D, Daar ES, Tierney C, Jahed NC, Tebas P, Myers L, Melbourne K, Ha B, Sax PE: **Bone mineral density and fractures in antiretroviral-naive persons randomized to receive abacavir-lamivudine or tenofovir disoproxil fumarate-emtricitabine along with efavirenz or atazanavir-ritonavir: aids clinical trials group A5224s, a substudy of ACTG A5202.** *J Infect Dis* 2011, **203**:1791–1801.
9. Bedimo R, Maalouf NM, Zhang S, Drechsler H, Tebas P: **Osteoporotic fracture risk associated with cumulative exposure to tenofovir and other antiretroviral agents.** *AIDS* 2012, **26**:825–831.
10. Choi AI, Vittinghoff E, Deeks SG, Weekley CC, Li Y, Shlipak MG: **Cardiovascular risks associated with abacavir and tenofovir exposure in HIV-infected persons.** *AIDS* 2011, **25**:1289–1298.
11. Worm SW, Sabin C, Weber R, Reiss P, El-Sadr W, Dabis F, De Wit S, Law M, Monforte AD, Friis-Moller N, *et al*: **Risk of myocardial infarction in patients with HIV infection exposed to specific individual antiretroviral drugs from the 3 major drug classes: the data collection on adverse events of anti-HIV drugs (D:A:D) study.** *J Infect Dis* 2010, **201**:318–330.
12. Martin A, Bloch M, Amin J, Baker D, Cooper DA, Emery S, Carr A: **Simplification of antiretroviral therapy with tenofovir-emtricitabine or abacavir-Lamivudine: a randomized, 96-week trial.** *Clin Infect Dis* 2009, **49**:1591–1601.
13. Costagliola D, Lang S, Mary-Krause M, Boccara F: **Abacavir and cardiovascular risk: reviewing the evidence.** *Curr HIV/AIDS Rep* 2010, **7**:127–133.
14. Mallal S, Phillips E, Carosi G, Molina JM, Workman C, Tomazic J, Jagel-Guedes E, Rugina S, Kozyrev O, Cid JF, *et al*: **HLA-B*5701 screening for hypersensitivity to abacavir.** *N Engl J Med* 2008, **358**:568–579.
15. Hosseinipour MC, van Oosterhout JJ, Weigel R, Phiri S, Kamwendo D, Parkin N, Fiscus SA, Nelson JA, Eron JJ, Kumwenda J: **The public health approach to identify antiretroviral therapy failure: high-level nucleoside reverse transcriptase inhibitor resistance among Malawians failing first-line antiretroviral therapy.** *AIDS* 2009, **23**:1127–1134.
16. Eron JJ, Young B, Cooper DA, Youle M, DeJesus E, Andrade-Villanueva J, Workman C, Zajdenverg R, Fätkenheuer G, Berger DS, *et al*: **Switch to a raltegravir-based regimen versus continuation of a lopinavir-ritonavir-based regimen in stable HIV-infected patients with suppressed viraemia (SWITCHMRK 1 and 2): two multicentre, double-blind, randomised controlled trials.** *Lancet* 2010, **375**:396–407.
17. Martinez E, Arnaiz JA, Podzamczer D, Dalmau D, Ribera E, Domingo P, Knobel H, Riera M, Pedrol E, Force L, *et al*: **Substitution of nevirapine, efavirenz, or abacavir for protease inhibitors in patients with human immunodeficiency virus infection.** *N Engl J Med* 2003, **349**:1036–1046.
18. Boyd MA, Kumarasamy N, Moore CL, Nwizu C, Losso MH, Mohapi L, Martin A, Kerr S, Sohn AH, Teppler H, *et al*: **Ritonavir-boosted lopinavir plus nucleoside or nucleotide reverse transcriptase inhibitors versus ritonavir-boosted lopinavir plus raltegravir for treatment of HIV-1 infection in adults with virological failure of a standard first-line ART regimen (SECOND-LINE): a randomised, open-label, non-inferiority study.** *Lancet* 2013, **381**:2091–2099.
19. Paton N, Kityo C, Hoppe A, Hakim J, van Oosterhout J, Siika A, Mwaba P, Kambugu A, Easterbrook, Boles J, Walker S, Mugyenyi P, EARNEST Trial Group: **A pragmatic randomised controlled strategy trial of three second-line treatment options for use in public health rollout programme settings: the Europe-Africa Research Network for Evaluation of Second-line Therapy (EARNEST) Trial [Abstract WELBB02].** In *7th International AIDS Conference on HIV Pathogenesis, Treatment and Prevention.* Kuala Lumpur, Malaysia; June-July 2013.
20. Tashima K, and OPTIONS Study group: **Omitting NRTI from ARV regimens is not inferior to adding NRTI in treatment-experienced HIV+ subjects failing a protease inhibitor regimen: the ACTG OPTIONS study [Abstract 153LB].** In *20th Conference on Retroviruses and Opportunistic Infections.* Atlanta, Georgia (USA); March 2013.
21. Imaz A, Llibre JM, Mora M, Mateo G, Camacho A, Blanco JR, Curran A, Santos JR, Caballero E, Bravo I, *et al*: **Efficacy and safety of nucleoside reverse transcriptase inhibitor-sparing salvage therapy for multidrug-resistant HIV-1 infection based on new-class and new-generation antiretrovirals [Erratum appears in].** *J Antimicrob Chemother* 2011, **66**(9):2194.
22. Nozza S, Galli L, Bigoloni A, Nicola G, Pogliaghi M, Cossarini F, Salpietro S, Galli A, Della Torre L, Tambussi G, *et al*: **Durability and safety of a novel salvage therapy in R5-tropic HIV-infected patients: maraviroc, raltegravir, etravirine.** *J Acquir Immune Defic Syndr* 2011, **56**:e113–e115.
23. Florence E, De Wit S, Castagna A, Ribera E, Hill A, Vanaken H, van Delft Y, Marks S: **HIV RNA suppression rates after 24 weeks of treatment with etravirine, darunavir/ritonavir and raltegravir in the etravirine early access programme.** *Int J STD AIDS* 2010, **21**:224–225.
24. Ruane P, Brinson C, Kumar P, De Jesus E, Ryan R, Cho M, Anderson D: **Intelence aNd pRezista Once A Day Study (INROADS): A Multicenter, Single-Arm, Open-Label Study of Once Daily Combination of Etravirine (ETR) and Darunavir/Ritonavir (DRV/r) as Dual Therapy in Early Treatment-Experienced Subjects (Abstract WEPE515).** In *7th International AIDS Conference on HIV Pathogenesis, Treatment and Prevention.* Kuala Lumpur, Malaysia; June-July 2013.
25. Hoy J, Martin A, Moore C, Mallon P, Emery S, Belloso W, Phanuphak P, Ferret S, Cooper D, Boyd M, SECOND LINE study team: **Changes in bone mineral density over 48 weeks among participants randomised to either lopinavir/ritonavir (LPV/r) + 2-3N(t)RTI or LPV/r + raltegravir as second-line therapy: a sub-study of the SECONDLINE trial.** In *7th IAS Conference on HIV Pathogenesis, Treatment and Prevention.* Kuala Lumpur, Malaysia; June-July 2013.
26. Ward DJ, O'Neil DJ: **Nucleoside-sparing antiretroviral regimens in clinical practice. [Abstract H-659].** In *the 53rd Interscience Conference on Antimicrobial Agents and Chemotherapy (ICAAC).* Denver USA; Sept. 2013.
27. Calin R, Valantin M, Simon A, Paris L, Tubiana R, Schneider L, Stitou H, Delanoe C, Wirden M, Agher R, Katlama C: **Raltegravir/etravirine dual therapy as a virologically safe treatment option in suppressed HIV-1-infected patients without previous NNRTI failure.** In *7th International AIDS Society Conference on HIV Pathogenesis Treatment and Prevention.* Kuala Lumpur, Malaysia; June-July 2013.
28. Katlama C, Assoumou L, Valantin M, Duvivier C, Soulie C, Chablais L, Pialoux G, Mercie P, Peytavin G, Marcelin A: **Maraviroc plus Raltegravir dual Therapy in Aviremic HIV infected Patients with Lipodystrophy: results from the ROCnRAL ANRS 157 Study.** In *20th Conference on Retroviruses and Opportunistic Infections.* Atlanta, GA; March 2013.
29. Cotte L, Durant J, Brochier C, André P, Cottalorda J, Pradat P, Vanhems P, Dellamonica P: **Safety and efficacy of a Maraviroc-Raltegravir combination following a 6 month induction phase with Maraviroc-Raltegravir-Tenofovir-Emtricitabine in naïve HIV-1 infected patients with CCR5 Virus: interim analysis of the No Nuc No Boost study [Abstract WEPE511].** In *7th International AIDS Society Conference on HIV Pathogenesis Treatment and Prevention.* Kuala Lumpur, Malaysia; June-July 2013.
30. Burgos J, Crespo M, Falco V, Curran A, Navarro J, Imaz A, Domingo P, Podzamczer D, Mateo MG, Villar S, *et al*: **Simplification to dual antiretroviral therapy including a ritonavir-boosted protease inhibitor in treatment-experienced HIV-1-infected patients.** *J Antimicrob Chemother* 2012, **67**:2479–2486.
31. Ofotokun I, Sheth AN, Sanford SE, Easley KA, Shenvi N, White K, Eaton ME, Del Rio C, Lennox JL: **A switch in therapy to a reverse transcriptase inhibitor sparing combination of lopinavir/ritonavir and raltegravir in virologically suppressed HIV-infected patients: a pilot randomized trial to assess efficacy and safety profile: the KITE study.** *AIDS Res Hum Retroviruses* 2012, **28**:1196–1206.
32. Carey D, Pett SL, Bloch M, Wand H, MacRae K, Beileiter K, Ray JE, Boyd MA, Emery S, Cooper DA: **A randomized study of pharmacokinetics, efficacy, and safety of 2 raltegravir plus atazanavir strategies in ART-treated adults.** *J Acquir Immune Defic Syndr* 2012, **60**:143–149.
33. Allavena C, Mounoury O, Rodallec A, Reliquet V, Billaud E, Raffi F: **Efficacy and safety of an NRTI-sparing dual regimen of raltegravir and ritonavir-boosted protease inhibitor in a triple antiretroviral class-experienced population.** *HIV Clin Trials* 2009, **10**:337–340.
34. Fischl MA, Collier AC, Mukherjee AL, Feinberg JE, Demeter LM, Tebas P, Giuliano M, Dehlinger M, Garren K, Brizz B, Bassett R: **Randomized open-label trial of two simplified, class-sparing regimens following a first suppressive three or four-drug regimen.** *AIDS* 2007, **21**:325–333.
35. Cordery DV, Hesse K, Amin J, Cooper DA: **Raltegravir and unboosted atazanavir dual therapy in virologically suppressed antiretroviral treatment-experienced HIV patients.** *Antivir Ther* 2010, **15**:1035–1038.
36. Monteiro P, Perez I, Laguno M, Martinez-Rebollar M, Gonzalez-Cordon A, Lonca M, Mallolas J, Blanco JL, Gatell JM, Martinez E: **Dual therapy with etravirine plus raltegravir for virologically suppressed HIV-infected**

patients: a pilot study. *J Antimicrob Chemother* 2013. Epub ahead of print] doi:10.1093/jac/dkt406.
37. Bierman WF, van Agtmael MA, Nijhuis M, Danner SA, Boucher CA: **HIV monotherapy with ritonavir-boosted protease inhibitors: a systematic review.** *AIDS* 2009, **23**:279–291.
38. Arribas JR, Doroana M, Turner D, Vandekerckhove L, Streinu-Cercel A: **Boosted protease inhibitor monotherapy in HIV-infected adults: outputs from a pan-European expert panel meeting.** *AIDS Res Ther* 2013, **10**:3.
39. Arribas JR, Delgado R, Arranz A, Munoz R, Portilla J, Pasquau J, Perez-Elias MJ, Iribarren JA, Rubio R, Ocampo A, *et al*: **Lopinavir-ritonavir monotherapy versus lopinavir-ritonavir and 2 nucleosides for maintenance therapy of HIV: 96-week analysis.** *J Acquir Immune Defic Syndr* 2009, **51**:147–152.
40. Clumeck N, Rieger A, Banhegyi D, Schmidt W, Hill A, Van Delft Y, Moecklinghoff C, Arribas J: **96 week results from the MONET trial: a randomized comparison of darunavir/ritonavir with versus without nucleoside analogues, for patients with HIV RNA <50 copies/mL at baseline.** *J Antimicrob Chemother* 2011, **66**:1878–1885.
41. Mills A, Mildvan D, Podzamczer D, Fatkenheuer G, Leal M, Than S, Valluri SR, Craig C, McFadyen L, Vourvahis M, *et al*: **Maraviroc once-daily nucleoside analog-sparing regimen in treatment-naive patients: randomized, open-label pilot study.** *J Acquir Immune Defic Syndr* 2013, **62**:164–170.
42. Reynes J, Trinh R, Pulido F, Soto-Malave R, Gathe J, Qaqish R, Tian M, Fredrick L, Podsadecki T, Norton M, Nilius A: **Lopinavir/ritonavir combined with raltegravir or tenofovir/emtricitabine in antiretroviral-naive subjects: 96-week results of the PROGRESS study.** *AIDS Res Hum Retroviruses* 2013, **29**:256–265.
43. Taiwo B, Swindells S, Berzins B, Acosta E, Ryscavage P, Lalezari J, Castro J, Adeyemi O, Yip B, Rathert M, Kuritzkes D, Eron J, MIDAS Study Team: **Week 48 results of the Maraviroc Plus Darunavir/ritonavir Study (MIDAS) for treatment-naive patients infected with R5-tropic HIV-1 [Abstract TUPE099].** In *19th International AIDS Conference*. Washington, DC (USA); July 2012.
44. Bedimo R, Drechsler H, Turner D, Moore T, Ghormley J, Jain M, Petersen T, Santos M, Farukhi I, Cutrell J: **RADAR study: Raltegravir combined with 656 boosted Darunavir has similar safety and antiviral efficacy as tenofovir/ emtricitabine combined with boosted darunavir in antiretroviral-naïve patients [Abstract MOPE214].** In *6th International AIDS Society Conference on HIV Pathogenesis, Treatment and Prevention*. Rome (Italy); July 2011.
45. Taiwo B, Zheng L, Gallien S, Matining RM, Kuritzkes DR, Wilson CC, Berzins BI, Acosta EP, Bastow B, Kim PS, *et al*: **Efficacy of a nucleoside-sparing regimen of darunavir/ritonavir plus raltegravir in treatment-naive HIV-1-infected patients (ACTG A5262).** *AIDS* 2011, **25**:2113–2122.
46. Riddler SA, Haubrich R, DiRienzo AG, Peeples L, Powderly WG, Klingman KL, Garren KW, George T, Rooney JF, Brizz B, *et al*: **Class-sparing regimens for initial treatment of HIV-1 infection.** *N Engl J Med* 2008, **358**:2095–2106.
47. Kozal MJ, Lupo S, DeJesus E, Molina JM, McDonald C, Raffi F, Benetucci J, Mancini M, Yang R, Wirtz V, *et al*: **A nucleoside- and ritonavir-sparing regimen containing atazanavir plus raltegravir in antiretroviral treatment-naive HIV-infected patients: SPARTAN study results.** *HIV Clin Trials* 2012, **13**:119–130.
48. Taiwo B, Acosta EP, Ryscavage P, Berzins B, Lu D, Lalezari J, Castro J, Adeyemi O, Kuritzkes DR, Eron JJ, *et al*: **Virologic response, early HIV-1 decay, and maraviroc pharmacokinetics with the nucleos(t)ide-free regimen of maraviroc plus darunavir/ritonavir in a pilot study.** *J Acquir Immune Defic Syndr* 2013, **64**:167–173.
49. The GARDEL Study Team: **Dual therapy with Lopinavir/ Ritonavir (LPV/r) and Lamivudine (3TC) is non-inferior to standard triple drug therapy in Naïve HIV-1 infected subjects: 48-week results of the GARDEL Study [Abstract LBPS7/6].** In *14th European AIDS Conference*. Brussels (Belgium); Sept. 2013.
50. Hill A, Sawyer W, Gazzard B: **Effects of first-line use of nucleoside analogues, efavirenz, and ritonavir-boosted protease inhibitors on lipid levels.** *HIV Clin Trials* 2009, **10**:1–12.
51. Achhra AC, Amin J, Hoy J, Tanuma J, Sirisanthana T, Nolan D, Merati T, Giles M: **Differences in lipid measurements by antiretroviral regimen exposure in cohorts from Asia and australia.** *AIDS Res Treat* 2012, **2012**:246280.
52. Sax P: *MODERN Study Stopped: An NRTI-Sparing, Two-Drug Initial Regimen Disappoints Again.* Available at http://blogs.jwatch.org/hiv-id-observations/index.php/modern-study-stopped-an-nrti-sparing-two-drug-initial-regimen-disappoints-again/2013/10/14/. Accessed on 30 October 2013.
53. Achhra AC, Boyd M, Law MG, Matthews G, Kelleher AD, Cooper DA: **Sequencing antiretroviral therapy to maximize patient safety: could we move away from Ritonavir, Abacavir, Tenofovir, and Efavirenz(RATE) - agents that concern prescribers and patients? A feasibility study and Call for a trial [Abstract: PE8/6].** In *14th European AIDS Conference*. Brussels (Belgium); Sept. 2013.
54. Gazzard B, Duvivier C, Zagler C, Castagna A, Hill A, van Delft Y, Marks S: **Phase 2 double-blind, randomized trial of etravirine versus efavirenz in treatment-naive patients: 48-week results.** *AIDS* 2011, **25**:2249–2258.

16

Should highly active antiretroviral therapy be prescribed in critically ill HIV-infected patients during the ICU stay?

Agnes Meybeck[1,3*], Lydie Lecomte[1], Michel Valette[2], Nicolas Van Grunderbeeck[1], Nicolas Boussekey[1], Arnaud Chiche[1], Hugues Georges[1], Yazdan Yazdanpanah[2] and Olivier Leroy[1]

Abstract

Background: The impact of highly active antiretroviral therapy (HAART) in HIV-infected patients admitted to the intensive care unit (ICU) remains controversial. We evaluate impact of HAART prescription in HIV-infected patients admitted to the ICU of Tourcoing Hospital from January 2000 to December 2009.

Results: There were 91 admissions concerning 85 HIV-infected patients. Reasons for ICU admission were an AIDS-related diagnosis in 46 cases (51%). Fifty two patients (57%) were on HAART at the time of ICU admission, leading to 21 immunovirologic successes (23%). During the ICU stay, HAART was continued in 29 patients (32%), and started in 3 patients (3%). Only one patient experienced an adverse event related to HAART. Mortality rate in ICU and 6 months after ICU admission were respectively 19% and 27%. Kaplan-Meier estimates of the cumulative unajusted survival probability over 6 months were higher in patients treated with HAART during the ICU stay (Log rank: $p = 0.04$). No benefit of HAART in ICU was seen in the adjusted survival proportion at 6 months or during ICU stay. Prescription of HAART during ICU was associated with a trend to lower incidence of new AIDS-related events at 6 months (respectively 17% and 34% with and without HAART, $p = 0.07$), and with higher incidence of antiretroviral resistance after ICU stay (respectively 25% and 7% with and without HAART, $p = 0.02$).

Conclusions: Our results suggest a lower death rate over 6 months in critically ill HIV-infected patients taking HAART during ICU stay. The optimal time to prescribe HAART in critically ill patients needs to be better defined.

Keywords: HIV, Intensive care, HAART

Background

Highly active antiretroviral therapy (HAART) has increased the life expectancy of patients who are infected with the human immunodeficiency virus (HIV) and has reduced the incidence of illnesses associated with the acquired immunodeficiency syndrome (AIDS). HIV-infected adults with CD4 cell count greater than 500 cells/mm3 on long-term combination antiretroviral therapy reach same mortality rates as the general population [1]. Survival of HIV-infected patients admitted to the intensive care unit (ICU) has been evaluated in a number of studies [2-6]. Most of these studies have shown improved survival since the late 1990s for HIV infected patients, associated with the advent of HAART. But whether or not the improved survival is dependent of the use of HAART remains controversial [5-7]. Changing practices of ICU care and decrease of AIDS-related admissions may explain survival improvement [2,8].

Very few previously published studies have reported data on the use of HAART in the ICU [9-11]. There are no randomized clinical trials and no consensus guidelines to assist in decisions regarding the use of HAART in the ICU [11]. Early prescription of HAART in ICU might decrease patient morbidity and mortality by restoring pathogen specific immune responses and speeding immune reconstitution. On the other hand, prescription of HAART in critically ill patients might result in higher morbidity and

* Correspondence: agnesmeybeck@yahoo.fr
[1]Service de Réanimation et Maladies Infectieuses, Hôpital de Tourcoing, 135 rue du Président Coty, Tourcoing BP 619, France
[3]Service de Réanimation et Maladies Infectieuses, Centre Hospitalier Dron, 128 rue du Président Coty, Tourcoing 59200, France

mortality by increasing toxicity of treatment, increasing drug-drug interactions, increasing the frequency of immune reconstitution and inflammatory syndrome (IRIS).

We conducted a retrospective cohort study of all consecutive cases of HIV-infected patients admitted to the ICU from January 2000 to December 2009 at Tourcoing Hospital. The aim of this study was to evaluate the impact of HAART prescription prior to ICU and during ICU stay.

Methods

Patients and hospital setting

We conducted a retrospective cohort study of all consecutive cases of HIV-infected patients admitted to the 16-bed ICU of Tourcoing Hospital from January 2000 to December 2009. As it was an observational retrospective study, in accordance with French law, neither approval of the ethics committee nor informed consent was required. If patients were admitted to the ICU more than one time during any hospitalisation, only data from admissions separated by > 90 days were considered independent events and were included in the analysis.

Data collection and baseline data

Data on HIV infection and on ICU stay were obtained retrospectively, using case-notes and computer database. Data obtained included age, sex, race, the indication(s) for ICU admission, underlying clinical conditions, presence of comorbidities, severity of illness at ICU admission. Admission was considered AIDS-related if the main admission diagnosis was an AIDS-defining condition (1993 Centers for Disease Control Classification System for HIV-Infected Adults) [12]. The underlying clinical conditions were classified according to the criteria proposed by McCabe and Jackson in 3 categories: non fatal (5 year survival not affect by underlying disease), ultimately fatal (not expected to survive more than 5 years), and rapidly fatal (not expected to survive more than 1 year) [13]. The severity of illness at the time of ICU admission was assessed by SAPS II and Glasgow Coma Score [14,15]. The SAPS II includes 12 physiology variables including Glasgow Coma Score, and age, type of admission (scheduled surgical, unscheduled surgical, or medical), and three underlying disease variable (acquired immunodeficiency syndrome, metastatic cancer, and hematologic malignancy). Neurological and mental status was stratified according to Glasgow Coma Score. The following therapeutic modalities in ICU were recorded: invasive or noninvasive mechanical ventilation, hemodialysis or hemofiltration, and use of vasoactive drugs.

The following data on HIV-infection were recorded for each case at ICU admission: risk factor for HIV, HIV disease staging according to CDC Classification System for HIV-Infected Adults (Category A: asymptomatic, acute HIV, or persistent generalized lymphadenopathy; Category B: symptomatic conditions not A or C; Category C: AIDS-indicator conditions), CD4 cell count and plasma HIV viral load if available within 6 months of admission. The mean time between determination of CD4 cell count and plasma HIV viral load and admission in ICU was 32 days. During ICU stay, we recorded new AIDS-defining event and IRIS occurence. IRIS was defined as a paradoxical deterioration in clinical status or laboratory findings after the initiation of antiretroviral therapy without another attribuable cause.

The following data on antiretroviral therapy were recorded: HAART prior and during ICU stay. We collected regimen, duration and adverse effects. HAART was defined as a combination of 3 or more antiretroviral drugs belonging to at least 2 classes among the following: protease inhibitors (PIs), nucleoside reverse transcriptase inhibitors (NRTIs), and nonnucleoside reverse transcriptase inhibitors (NNRTIs). No other antiretroviral combination than HAART was prescribed in our cohort.

After the ICU stay, the following data were recorded: CD4 cell count and viral load at 3, 6, and 12 months after ICU admission, occurence of a new AIDS defining event, occurence of IRIS, change in HAART prescription, emergence of antiretroviral-resistance at any time during a 12 months period following ICU admission.

Outcome measures

Our primary outcomes of interest were in ICU and 6-month mortality. Secondary outcomes of interest were the occurrence of a new AIDS related event, immunovirological response, adverse event of antiretroviral therapy, emergence of resistance. Immunovirological success was defined as viral load < 200 copies/ml and CD4 > 200 cells/mm^3.

Statistical analyses

Analyses were performed to identify predictive factors of ICU and 6-month mortality. All collected variables concerning underlying disease, severity of illness, care in ICU, and HIV-infection were analysed. Categorical variables were compared using Chi-square test or Fisher's exact test when Chi-square was not appropriate. Continuous variables were compared using Student's t test or Mann–Whitney test when appropriate. All variables attaining an α value of 0.05 were included in a multiple logistic regression analysis model with a stepwise selection of variables to identify predictive factors of ICU and 6-month mortality. Variables that originate a multicolinearity were eliminated. The quality of the model was evaluated through its measures of sensitivity and specificity with establishment of a ROC curve. Kaplan Meier survival analysis was used to estimate cumulative mortality over 6 months. Log rank test was used to compare differences in survival between two groups (no HAART use in ICU vs HAART use in ICU). Differences between groups were considered to be significant for variables yielding a p value ≤ 0.05.

Results

Demographic and clinical characteristics

There were 91 ICU admissions concerning 85 HIV-infected patients. Demographic and clinical characteristics of our patients are shown Table 1. The majority of the ICU cohort consisted of men (n = 61, 67%), and was ever diagnosed with AIDS (n = 69, 76%). Patients were equally likely to be heterosexual (n = 31, 34%), or homosexual (n = 31, 34%). Median CD4 cell count at ICU admission was 112/mm^3 [1–935]. The ICU admission represented the initial HIV diagnosis for 19% of the cases. Respiratory failure and neurologic disorder were the most frequent reasons for ICU admission (51% and 27% respectively). The ICU admissions were motivated by AIDS-associated diagnosis in 46 patients (51%). HAART adverse events led to ICU admission in 4 patients. Mechanical ventilation was needed in 45 patients (49%) for a mean duration of 5 ± 10 days. The mean length of ICU stay was 8 ± 10 days.

Patients who received HAART in ICU were similar to those who did not with respect to age, gender, mean SAPS II, and Glasgow score. Patients who received HAART in ICU were less likely to be ignorant of their

Table 1 Characteristics of the patients and clinical data depending on HAART use during ICU stay*

Characteristics and clinical data	Total (n = 91)	without HAART (n = 59)	with HAART (n = 32)	p
Characteristics				
Age (in years)	42 ± 10	42 ± 9	43 ± 11	0.98
Sex (M/F)	61/30	40/19	21/11	0.99
SAPS II on admission	47 ± 20	48 ± 21	46 ± 17	0.83
Glasgow score	12 ± 4	12 ± 5	13 ± 4	0.24
Main reasons for ICU admission				
Respiratory	46 (51)	28 (47)	18 (56)	0.51
Neurologic	25 (27)	16 (27)	9 (28)	0.99
Shock	10 (11)	6 (10)	4 (13)	0.99
Others	10 (11)	9 (15)	1 (3)	0.09
HIV infection				
Initial HIV diagnosis	17 (19)	16 (27)	1 (3)	**0.004**
Stage C	69 (76)	43 (73)	26 (81)	0.85
CD4 count at admission (cells/mm^3)	112 [1–935]	100 [2–935]	161 [1–822]	0.68
Viral load at admission (log10)	3.38 ± 1.60	3.86 ± 1.51	2.63 ± 1.45	**0.0005**
AIDS related diagnosis at ICU admission	46 (51)	33 (56)	13 (41)	0.25
Opportunistic infections				
Pneumocystis jirovecii	12	10	2	0.2
Toxoplasmosis	7	5	2	0.99
Mycobacterial infections	7	4	3	0.69
Pneumonia	3	2	1	0.99
Others	5	3	2	0.99
Care in ICU				
Mechanical ventilation (MV)	45 (49)	29 (49)	16 (32)	0.87
Duration of ventilation (days)	5 ± 10	5 ± 11	5 ± 9	0.81
Renal replacement	7 (8)	3 (5)	4 (13)	0.33
Vasoactive drugs	22 (24)	15 (25)	7 (22)	0.99
Duration of vasoactive drugs (days)	1 ± 2	1 ± 2	1 ± 2	0.99
ICU length of stay (days)	8 ± 10	8 ± 11	8 ± 9	0.43
Death in ICU	17 (19)	12 (20)	5 (16)	0.78

*Data are presented as No. (%) or mean ± SD, except for CD4 cell count which are expressed as median [range].

HIV infection (3% vs 27%, p = 0.004) and had significantly lower mean log viral load (2.63 ± 1.45 log copies/ml vs 3.86 ± 1.51 log copies/ml, p = 0.0005). Median CD4 cell count at admission was similar in both groups.

Risk factors for mortality

Mortality rate in ICU, and 6 months after ICU admission were respectively 19% and 27%. Results for univariate analysis for ICU and 6-month outcomes are presented respectively in Table 2 and Table 3.

By univariate analysis, the factors associated with ICU mortality were high SAPS II score, low Glasgow score, use of mechanical ventilation, prolonged duration of mechanical ventilation, and of catecholamine prescription. Patient with undiagnosed HIV were more likely to die in ICU. By univariate analysis, the factors associated with 6-month mortality were similar to those associated with ICU mortality. Neither history of HAART use prior to ICU admission, nor use of HAART during ICU stay was associated with ICU and 6-month survival.

Results for multivariate analysis for ICU and 6-month mortality are presented respectively in Table 4 and Table 5. By multivariate analysis, the only factor independently associated with ICU mortality was SAPS II score (OR = 1.05 per point; 95%CI: 1.02-1.08; p = 0.001). SAPS II score and AIDS-associated diagnosis were independently associated with 6-month mortality (respectively OR = 1.05 per point; 95%CI: 1.01-1.06; p = 0.001 and OR = 2.9, 95%CI: 1.01-8.31; p = 0.04). The quality of the model has been evaluated through its measures of sensitivity and specificity with establishment of a ROC curve, the area under the curve being 0.739 (Figure 1).

Table 2 Univariate predictors of ICU survival*

Characteristics	Non survivors n = 17 (19)	Survivors n = 74 (81)	p
Characteristics at ICU admission			
Age (in years)	40 ± 9	43 ± 10	0.13
Sex (M/F)	7/10	23/51	0.57
Glasgow score	8 ± 5	13 ± 4	**0.0003**
HIV infection			
Initial HIV diagnosis	7 (37)	10 (14)	**0.015**
Stage C	13 (76)	56 (76)	0.99
CD4 count at admission (cells/mm3)	120 ± 98	206 ± 209	0.38
AIDS related diagnosis at ICU admission	11 (65)	35 (47)	0.28
Care in ICU			
Mechanical ventilation	17 (100)	28 (38)	**<0.0001**
Duration of ventilation (days)	12 ± 13	4 ± 9	**<0.0001**
Vasoactive drugs	5 (29)	8 (11)	0.06
Duration of vasoactive drugs use (days)	2.5 ± 2.7	0.7 ± 1.7	**<0.0001**
Use of HAART			
HAART at ICU admission	6 (38)	46 (62)	0.09
§ immunovirological success at ICU admission	2 (12)	19 (26)	0.34
HAART during ICU stay	5 (29)	27 (36)	0.78

*Data are presented as No. (%) or mean ± SD. §Immunovirological success was defined as viral load < 200 copies/ml and CD4 > 200 cells/mm^3.

Table 3 Univariate predictors of 6-month survival*

Characteristics	Non survivors n = 25	Survivors n = 55	p
Characteristics at ICU admission			
Age	40 ± 9	42 ± 9	0.19
Sex (M/F)	8/17	19/36	0.99
SAPSII on admission	55 ± 25	42 ± 16	**0.02**
Glasgow on admission	10 ± 5	13 ± 4	**0.05**
HIV infection			
Initial HIV diagnosis	8 (32)	6 (11)	**0.03**
Stage C	20 (80)	43 (78)	0.99
CD4 count at admission (/mm3)	154 ± 201	215 ± 198	0.21
AIDS related diagnosis at ICU admission	16 (64)	24 (44)	0.15
Care in ICU			
Mechanical ventilation	19 (76)	20 (36)	**0.0015**
Duration of ventilation (days)	10 ± 13	3 ± 8	**0.0001**
Vasoactive drugs	6 (24)	5 (9)	0.09
Duration of vasoactive drugs use (days)	1.7 ± 2.5	0.6 ± 1.3	**0.006**
Use of HAART			
HAART at ICU admission	11 (44)	35 (64)	0.14
immunovirological success at ICU admission	3 (12)	17 (31)	0.096
HAART during ICU stay	9 (36)	21 (38)	0.99

*Data are presented as No. (%) or mean ± SD.

Use of HAART

At the time of ICU admission, 52/91 (57%) of patients were on HAART, leading to only 21 (23%) immunovirological successes. A combination of two nucleoside/nucleotide reverse transcriptase inhibitor (NRTI) and one protease inhibitor (PI) was the most common prescribed regimen (n = 31/52, 59%).

Table 4 Multivariate predictors of ICU survival*

Variables	Adjusted OR (95% CI)	p value
SAPS II on admission (per 1 point of increment)	1.05 (1.02-1.08)	0.001

*The retained variables for the multivariate analysis were those the adjustment of which had a medical or biological meaning, eliminating that originate a multicolinearity. Variables were retained when their effect had a P value less than 0.05.

Table 5 Multivariate predictors of 6-month survival*

Variables	Adjusted OR (95% CI)	p value
SAPS II on admission (per 1 point of increment)	1.05 (1.01-1.06)	0.001
AIDS related diagnosis	2.9 (1.01-8.31)	0.04

*The retained variables for the multivariate analysis were those the adjustment of which had a medical or biological meaning, eliminating that originate a multicolinearity. Variables were retained when their effect had a P value less than 0.05.

During ICU stay, antiretroviral therapy was continued in 32 patients (35%), and initiated in ICU in 3 patients (3%). In patients already receiving antiretroviral therapy at ICU admission, HAART was continued in 26 patients (50%), modified in 3 patients (6%), stopped in 23 patients (44%). HAART interruption was motivated by a severe side effect in 4 patients. In 19 patients, no justification for HAART discontinuation was found in the patient chart. HAART was stopped despite immunovirological success in 9 patients. The 3 patients who changed HAART, replaced another boosted protease inhibitor by the combination lopinavir-norvir, available in liquid form. The median delay between ICU admission and HAART prescription was 0 day [0–38]. In case of HAART initiation in ICU, this delay was prolonged: 19 [2–38] days. The duration of HAART in ICU was 5 ± 4 days. Patients treated with HAART in ICU spent 76% of their ICU stay on HAART. The most commonly prescribed regimen in ICU was the combination of two NRTI and one PI (n = 24/32, 75%).

All patients who received HAART during ICU stay continued HAART after ICU stay. After ICU discharge, antiretroviral combination was modified in 8 patients, because of drug interaction in 3 patients, adverse event occurence in 2 patients, virological failure in one patient, addition of enfuvirtide in one patient. No motivation was found in one patient. HAART was initiated (n = 14) or reintroduced (n = 15) in patients not treated in ICU after a mean delay of 19 ± 22 days after ICU release. The most common prescribed regimen after ICU stay was the combination of two NRTI and one PI (n = 38/61, 62%).

Impact of HAART on survival

The mortality rate was not significantly different at ICU discharge and at 6 months according to the use of HAART during the ICU stay: respectively 16% vs 20% with and without HAART at ICU discharge, and 28% vs 27% respectively with and without HAART at 6 months. Kaplan-Meier estimates of the cumulative unadjusted survival probability over 6 months were significantly higher in the group of patients treated with HAART during the ICU stay (Log rank test, p = 0.04) (Figure 2). But, no benefit of HAART was seen specifically in the adjusted survival proportion at 6 months or during ICU stay (Table 2 and Table 4).

Impact of HAART on AIDS progression and immunovirologial response

During ICU stay, a new AIDS related event was diagnosed in 3 patients (9%) treated with HAART, and in 5 patients (8%) not treated with HAART. At 6 months, new AIDS related events tended to be less frequent in the group of patients treated with HAART in ICU, respectively 17% vs 34% with and without HAART (p = 0.07).

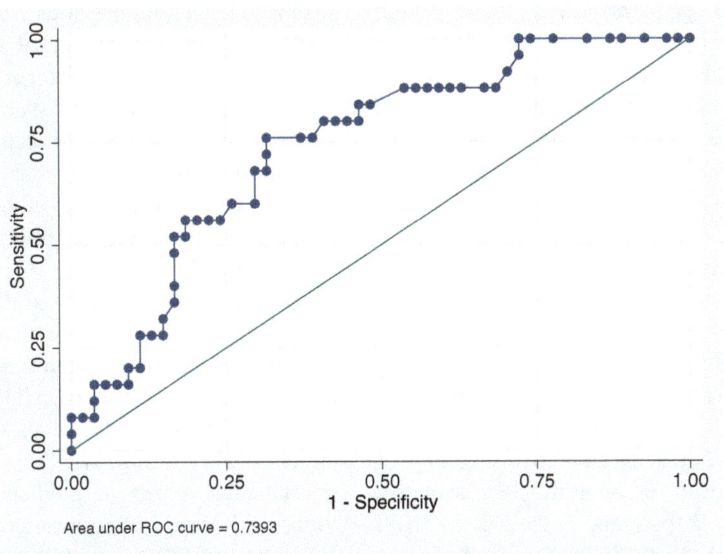

Figure 1 ROC curve evaluating quality of the model including SAPS II and AIDS-related diagnosis to determine 6-month mortality risk. The quality of the multiple logistic regression analysis model was evaluated through its measures of sensitivity and specificity with establishment of a ROC curve. Aera under the ROC curve was 0.7393.

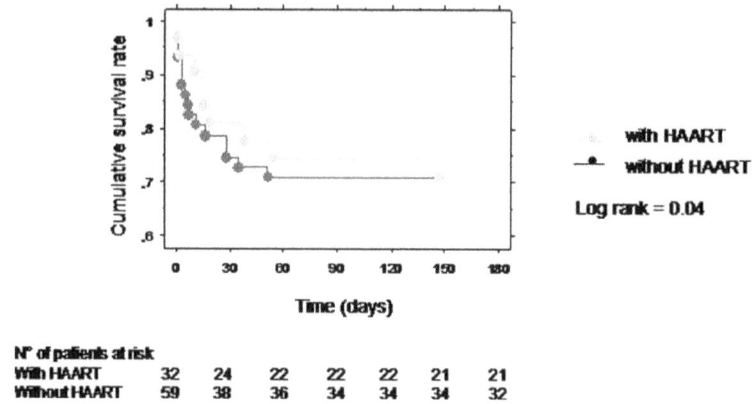

Figure 2 The effect of the prescription of antiretroviral therapy in ICU on 6-month cumulative survival. Kaplan-Meier estimates of the cumulative unajusted survival probability over 6 months were higher in patients with HAART (grey line) vs without HAART(black line) during the ICU stay (Log rank: p = 0.04).

When comparing mean CD4 cell count, there was no significant difference between the two groups (with vs without HAART) at any time of the year following ICU admission. Median CD4 cell count at 12 months reached 1309 [365–2254] cells/mm^3 and 385 [99–605] cells/mm^3 respectively with and without HAART (p = 0.23). Mean log10 viral load was significantly lower at 3 and 6 months in patients treated with HAART while in ICU (2.06 ± 0.78 vs 3.16 ± 1.46 copies/ml with and without HAART at 3 months, p = 0.02, and 2.42 ± 0.68 vs 3.37 ± 1.36 copies/ml with and without HAART at 6 months, p = 0.03). One year after ICU admission, immunovirological success was achieved in 25% of patients treated with HAART and in 16% of patients not treated with HAART (p = 0.25).

A resistance to an antiretroviral molecule was diagnosed after ICU in 8 patients (25%) treated with HAART, and in 4 patients (7%) not treated with HAART (p = 0.02). A history of HAART prior to ICU and an immunovirologic failure at ICU admission were reported respectively in 12 and 5 patients diagnosed with antiretroviral resistance after ICU.

Tolerance of HAART

In ICU, a side effect motivating interruption of HAART was reported in one patient, who suffered from severe anemia while treated with zidovudine. After ICU stay, 21 adverse events motivating interruption or change of HAART were reported after a mean duration of treatment of 107 ± 112 days. The incidence of adverse events after ICU was not different according to the timing of HAART prescription, during or after the ICU stay. An IRIS was diagnosed in 2 patients (2.2%). Both IRIS occured after ICU stay, respectively 25 days and 45 days after ICU admission. One patient received HAART in ICU. The other one began HAART the day he left the ICU, 7 days after his admission.

Discussion

In our cohort of HIV-infected patients admitted to the ICU, the only independent predictor of ICU outcome was severity of acute illness assessed by SAPS II score at ICU admission. Two factors were independent predictors of decreased 6-month survival: SAPS II score and AIDS-associated diagnosis at ICU admission. Use of HAART during ICU stay improved unadjusted survival at 6 months. But no benefit was seen specifically in the adjusted survival proportion at 6 months or during ICU stay. Use of HAART during ICU stay tended to reduce AIDS progression. Tolerance of HAART in ICU was good. IRIS was rare. Prescription of HAART during ICU stay was associated with higher incidence of antiretroviral resistance after ICU stay.

In our cohort, risk factors for ICU mortality were consistent with factors previously identified in the literature; these relate to the extent of organ dysfunction rather than HIV-related characteristics [6,7,16]. Severity of acute illness assessed by various scores (APACHE-II score, SAPS-II), need for mechanical ventilation, or catecholamine predicted higher mortality rate in ICU [2,3,6,7,16,17]. Low serum albumin level has been associated with increased mortality rate in ICU in several studies [6,7,17,18].

In our series, AIDS-related disease at the time of ICU admission was associated with a higher 6-month mortality rate. Other previous reports demonstrated an impact on long term survival of AIDS-associated diagnosis in the ICU [2,6,17]. Morris A et al. reported that the patients with a non-AIDS-associated diagnosis had a dramatically improved median survival compared with those with an AIDS-associated diagnosis [6]. Khouli H et al. showed HIV-related illness to be a significant independent predictor of increased hospital mortality [17]. Among the HIV-related characteristics, the CD4 cell count may be a predictor of long-term outcome [19].

But, several authors, like us, did not report any significant relationship between the CD4 cell count and survival [4,6,20].

Concerning HAART prescription, almost two thirds of our patients were on HAART at the time of ICU admission. But only 23% of the patients have achieved immunovirological success. Prior HAART was continued in ICU in only 53% of the patients, and HAART was almost never initiated in ICU. By multivariate analysis, the use of HAART prior to ICU admission and during ICU stay did not independently affect ICU or 6-month survival. But the log rank test suggests a lower death rate over 6-months in patients treated with HAART in ICU. The discrepancy between log-rank curves and the multivariate analysis may be due to potential confounders. Patients without HAART in ICU were more likely to be ignorant of their HIV infection and tended to suffer more often from an opportunistic disease. This could influence the prognosis. Patients with HAART in ICU tended to experience fewer AIDS-associated diagnosis during the 6-month follow-up period. Improved immune function and increased CD4 cell count following HAART could explain the reduction of AIDS progression in case of HAART use in ICU. Published data that have assessed the impact of HAART in ICU are few. Several retrospective studies have reported an improvement of survival of HIV-infected patients admitted in ICU in the last decade, since the advent of HAART [2,4,6]. But the impact of HAART on survival is intringuing. The decrease in mortality could be a result of a change in the spectrum of admission diagnosis as non AIDS-associated diagnosis became more common and were associated with a better survival than AIDS-associated diagnosis. Powell K. et al. examined survival to hospital discharge of HIV-infected patients admitted to the ICU since the year 2000 [7]. They reported that survival for critically ill HIV-infected patients continues to improve in the current era of HAART. This improvement appeared to be independent of the use of HAART. Many advances in critical care practice (e.g., low tidal volumes for patients with respiratory failure, tight glycemic control, adjuvant corticosteroïds for certain conditions, early goal-directed therapy for sepsis) have been made across this last decade [21-23]. They could contribute to outcome improvement of HIV infected patients admitted in ICU.

None of these observational studies reported data on the prescription of HAART during the ICU stay. Only three retrospective studies have assessed the potential benefit associated with administrating HAART in the ICU. Morris et al. performed a retrospective study of 58 patients admitted to the ICU with *Pneumocystis jirovecii* between 1996 and 2001 [24]. They found that patients who were receiving HAART at the time of ICU admission or had HAART started during the ICU stay had a reduced mortality rate compared to those who did not receive HAART. Another retrospective study conducted in a Mexican ICU found HAART prior to admission or starting within one month after ICU discharge to be the major protective factor for death [9]. In their cohort, Croda et al. reported a significantly better survival of patients who began HAART during ICU stay compared to patients without HAART during ICU stay [10]. The potential benefit of HAART found in these three studies could reflect the impact of early prescription of HAART in the context of AIDS-defining diagnosis. An AIDS-defining diagnosis motivated ICU admission in 51% of patients in our cohort and in up to 80% of patients in the last study mentioned. But, in our population, only 19% of patients had not been diagnosed with HIV infection prior to their admission in ICU. A majority of our patients had history of HAART. The very small proportion of patients initiating HAART in our cohort could explain the lack of significant impact of HAART prescription on prognosis. Recently, Zolopa et al. conducted a prospective randomized study to compared immediate HAART (within two days of study enrollment) to deferred HAART (between week 6 and week 12) in HIV-patients diagnosed with acute AIDS-related opportunistic infection [25]. Early HAART resulted in less AIDS progression and death compared to deferred HAART. Concurrent treatment of the opportunistic infection and HIV might increase the frequency of IRIS and have a deleterious impact on outcomes. Incidence and consequences of IRIS vary by opportunistic infections and corticoid use [25-27]. In case of cryptococcal meningitis, early initiation of HAART resulted in increased rate of IRIS, and increased mortality [26]. In case of tuberculosis, HAART started during tuberculosis therapy resulted in lower mortality despite higher incidence of IRIS [27]. In the setting of the opportunistic infections observed in our cohort, most particularly *Pneumocystis* pneumonia, IRIS occurence was rare. Only one previous study conducted in ICU has reported data on IRIS [10]. Among 278 HIV-infected patients admitted in ICU, three patients with tuberculosis developed IRIS during their ICU stay.

Our study is the first to report data on the use of HAART after the ICU stay. In our cohort, patients not receiving HAART in ICU initiated or restarted HAART after a median delay of three weeks after ICU release. This relatively short delay could have reduced the impact of HAART prescription in ICU. The optimal time to prescribe HAART in ICU patients (immediate treatment vs early treatment after ICU discharge) needs to be defined. The decision regarding when to administrate antiretroviral therapy in critically ill HIV-patients must balance the risk of HIV disease progression with the potential risk of drug toxicities. In our cohort, tolerance of HAART in ICU was good with only one patient (3%) suffering from a side effect motivating interruption of HAART. After ICU discharge, the incidence of adverse events was not different according to the timing of HAART prescription, during or after the ICU stay. Only one previous study conducted in ICU has reported data on HAART adverse effects. The incidence of side effects demanding either switch in or discontinuation of HAART was 18% [10]. Occurence of an adverse effect had no impact on mortality.

Another concern about HAART prescription in ICU is drug delivery. Most drugs are only available orally with few liquid medications, and absorption is often unpredictable in seriously ill patients. Multiple drug interactions with HAART can result in either toxic or subtherapeutic antiretroviral drug levels. In our cohort, we did not practice any drug monitoring. But we observed a higher proportion of antiretroviral drug resistance after ICU discharge in patients treated with HAART in ICU. Low antiretoviral drug concentrations in critically ill patients could lead to selection of resistant virus. Non compliance to HAART before ICU admission could have contributed to the resistance. All patients diagnosed with resistance after ICU have been exposed to HAART. But we did not specifically evaluate adherence to HAART.

Our study has several limitations in interpretation and the ability to generalize from its results. We conducted our study at a single institution. Clinical practice and demographics may differ across institutions, and countries. As in any observational retrospective study, the missing data could have reduced the strength of our observations. Because of the study's retrospective nature, it is possible that patients receiving HAART differ in some systematic way beyond the direct effects of the medications. In our cohort, patients who received HAART in ICU were less likely to be ignorant of their HIV infection. Confounders may have affected our observations. But the major limitations of our study are the small size and heterogeneity of patients groups that prevent adequate statistical analysis. Nevertheless, the relatively short duration of inclusion time allowed standardized ICU care. All patients were admitted in ICU during an era including tight glycemic control, protective ventilation in case of acute respiratory distress syndrome, corticosteroids in case of *Pneumocystis* pneumonia or septic shock [21-23].

Conclusion

In our cohort of critically ill HIV-infected patients, benefit of HAART administration during ICU stay was limited. The reticence of intensivists to use HAART and the early prescription of HAART after ICU discharge may have reduced the impact of HAART use in ICU. Our results support the need for prospective randomized clinical trials to address the optimal timing to prescribe HAART in critically ill patients. Future trials should provide antiretroviral drug monitoring and data on compliance to HAART after ICU discharge.

Abbreviations

AIDS: Acquired immunodeficiency syndrome; CI: Confidence interval; HAART: Highly active antiretroviral therapy; HIV: Human immunodeficiency virus; ICU: Intensive care unit; IRIS: Immune reconstitution and inflammatory syndrome; NRTI: Nucleoside/Nucleotide reverse transcriptase inhibitor; PI: Protease inhibitor; OR: Odds ratio; SAPS: Simplified acute physiology score.

Competing interests

The authors declare that they have no competing interests.

Authors' contributions

AM, LL have contributed to study design, analysis and interpretation of data. MV has performed statistical analysis. NV has contributed to interpretation of data and has revised critically the manuscript. NB, AC, HG drafted the manuscript. YY, OL have participated in data interpretation and manuscript drafting. All authors read and approved the final manuscript.

Author details

[1]Service de Réanimation et Maladies Infectieuses, Hôpital de Tourcoing, 135 rue du Président Coty, Tourcoing BP 619, France. [2]Service des Maladies Infectieuses et du Voyageur, Hôpital de Tourcoing, 135 rue du Président Coty, Tourcoing BP 619, France. [3]Service de Réanimation et Maladies Infectieuses, Centre Hospitalier Dron, 128 rue du Président Coty, Tourcoing 59200, France.

References

1. Lewden C, Chene G, Morlat P, Raffi F, Dupon M, Dellamonica P, Pellegrin JL, Katlama C, Dabis F, Leport C, Agence Nationale de Recherches sur le Sida et les Hepatites Virales (ANRS) CO8 APROCO-COPILOTE Study Group; Agence Nationale de Recherches sur le Sida et les Hepatites Virales (ANRS) CO3 AQUITAINE Study Group: **HIV-infected adults with CD4 cell count greater than 500 cells/mm3 on long-term combination antiretroviral therapy reach same mortality rates as the general population.** *J Acquir Defic Syndr* 2007, **46:**72–77.
2. Casalino E, Wolff M, Ravaud P, Choquet C, Bruneel F, Regnier B: **Impact of HAART advent on admission patterns and survival in HIV-infected patients admitted to an intensive care unit.** *AIDS* 2004, **18:**1429–1433.
3. Palacios R, Hidalgo A, Reina C, de la Torre MV, Marquez M, Santos J: **Effect of antiretroviral therapy on admissions of HIV-infected patients to an intensive care unit.** *HIV Medicine* 2006, **7:**193–196.
4. Narasimhan M, Posner AJ, DePalo VA, Mayo PH, Rosen MJ: **Intensive care in patients with HIV infection in the era of higly active antiretroviral therapy.** *Chest* 2004, **125:**1800–1804.
5. Vargas-Infante YA, Lourdes Guerrero M, Ruiz-Palacios GM, Sot-Ramirez LE, Del Rio C, Carranza J, Dominguez-Cherit G, Sierra-Madero JG: **Improving outcome of human immunodeficiency virus-infected patients in a mexican intensive care unit.** *Arch Med Res* 2007, **38:**827–833.
6. Morris A, Creasman J, Turner J, Luce JM, Wachter RM, Huang L: **Intensive care of human immunodeficiency virus-infected patients during the era of highly active antiretrovial therapy.** *Am J Respir Crit Care Med* 2002, **166:**262–267.
7. Powell K, Lucian Davis J, Morris AM, Chi A, Bensley MR, Huang L: **Survival for patients with human immunodeficiency virus admitted to the intensive care unit continues to improve in the current era of highly active antiretroviral therapy.** *Chest* 2009, **135:**11–17.
8. Davis JL, Morris A, Kallet RH, Powell K, Chi AS, Bensley M, Luce JM, Huang L: **Low tidal volume ventilation is associated with reduced mortality in HIV-infected patients with acute lung injury.** *Thorax* 2008, **63:**988–993.
9. Vargas-Infante YA, Guerrero ML, Ruiz-Palacios GM, Soto-Ramirez LE, Carranza J, Dominguez-Cherit G, Sierra-Madero JG: **Improving outcome of human**

immunodeficiency virus-infected patients in a Mexican intensive care unit. *Arch Med Res* 2007, **38**:827–833.
10. Croda J, Garcia Croda M, Neves A, De Sousa dos Santos S: Benefit of antiretroviral therapy on survival of human immunodeficiency virus-infected patients admitted to an intensive care unit. *Crit Care Med* 2009, **37**:1605–1611.
11. Huang L, Quartin A, Jones D, Havlir DV: Intensive care of patients with HIV infection. *N Engl J Med* 2006, **355**:173–181.
12. From the Center for Disease Control and prevention: 1993 revised classification system for HIV infection and expanded surveillance case definition for AIDS among adolescents and adults. *JAMA* 1993, **269**:729–730.
13. McCabe WR, Jackson CG: Gram-negative bacteremia: etiology and ecology. *Arch Intern Med* 1962, **110**:847–855.
14. Le Gall JR, Lemeshow S, Saulnier F: A new simplified acute physiology score (SAPS II) based on a European/North American multicenter study. *JAMA* 1993, **270**:2957–2963.
15. Teasdale G, Murray G, Parker L, Jennett B: Adding up the Glasgow Coma Score. *Acta Neurochir* 1979, **28**(Suppl):13–16.
16. Watcher RM, Luce JM, Hopewell PC: Critical care of patients with AIDS. *JAMA* 1992, **267**:541–547.
17. Khouli H, Afrasiabi A, Shibli M, Hajal R, Barrett CR, Homel P: Outcome of critically ill human immunodeficiency virus-infected patients in the era of highly active antiretroviral therapy. *J Intensive Care Med* 2005, **20**:327–333.
18. Casalino E, Mendoza-Sassi G, Wolff M, Bedos JP, Gaudebout C, Regnier B, Vachon F: Predictors of short- and long-term survival in HIV-infected patients admitted to the ICU. *Chest* 1998, **113**:421–429.
19. Nickas G, Watcher RM: Outcomes of intensive care of patients with human immunodeficiency virus infection. *Arch Intern Med* 2000, **160**:541–547.
20. Afessa B, Green B: Clinical course, prognostic factors, and outcome prediction for HIV patients in the ICU: the PIP (Pulmonary complications, ICU support, and prognostic factors in hospitalized patients with HIV) study. *Chest* 2000, **118**:138–145.
21. Van den Berghe G, Wouters P, Weekers F, Verwaest C, Bruyninckx F, Schetz M, Vlasselaers D, Ferdinande P, Lauwers P, Bouillon R: Intensive insulin therapy in critically ill patients. *N Engl J Med* 2001, **345**:1359–1367.
22. The Acute Respiratory Distress Syndrome Network: Ventilation with lower tidal volumes for acute lung injury and the acute respiratory distress syndrome. *N Engl J Med* 2000, **342**:1301–1308.
23. Rivers E, Nguyen B, Havstad S, Ressler J, Muzzin A, Knoblich B, Peterson E, Tomlanovich M: Early Goal-Directed Therapy Collaborative Group: Goal-directed therapy in the treatment of severe sepsis and septic shock. *N Engl J Med* 2001, **345**:1368–1377.
24. Morris A, Watcher RM, Luce J, Turner J, Huang L: Improved survival with highly active antiretroviral therapy in HIV-infected patients with severe Pneumocystis carinii pneumonia. *AIDS* 2003, **17**:73–80.
25. Zolopa AR, Andersen J, Komarow L, Sanne I, Sanchez A, Hogg E, Sckow C, Powderly W, For the ACTG A5164 study team: Early antiretroviral therapy reduces AIDS progression/death in individuals with acute opportunistic infections: a multicenter randomized strategy trial. *PLoS One* 2009, **4**:e5575.
26. Makadzange AT, Ndhlovu CE, Takarinda K, Reid M, Kurangwa M, Gona P, Hakim JG: Early versus delayed initiation of antiretroviral therapy for concurrent HIV infection and cryptococcal meningitis in Sub-Saharan Africa. *Clinical Infect Dis* 2010, **50**:1532–1538.
27. Abdool Karim SS, Naidoo K, Grobler A, Padayatchi N, Baxter C, Gray A, Gengiah T, Nair G, Bamber S, Singh A, Khan M, Pienaar J, El-Sadr W, Friedland G, Abdool Karim Q: Timing of initiation of antiretroviral drugs during tuberculosis therapy. *N Engl J Med* 2010, **362**:697–706.

17

Greater frequency of CD5-negative CD8$^+$ T cells against human immunodeficiency virus type 1 than other viruses is consistent with adaptation to antigenic variation

Stephen J Penney[1], Maureen E Gallant[1] and Michael D Grant[1,2*]

Abstract

Background: The CD5 protein antagonizes phosphorylation events downstream of T cell receptor (TCR) engagement to decrease T cell responsiveness. CD5-negative T cell clones respond preferentially over their CD5$^+$ counterparts against cells with low human histocompatibility-linked leukocyte antigen (HLA) levels. In human immunodeficiency virus type 1 (HIV-1) infection, CD5$^-$CD8$^+$ T cells increase in prevalence with disease progression.

Methods: To investigate potential causes of this expansion of CD5$^-$CD8$^+$ T cells in HIV-1 infection, we compared CD5 expression on CD8$^+$ T cells reactive against HIV-1 peptides, common viral peptides and a self peptide that together span a broad range of TCR avidities in the context of the common HLA-A2 class I restriction molecule. Following stimulation, CD5 expression on peptide-specific CD8$^+$ T cells was assessed by flow cytometry.

Results: In healthy controls, there was no significant difference in the CD5$^+$ percentage of CD8$^+$ T cells specific for common viral peptides, but a lower percentage of those responding against a common self peptide expressed CD5. The same relationship occurred in HIV-infected individuals, however, a lower percentage of HIV peptide-specific CD8$^+$ T cells than other viral peptide-specific CD8$^+$ T cells expressed CD5. In terms of overall CD5 expression level at the peptide-specific responder population level, HIV-specific CD8$^+$ T cells resembled those responsive against the self peptide, despite much higher avidity TCR/HLA/peptide interactions.

Conclusions: This deficit in CD5 expression selective for HIV-specific CD8$^+$ T cells is consistent with *in vivo* adaptation to low avidity HIV peptide variants and has potential consequences for CD8$^+$ T cell expansion, cross-reactivity and autoreactivity.

Keywords: CD5, CD8$^+$ T cell, HIV, T cell receptor, Peptide, Avidity, HLA class I

Background

Selective recognition of peptides within particular major histocompatibility complex (MHC) molecules by clonotypic T cell receptors (TCR) underlies both the specificity and mechanics of T cell activation. While the overall strength or avidity of the cognate TCR/peptide/MHC interaction must itself exceed a certain threshold, non-polymorphic accessory, co-receptor and other molecules can modulate the tenor of signal transduction and sway the outcome of antigen-specific recognition. The group B cysteine-rich scavenger receptor CD5 modulates antigen-specific signaling on virtually all T cells in a ligand-independent manner [1-5]. When T cells form conjugates with antigen-presenting cells, CD5 colocalizes with TCRs engaging cognate MHC/peptide complexes within the immunological synapse and recruits SHP phosphatases to the area through its cytoplasmic tyrosine inhibitory motif (ITIM), [3,6]. Thus, localized antagonism of phosphorylation events by CD5 diminishes TCR-derived activation signals [7]. With higher levels of CD5, the interaction between TCR and MHC/

* Correspondence: mgrant@mun.ca
[1]Immunology and Infectious Diseases Program, Division of BioMedical Sciences, Faculty of Medicine, Memorial University of Newfoundland, St. John's, NL A1B 3 V6, Canada
[2]H1803-Immunology, Faculty of Medicine, Memorial University of Newfoundland, 300 Prince Philip Drive, St. John's, NL A1B 3 V6, Canada

peptide complex must be stronger to overcome such inhibition. This implies a relationship where the level of CD5 expression on a T cell could fine tune the avidity of cognate TCR/MHC/peptide complex interactions required for T cell activation [8].

The first direct evidence that CD5 represses T cell activation was hyperresponsiveness of thymocytes from CD5-knockout mice to TCR signaling, implicating thymic selection in tuning CD5 expression levels to TCR avidity [4,9]. As thymocytes mature, CD5 and TCR levels increase in parallel, which should facilitate early positive selection of $CD5^{low}$ thymocytes by lower avidity interactions and hinder late negative selection of $CD5^{high}$ thymocytes by higher avidity interactions [10]. The modulating effect of CD5 during thymic selection and tuning of CD5 levels potentially extends the overall avidity range of the selected TCR repertoire, especially at the higher end. In TCR transgenic mice, autoreactive T cells with high levels of CD5 expression escape negative thymic selection, but peripheral downregulation of CD5 releases their autoreactivity [11-13]. There is also a striking difference in vitro in the behaviour of T cell clones derived from tumour-infiltrating lymphocytes in that only CD5-negative clones are activated by tumour cells expressing low levels of cognate MHC/peptide complexes [14]. Since the clones have identical TCR, CD5 expression is not inexorably hard-wired to TCR avidity and under certain conditions, adapts to the antigenic environment or to homeostatic pressures to either increase or decrease T cell responsiveness [15-17]. However, the role that CD5 expression plays in shaping peripheral T cell responses against foreign antigens in non-transgenic animals is completely obscure.

Substantial increases in CD5-negative T cells were reported in human immunodeficiency virus type 1 (HIV-1) infection, especially in its later stages [18]. These data predate the introduction of highly active antiretroviral therapy (HAART), suggesting a relationship between robust HIV replication and selective expansion of CD5-negative T cells. The CD5-negative T cells observed were predominantly $CD8^+$, but neither their specificity nor function was investigated [18]. Subsequent studies of $CD8^+$ T cells in HIV infection have reported abnormal promiscuity amongst HIV peptide-specific $CD8^+$ T cells, including unexpected cross-reactivity against multiple HIV peptides, other viral peptides and self peptides [19-21]. The high mutation rate of HIV generates multiple variants of the peptide epitopes activating HIV-specific $CD8^+$ T cells. While some are escape mutants, many variants will bind the same class I MHC protein, but mediate higher or lower avidity interactions with the TCR of $CD8^+$ T cells initially activated by the wild type peptide. In this setting, downregulation of CD5 could compensate for loss of avidity, selectively reduce the percentage of HIV-specific $CD8^+$ T cells expressing CD5 and increase the likelihood of $CD8^+$ T cell cross-reactivity and autoreactivity.

To investigate the possibility of selective reduction in the percentage of HIV peptide-specific $CD8^+$ T cells expressing CD5, we compared $CD8^+$ T cells specific for HIV peptides, non-HIV viral peptides, and a low avidity self peptide in HIV-infected individuals and healthy controls. Our rationale was that $CD8^+$ T cells reactive against peptides from viruses with much less variation than HIV would not undergo selection for CD5-downregulation and a higher percentage would express CD5. Dominant $CD8^+$ T cell epitopes from common influenza (flu), cytomegalovirus (CMV) and Epstein-Barr virus (EBV) viruses were selected for comparison with dominant $CD8^+$ T cell epitopes from HIV and the common self peptide. We chose these particular viruses and epitopes restricted to HLA-A2 because widespread exposure of the general population to flu, CMV and EBV and the high frequency of HLA-A2 in the population make the comparison feasible with less subject screening. Healthy controls expressing HLA-A2 were initially screened by interferon-gamma (IFN-γ) ELIspot assay for reactivity against the common viral peptides and self peptide, while HIV-infected individuals expressing HLA-A2 were screened against the common viral peptides, HIV peptides and common self peptide. For those individuals reactive by ELIspot, we followed up with $CD8^+$ T cell proliferation assays, which allowed us to assess by flow cytometry the percentage of $CD8^+$ T cells expressing CD5 in the population responding to the peptide. The percentage of $CD8^+$ T cells expressing CD5 varies with their specificity and with the underlying avidity of TCR/peptide/MHC interactions.

Results

Percentage of circulating $CD8^+$ T cells expressing CD5 in HIV-infected and uninfected individuals

Before assessing the percentages of peptide-specific $CD8^+$ T cells expressing CD5 in HIV-infected individuals and healthy controls, we measured the percentage of $CD8^+$ T cells expressing CD5 in the general $CD8^+$ T cell populations of 32 HIV-infected individuals and 17 healthy controls by flow cytometry. The median percentage of $CD8^+$ T cells expressing CD5 was significantly lower for the HIV-infected individuals (median = 95.3, interquartile range 93.5-96.6 versus median 98.6, interquartile range 97.1-99.5, $p < 0.0001$, Mann Whitney test). While HIV-infection significantly reduces the proportion of $CD8^+$ T cells expressing CD5, a median of > 95% of all $CD8^+$ T cells expressed CD5 in both groups (Figure 1). Thus, in the post-HAART era, with HIV replication effectively suppressed, a small subset of $CD8^+$ T cells is selectively affected by HIV infection in terms of CD5 expression. Subsequent experiments addressed the potential contribution of different $CD8^+$ T cell specificities to this effect.

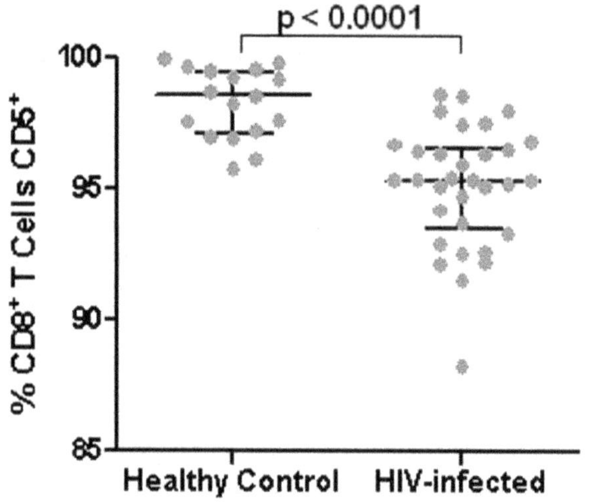

Figure 1 Comparison of the percentage of circulating CD8$^+$ T cells expressing CD5 in HIV-infected individuals and healthy controls. The median percentage of circulating CD8$^+$ T cells expressing CD5 measured by flow cytometry is shown for each group by a horizontal line bisecting the data points with upper and lower horizontal lines in each group indicating interquartile range. Significant difference between the medians is indicated by the p value above the line spanning the data sets (Mann–Whitney test).

Percentage of CMV, EBV, flu and IP-30 self peptide-specific CD8$^+$ T cells expressing CD5 in healthy controls

We first analyzed CD8$^+$ T cells proliferating in response to the common non-HIV viral peptides and IP-30 self-peptide in HLA-A2$^+$ healthy controls to test if a general relationship between avidity of peptide/TCR interactions and the percentage of responding CD8$^+$ T cells expressing CD5 was apparent. Avidities of the non HIV and HIV peptides used in this study are listed in Table 1. The percentage of peptide-specific CD8$^+$ T cells expressing CD5 was estimated by flow cytometry after gating on CD8$^+$CD3$^+$ cells and visualizing CD5 expression on CFSE^{low} cells as shown for representative examples in Figure 2. For the 3 foreign peptides, medians of 97.0%, 96.3% and 95.3% of CMV, EBV and flu peptide-specific CD8$^+$ T cells respectively, expressed CD5, with no significant difference between medians (Figure 3a). Only 4 of 24 uninfected controls tested had CD8$^+$ T cell proliferation stimulated by the low avidity IP-30 self peptide, with a median of 86.5% of the responding CD8$^+$ T cells expressing CD5. While the non-HIV viral peptides tested varied from 1.0 to 500 nM in TCR avidity, the avidity difference over this range was not reflected in significantly different percentages of responding CD8$^+$ T cells expressing CD5. However, a significantly lower percentage of CD8$^+$ T cells responding against the IP-30 self peptide (avidity = 2.0 μM) expressed CD5 compared to the CD8$^+$ T cells responding against the highest avidity CMV peptide ($p < 0.02$, Mann–Whitney test). The small number of responses to the IP-30 peptide in the non-HIV-infected population limited the significant difference to CMV-specific CD8$^+$ T cells when individual comparisons between peptide-specific CD8$^+$ T cells were done, but when grouped together, a significantly higher percentage of the CMV, EBV and flu peptide-specific CD8$^+$ T cells expressed CD5 than the IP-30 peptide-specific CD8$^+$ T cells ($p < 0.02$, Mann–Whitney test). These data indicate an increase in the percentage of CD5-negative peptide-specific CD8$^+$ T cells in association with a low avidity TCR/peptide/MHC interaction in non-HIV-infected healthy control subjects.

Table 1 Selected peptides and corresponding avidities of TCR/HLA-A2/peptide interaction

Peptide	Protein and location	Sequence	Avidity
CMV	pp65 495-503	NLVPMVATV	1.0 nM
Flu	Matrix 55-63	GILGFVFTL	250 nM
EBV	BMLF1 280-288	GLCTLVAML	500 nM
IP-30	IP-30 -11 to -3	LLDVPTAAV	2.0 μM
Gag	p17 77-85	SLYNTVATL	50 nM
RT_1	RT 33-41	ALVEICTEM	10 nM
RT_2	RT 179-187	VIYQYMDDL	10 nM
PR	PR 76-84	LVGPTPVNI	0.1 nM

Percentage of CMV, EBV, flu and IP-30 peptide-specific CD8$^+$ T cells expressing CD5 in HIV infection

Data collected in the previous section allows us to test whether the overall reduction in percentage of CD8$^+$ T cells expressing CD5 in HIV-infected individuals was reflected in non-HIV peptide-specific CD8$^+$ T cells. To address this possibility, we next analyzed CD8$^+$ T cells responding to non-HIV viral peptides and the IP-30 self-peptide in HIV-infected individuals. General characteristics of the HIV-infected study subjects are listed in Table 2. All subjects selected for testing were previously identified as expressing HLA-A2. For the 3 foreign peptides, medians of 98.4%, 97.6% and 96.7% of CMV, flu and EBV peptide-specific CD8$^+$ T cells respectively from HIV-infected individuals expressed CD5, with no significant differences between peptides (Figure 3b). The percentage of CD8$^+$ T cells reacting against the IP-30 self peptide that expressed CD5 (median = 88.4%) was significantly less than the percentages of CD8$^+$ T cells reacting against the CMV, EBV and flu peptides either individually ($p = 0.0004$, $p < 0.02$ and $p = 0.004$ respectively, Mann–Whitney test) or grouped together ($p = 0.0004$, Mann–Whitney test). The percentages of CMV, EBV, flu and IP-30 peptide-specific CD8$^+$ T cells expressing CD5 were not significantly different between the HIV-infected and healthy control groups, either when compared individually or grouped together as non-HIV viral peptide-specific CD8$^+$ T cells. Therefore,

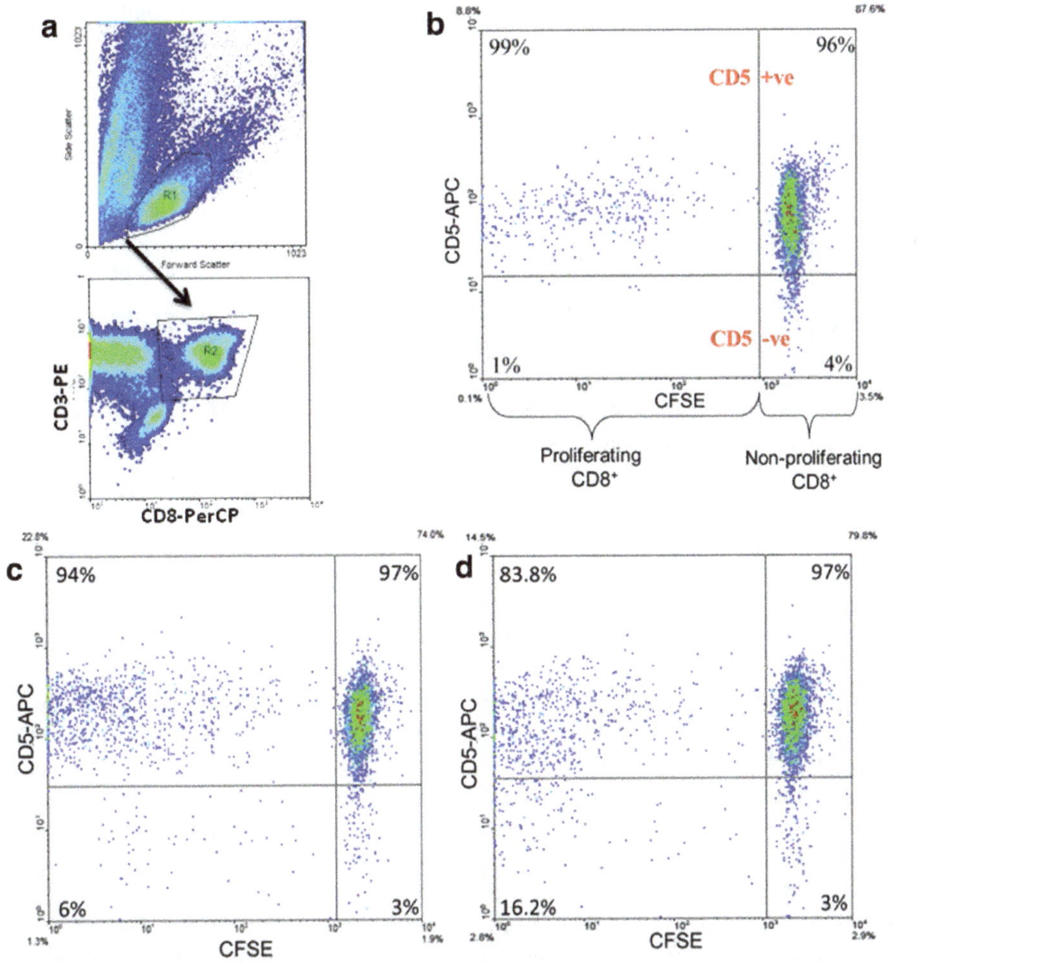

Figure 2 Assessment of the percentage of peptide-specific CD8$^+$ T cells expressing CD5. Responder cells were labeled with CFSE, stimulated with the desired peptides for 7 days, surface stained for CD3, CD8 and CD5 and then analyzed by flow cytometry. CD3$^+$CD8$^+$ lymphocytes were positively gated from the live lymphocyte population **(a)** and the fraction of proliferating cells expressing CD5 was calculated by visualizing CFSE fluorescence intensity versus CD5 in plots **b-d**. Proliferating, peptide responsive cells have lower CFSE fluorescence intensity than the parental non-responding, non proliferating population **(b)**. Numbers in the quadrants of plots **(b-d)** represent CD5$^+$ (upper quadrants) and CD5-negative (lower quadrants) percentages of the non-responding (right hand quadrants) and peptide responsive CD8$^+$ T cell populations (left hand quadrants). Representative examples where the percentage of peptide-responsive, proliferating cells not expressing CD5 spans a range of 1% **(b)** to 16% **(d)** are shown for CD8$^+$ T cell responses to the CMV **(b)** PR **(c)** and Gag **(d)** peptides described in Table 1.

HIV infection itself had no effect on CD8$^+$ T cells specific for non-HIV viral peptides in terms of the percentage expressing CD5. As in the uninfected group, an increase in the percentage of CD5-negative T cells was associated with a low avidity TCR/peptide/MHC interaction involving a self peptide relative to those CD8$^+$ T cells with higher avidity TCR/peptide/MHC interactions involving non-HIV viral peptides.

Percentage of HIV peptide-specific CD8$^+$ T cells expressing CD5

Next, we analyzed CD5 expression on CD8$^+$ T cells responding to HIV peptides. The percentages expressing CD5 were generally lower than for CD8$^+$ T cells responding to non-HIV peptides and similar to the percentages of CD8$^+$ T cells reacting against the low avidity IP-30 self peptide (Figure 4a). There was no significant difference in the percentage of CD8$^+$ T cells expressing CD5 between the 4 HIV peptides themselves, nor between any of the 4 HIV peptides, individually or in aggregate, and the IP-30 self peptide. Since there was no significant difference between CD5 expression levels of the individual HIV peptide-specific CD8$^+$ T cell populations, we grouped them together for comparison with the non-HIV viral peptide and IP-30 peptide-specific CD8$^+$ T cell populations of the HIV-infected and uninfected groups. A significantly lower percentage of HIV-specific CD8$^+$ T cells expressed CD5 compared to the non-HIV viral peptide specific CD8$^+$ T cells of HIV-infected ($p = 0.0007$, Mann–Whitney test) and healthy control ($p = 0.02$, Mann–Whitney test)

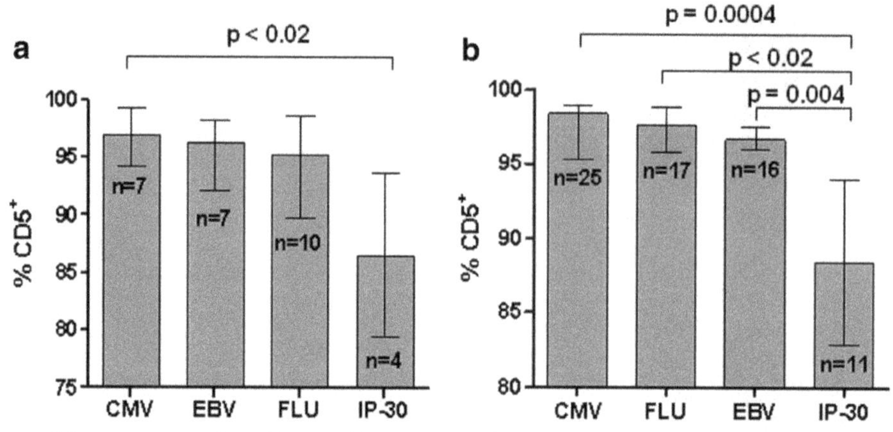

Figure 3 Comparison of the percentage of non-HIV peptide-specific CD8$^+$ T cells expressing CD5 for healthy controls and HIV-infected individuals. Solid columns represent median values of the percentage of peptide-specific CD8$^+$ T cells expressing CD5 for each individual peptide (identified below the column) with error bars showing interquartile range for healthy controls **(a)** and HIV-infected individuals **(b)**. The number of individuals in each group with specific proliferation against each individual peptide is indicated by the n value within the column. Significant differences between medians are shown by p values above lines bracketing the relevant groups (Mann–Whitney test).

groups (Figure 4b). The individual variability in the percentage of HIV peptide-responsive CD8$^+$ T cells expressing CD5 was greater than for the non-HIV viral peptide-specific CD8$^+$ T cells in either the HIV-infected or uninfected group (Figure 4b). These data indicate a broader range and selective reduction of the percentage of CD8$^+$ T cells expressing CD5 within the HIV-specific CD8$^+$ T cell population relative to the CD8$^+$ T cells specific for other viral peptides in both the HIV-infected and healthy control groups. Features of the HIV-specific CD8$^+$ T cells in terms of the range and median percentage expressing CD5 were similar to those of the self-peptide reactive CD8$^+$ T cells.

IP-30 self peptide reactivity

Since downregulation of CD5 on transgenic T cells is associated with manifestation of autoreactivity, we compared the frequency and levels of CD8$^+$ T cell reactivity against the IP-30 self peptide in healthy control and HIV-infected study groups [14]. Proliferative CD8$^+$ T cell responses against the IP-30 self peptide occurred in both the healthy control (4/24) and HIV-infected groups (13/36). There was a trend towards more frequent IP-30 self-peptide reactivity in HIV infection ($p = 0.051$, χ^2 test) and several individuals in the HIV-infected group had notably strong proliferative responses to the IP-30 self peptide, but there was no significant difference in the median percentage of CFSE^{low} cells between IP-30 peptide responders in the HIV-infected versus healthy control groups (Figure 5).

Discussion

The role of CD5 as a negative regulator of TCR signaling is well established and selective activation of variant CD5-negative T cell clones by tumour cells expressing low levels of HLA-class I/antigenic peptide complexes illustrates its biological relevance [15]. While modulation of CD5 under various conditions on transgenic T cells and selective expansion of CD5-negative T cells in HIV infection have been described, this is the first study comparing the percentage of CD5$^+$ T cells from extended T cell repertoires responding against different peptides ranging in TCR avidity. The mean CD5-negative percentage of CD8$^+$ T cells responding to three peptides from common viruses was low (6% or less) for both HIV-infected and control groups. There were no significant differences in the percentage of CD8$^+$ T cells expressing CD5 between responses to the different peptides, despite TCR avidities ranging from 1.0-500 nM. There was also no significant difference between the HIV-infected and control groups for the three non-HIV viral peptides, either individually or in unison. However, in both the HIV-infected and control groups, the median percentage of CD5-negative CD8$^+$ T cells responding to stimulation with a low TCR avidity (2.0 μM) self peptide was significantly higher than it was for the three peptides from common viruses. Although the four HIV peptides used for these studies had TCR avidities comparable to, or higher than the three non-HIV viral peptides, the median percentage of CD5-negative CD8$^+$ T cells responding to stimulation with the HIV peptides was also significantly higher, and similar to the CD8$^+$ T cell responses against the low avidity self peptide. This was not related to HIV infection itself as responses against non-HIV viral peptides were similar to uninfected controls in terms of the percentage of CD5-negative CD8$^+$ T cells and the percentage of the general CD8$^+$ T cell population of HIV-infected individuals expressing CD5 was significantly higher than in the CD8$^+$ T cell responses against either the HIV peptides or self

Table 2 General characteristics of HIV-infected study subjects

ID	Age (years)	Sex	Duration of HIV infection (years)	$CD4^+$ T cells/μL peripheral blood	Virus load[a]	Treatment[b]
11	44	Female	>20	200	2.81	cART
12	40	Male	>20	518	<1.6	cART
18	37	Male	>20	729	1.97	cART
28	45	Male	>20	144	4.94	None
30	50	Male	>20	884	<1.6	cART
34	37	Female	>20	450	3.26	cART
35	52	Male	>25	882	1.6	cART
39	38	Female	>20	506	2.74	cART
43	49	Male	>20	450	4.15	None
45	42	Female	>20	456	<1.6	cART
62	38	Female	>20	720	<1.6	cART
65	54	Female	>20	306	<1.6	cART
71	38	Female	>20	860	<1.6	cART
78	41	Male	>20	150	2.73	cART
90	42	Female	>10	315	<1.6	cART
92	36	Female	>15	325	5.5	None
96	44	Female	>15	812	<1.6	cART
105	46	Male	>10	527	2.15	cART
115	44	Female	>10	704	<1.6	cART
117	45	Male	>15	322	<1.6	cART
125	51	Male	>10	420	<1.6	cART
126	50	Male	>10	754	<1.6	cART
132	37	Female	>15	30	5.53	None
134	44	Female	>20	780	<1.6	cART
151	54	Male	>10	360	<1.6	cART
154	47	Male	>20	442	<1.6	cART
155	41	Female	>5	500	<1.6	cART
179	44	Male	>5	984	<1.6	cART
181	39	Male	>20	104	4.79	None
193	43	Female	>5	420	<1.6	cART
196	54	Male	>5	273	<1.6	cART
197	59	Male	>5	616	<1.6	cART
201	52	Male	>5	434	<1.6	cART
204	42	Female	>20	437	<1.6	cART
213	55	Female	>5	561	<1.6	cART

[a]Virus load is expressed in $\log_{10}$ copies HIV RNA/ml plasma.
[b]Combination antiretroviral therapy (cART) represents various two or three class highly active antiretroviral drug regimens.

peptide. These data suggest that a general relationship between the percentage of CD5-negative $CD8^+$ T cells responding against a peptide and TCR avidity may be apparent in responses against very low avidity self peptides, but not across a relatively broad range of avidities associated with peptides from three common viruses with low mutation rates compared to HIV. In contrast, the percentage of CD5-negative, HIV-specific $CD8^+$ T cells responding against HIV peptides was inconsistent with their TCR avidities relative to the other viral peptides and similar to that seen in responses against the low avidity self peptide.

While $CD8^+$ T cell responses to only a few peptides and viruses in the context of just one HLA-restriction molecule (HLA-A2) were studied, we speculate that this apparent inconsistency in CD5 expression levels could

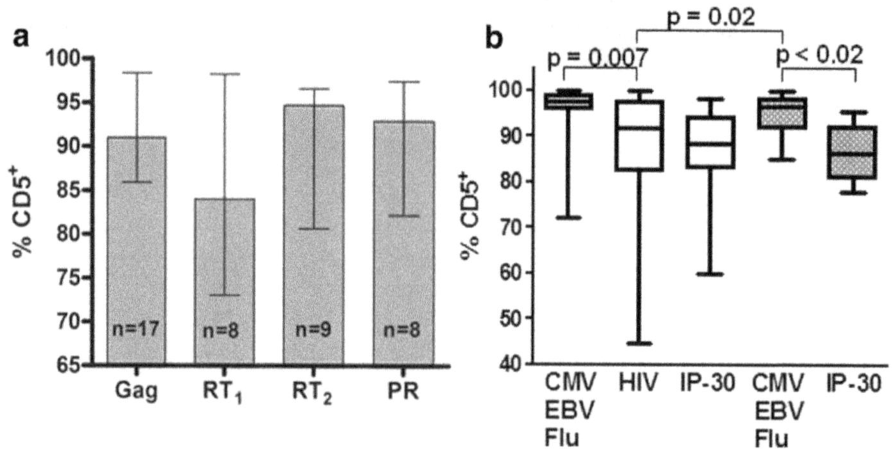

Figure 4 The percentage of HIV peptide-specific CD8⁺ T cells expressing CD5 and comparison to other virus peptide and self-peptide-specific CD8⁺ T cells. (a) Solid columns represent median values for each individual peptide (identified below the column) with error bars showing interquartile range and n within each column indicating the number of individuals with specific proliferation against each individual peptide. **(b)** Box and whisker plots showing median percentages of non-HIV viral peptide, HIV peptide and self peptide-specific $CD8^+$ T cells expressing CD5 for healthy controls (grey boxes) and HIV-infected individuals (white boxes). Horizontal lines within the box represent the median, with boxes illustrating interquartile range and vertical error bars indicating overall range. Significant differences between medians are shown by p values above lines bracketing the relevant groups (Mann–Whitney test).

reflect the diverse in vivo representation of HIV peptides within viral quasispecies. The sequence of wild-type or reference peptides used for in vitro stimulation is actually based on a consensus drawn from multiple variants. Sequence variation generated in vivo probably goes well beyond that observed in the viruses that successfully achieve some level of prominence. Thus, for each HIV peptide epitope defined by a reported consensus sequence, the $CD8^+$ T cells of an infected individual are most likely exposed to multiple variants in vivo, many of which will continue to be presented by the relevant HLA class I molecule. Rather than a single TCR/MHC peptide interaction with a unique associated avidity, this would produce a spectrum of interactions and avidities imposing different constraints on CD5 expression levels compatible with T cell activation. In vivo adaptation to the many variants producing a generally lower and individually more variable percentage of CD5-expressing $CD8^+$ T cells responding to the wild-type peptide in vitro is one possible explanation for the results observed in our study.

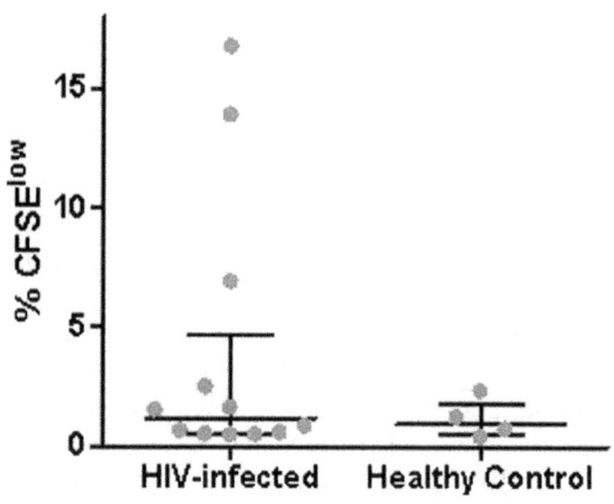

Figure 5 Proliferative responses against IP-30 self peptide in healthy controls and HIV-infected individuals. The percentage of $CD8^+$ T cells proliferating in response to the IP-30 self peptide is shown for each of 4/24 healthy controls and 13/36 HIV-infected individuals with positive proliferative responses to the self peptide.

Such in vivo adaptation in the percentage of responding cells expressing CD5 could have positive and negative implications. Cells lacking CD5 would be selectively activated and mediate broader recognition of variant peptides arising in vivo than their CD5 expressing counterparts. However, transgenic TCR studies suggest the CD5-negative $CD8^+$ T cells would also be more likely to mediate autoimmunity by reacting against self-peptides with low avidity TCR interactions and to skew the T cell repertoire through a selective advantage for homeostatic proliferation [12,13,16]. This feature might underlie the more substantial fractional expansion of CD5-negative $CD8^+$ T cells reported in HIV-infected individuals in the study carried out prior to the introduction of HAART [18]. In secondary haemophagocytic lymphohistiocytosis, often driven by EBV infection, there is a rapid and profound oligoclonal expansion of activated CD5-negative T cells expressing EBV RNA [22,23]. The oligoclonality of the CD5-negative cells suggests they may be involved in the immune response against EBV and that downregulation of CD5 facilitates their rapid expansion. This may facilitate rapid generation of a massive oligoclonal response that effectively suppresses replication of a relatively stable DNA virus like EBV. In this case, down-regulation of CD5 could be an effective antiviral adaptation to amplify the immune response, with only a transient effect on the $CD8^+$ T cell population due to heightened sensitivity of CD5-negative $CD8^+$ T cells to apoptosis [24]. In this scenario, down-regulation of CD5 could also be advantageous for tumour infiltrating lymphocytes. However, the association between EBV infection and CD5 down-regulation could actually reflect direct infection of the $CD8^+$ T cells with EBV rather than the immune response against EBV [22,23].

Adaptive regulation of CD5 expression on T cells may amplify the immune response in certain settings and conversely, activate Treg cells in others [25]. The Ets family E47 transcription factor and IL-7 negatively regulate CD5 expression through poorly understood mechanisms [12,26,27]. Better understanding of the impact, molecular basis and dynamics of CD5 regulation on different T cell subsets could reveal new methods to modulate immunity in pathological settings.

Conclusions

There is a general relationship between a reduced percentage of responding $CD8^+$ T cells expressing CD5 and reactivity against the common HLA-A2-restricted low avidity self peptide used in this study. While this relationship was not seen across a set of common viral peptides spanning a 500 nM range of avidity, we also observed reduced CD5 expression on $CD8^+$ T cells reactive against four HIV peptides similar to that seen with $CD8^+$ T cells responding against the low avidity self peptide. Since HIV mutates extensively, one possible explanation is that down-regulation of CD5 on HIV-specific $CD8^+$ T cells represents in vivo adaptation to HIV variant peptides with lower avidities than the reference peptides used to assess reactivity. This adaptation would have potential for positive consequences in terms of functional recognition of a broader set of viral variants, but also for negative consequences related to autoreactivity and narrowing of the T cell repertoire.

Methods

Subjects

Healthy controls were recruited from laboratory and hospital personnel and HIV-1-infected subjects recruited through the Newfoundland and Labrador Provincial HIV Clinic in St. John's, Newfoundland. Ethical approval for this study was granted by the Newfoundland and Labrador Health Ethics Research Authority and all participants provided written informed consent for blood collection and immunological studies. Peripheral blood was obtained by forearm venipuncture into vacutainers with acid citrate dextrose anticoagulant (Becton Dickinson) and peripheral blood mononuclear cells (PBMC) were isolated by ficoll-hypaque plus (GE Healthcare) density gradient centrifugation. Isolated PBMC were washed and resuspended in lymphocyte medium consisting of Roswell Park Memorial Institute (RPMI) 1640, 10% fetal calf serum (FCS), 10 mM HEPES, 2 mM L-glutamine, 100 IU/mL penicillin, 100 µg/mL streptomycin and 2×10^{-5} M 2-mercaptoethanol (all from Invitrogen). The cells were then counted and used directly for human leukocyte histocompatibility-linked antigen (HLA) typing with the remaining cells resuspended at 1.0×10^7/mL in medium with 20% FCS and 10% dimethylsulfoxide (Sigma) for preservation in liquid N_2 until use. All subjects were typed for class I A and B HLA antigens by serologic assay as previously described and those expressing HLA-A2 chosen for further study [28].

Peptide selection

A selection of peptides presented to $CD8^+$ T cells by HLA-A2 were used in this study, including immunodominant peptides from common viruses to which most individuals are exposed: cytomegalovirus (CMV) pp65 495–503 (NLVPMVATV); Epstein-Barr virus (EBV) BMLF1 280–288 (GLCTLVAML); influenza (flu) A Matrix 55–63 (GILGFVFTL), interferon inducible protein (IP)-30 -11 to -3 (LLDVPTAAV) self-peptide; HIV-1 peptides commonly recognized by subjects in our cohort; Gag P17 77–85 (SLYNTVATL); Pol reverse transcriptase (RT_1) 33–41 (ALVEICTEM); Pol RT_2 179–187 (VIYQYMDDL); Pol protease (PR) 76–84 (LVGPTPVNI). The TCR avidities of these peptides reported in the literature span a 3 log range, which we confirmed with our own reactive samples. Peptides were synthesized and purified to > 95% purity by EZBiolab.

ELISPOT assays

Twenty-four HLA-A2 healthy control individuals were tested by interferon-gamma (IFN-γ) ELISPOT for $CD8^+$ T cells specific for the CMV, flu, EBV and IP-30 self peptides. Multiscreen microtitre plates (Millipore) were coated overnight at 4°C with 100 µL/well of 7.5 µg/ml anti-IFN-γ monoclonal antibody (mAb) 1-D1K (MAbtech) and then washed 3 times with phosphate-buffered saline (PBS). Duplicate wells were incubated overnight with 200 µL total volume lymphocyte medium containing 4 µg/mL of either CMV, EBV, flu or IP-30 peptide and 1×10^5 PBMC from the subject being tested. Cells recovered from liquid N_2 were cultured overnight before counting to ensure viability. Medium alone served as negative control and 5 µg/mL phytohemagluttinin (PHA, MP Biomedicals) as positive control. After overnight (16 hr) incubation, PBMC were removed from the wells, the plates washed 6 times and 100 µL of 1 µg/mL biotinylated anti-IFN-γ mAb 7-B6-1 (MAbtech) added for 2 h. Plates were washed 6 more times and 100 μL/well of a 1/1000 dilution of streptavidin-alkaline phosphatase (AP) (MAbtech) added for 1 h. Plates were washed 6 more times and 100 μL/well chromogenic AP substrate (BioRad) added. After spots developed (~30 min), plates were washed with tap water to stop reactions and then air-dried. Spots corresponding to cytokine-producing T cells were counted on a Cellular Technology Limited Immunoscan reader. Subjects were considered to have detectable memory $CD8^+$ T cells against the relevant peptides when the number of spot forming cells (sfc) was > $200/10^6$ PBMC after subtraction of background spots in negative control wells. Thirty-six HIV-infected subjects expressing HLA-A2 were tested by ELISPOT as above for $CD8^+$ T cell reactivity with the non-HIV peptides and with the 4 common HIV-1 peptides also presented by HLA-A2 and listed above.

Avidity determination

Avidity levels reported in the literature for TCR interactions with the relevant peptide/HLA-A2 complexes were confirmed as previously described by serial dilution of the peptides in cell-mediated cytotoxicity assays [21]. Briefly, cytotoxic T cells (CTL) specific for the peptide were generated by incubating 5×10^6 PBMC from a reactive subject in a small volume of medium for 1 hr with 100 μM peptide and then culturing the cells at 2.5×10^6/mL in medium supplemented with 25 ng/mL recombinant interleukin-7 (R&D Systems). After 3 days, interleukin-2 (Roche) was added to 10 U/mL and the cells expanded for a further 7 days. The effector cells were first tested against autologous or HLA-A2 matched ^{51}Cr-labelled BLCL pulsed for 1 hr with 10 μM peptide as in reference [20] to determine an appropriate effector-to-target (E:T) ratio and then were tested against target cells pulsed with a serial dilutions of the test peptide beginning at 1 μM and progressing through 5 fold dilutions to < 0.02 nM. The avidity of the TCR/peptide-Class I HLA complex interaction was determined by graphing percent specific cytotoxicity against peptide concentration and estimating the concentration of peptide at which specific cytotoxicity fell to 50% of maximum cytotoxicity observed.

Proliferation assays

To evaluate CD5 expression on peptide-specific $CD8^+$ T cells, 2×10^6 PBMC were labeled with 1 μM carboxyfluorescein succinimidyl ester (CFSE, Invitrogen) as per the manufacturer's instructions, washed, and incubated in a small volume with either lymphocyte medium alone or 100 μM peptide of interest for 1 hour, then resuspended and cultured in 1 mL lymphocyte medium (with human serum substituted for FCS) for 7 days. Peptide-specific T cells were identified by CFSE fluorescence intensity dilution using a Becton Dickinson FacsScan flow cytometer. $CD8^+CD3^+$ cells were identified using phycoerythrin (PE)-conjugated anti-CD3 and peridinyl chlorophyll protein (PerCP)-conjugated anti-CD8 (clones UCHT1 and HIT8a respectively, BioLegend). The fraction of proliferating cells expressing CD5 was estimated by co-staining the cells with allophycocyanin-conjugated anti-CD5 (clone L17F12, eBioscience), gating on $CD8^+CD3^+$ cells and plotting CD5 versus CFSE intensity. Positive peptide-specific proliferation was defined as at least twice the percentage of proliferating cells compared to the control culture. If background proliferation in the absence of stimulation was > 2.5%, results were excluded. The baseline fraction of $CD8^+$ T cells expressing CD5 was measured by flow cytometry with fresh PBMC using the same antibodies.

Statistical analysis

Data analysis and graphical representation was done with GraphPad Prism software, v4.03. Normality of data distribution was assessed by Kolmogorov-Smirnoff and D'Agostino Pearson tests, but medians with interquartile range were shown since not all data sets in any of the comparisons had normal distributions. Differences in the median percentages of different $CD8^+$ T cell populations expressing CD5 were assessed with the two tailed non-parametric Mann–Whitney test.

Competing interests

The authors declare that they have no competing interests.

Authors' contributions

SJP carried out the research described in this manuscript, analyzed the data and contributed to drafting the manuscript. MEG processed samples, carried out the HLA typing and collected some of the data presented in this manuscript. MDG conceived and designed the study, directed the research, modified the figures for presentation and finalized the manuscript for submission. All authors read and approved the final manuscript.

Acknowledgements

The authors would like to thank all the individuals who donated blood for the study and thank Kim Burt, the nurse practitioner with the Newfoundland and Labrador Provincial HIV clinic for scheduling bloodwork. This study was supported by a research grant (HOP 111725) from the Canadian Institutes of Health Research (CIHR) awarded to M. Gr. S.P. was supported by CIHR, Memorial University of Newfoundland's School of Graduate Studies and Memorial University of Newfoundland's Faculty of Medicine.

References

1. McAlister MS, Brown MH, Willis AC, Rudd PM, Harvey DJ, Aplin R, Shotton DM, Dwek RA, Barclay AN, Driscoll PC: **Structural analysis of the CD5 antigen–expression, disulphide bond analysis and physical characterisation of CD5 scavenger receptor superfamily domain 1.** *Eur J Biochem* 1998, **257**:131–141.
2. Reinherz EL, Kung PC, Goldstein G, Schlossman SF: **A monoclonal antibody with selective reactivity with functionally mature human thymocytes and all peripheral human T cells.** *J Immunol* 1979, **123**:1312–1317.
3. Perez-Villar JJ, Whitney GS, Bowen MA, Hewgill DH, Aruffo AA, Kanner SB: **CD5 negatively regulates the T-cell antigen receptor signal transduction pathway: involvement of SH2-containing phosphotyrosine phosphatase SHP-1.** *Mol Cell Biol* 1999, **19**:2903–2912.

4. Bhandoola A, Bosselut R, Yu Q, Cowan ML, Feigenbaum L, Love PE, Singer A: **CD5-mediated inhibition of TCR signaling during intrathymic selection and development does not require the CD5 extracellular domain.** *Eur J Immunol* 2002, **32:**1811–1817.
5. Rodamilans B, Munoz IG, Bragado-Nilsson E, Sarrias MR, Padilla O, Blanco FJ, Lozano F, Montoya G: **Crystal structure of the third extracellular domain of CD5 reveals the fold of a group B scavenger cysteine-rich receptor domain.** *J Biol Chem* 2007, **282:**12669–12677.
6. Vila JM, Gimferrer I, Padilla O, Arman M, Places L, Simarro M, Vives J, Lozano F: **Residues Y429 and Y463 of the human CD5 are targeted by protein tyrosine kinases.** *Eur J Immunol* 2001, **31:**1191–1198.
7. Neel BG: **Role of phosphatases in lymphocyte activation.** *Curr Opin Immunol* 1997, **9:**405–420.
8. Azzam HS, DeJarnette JB, Huang K, Emmons R, Park CS, Sommers CL, El-Khoury D, Shores EW, Love PE: **Fine tuning of TCR signaling by CD5.** *J Immunol* 2001, **166:**5464–5472.
9. Tarakhovsky A, Kanner SB, Hombach J, Ledbetter JA, Muller W, Killeen N, Rajewsky K: **A role for CD5 in TCR-mediated signal transduction and thymocyte selection.** *Science* 1995, **269:**535–537.
10. Azzam HS, Grinberg A, Lui K, Shen H, Shores EW, Love PE: **CD5 expression is developmentally regulated by T cell receptor (TCR) signals and TCR avidity.** *J Exp Med* 1998, **188:**2301–2311.
11. Marquez ME, Ellmeier W, Sanchez-Guajardo V, Freitas AA, Acuto O, Di Bartolo V: **CD8 T cell sensory adaptation dependent on TCR avidity for self-antigens.** *J Immunol* 2005, **175:**7388–7397.
12. Gagnon J, Chen XL, Forand-Boulerice M, Leblanc C, Raman C, Ramanathan S, Ilangumaran S: **Increased antigen responsiveness of naive CD8 T cells exposed to IL-7 and IL-21 is associated with decreased CD5 expression.** *Immunol Cell Biol* 2009, **88:**451–460.
13. Ramanathan S, Dubois S, Chen XL, Leblanc C, Ohashi PS, Ilangumaran S: **Exposure to IL-15 and IL-21 enables autoreactive CD8 T cells to respond to weak antigens and cause disease in a mouse model of autoimmune diabetes.** *J Immunol* 2011, **186:**5131–5141.
14. Dorothee G, Vergnon I, El Hage F, Le Maux Chansac B, Ferrand V, Lecluse Y, Opolon P, Chouaib S, Bismuth G, Mami-Chouaib F: **In situ sensory adaptation of tumor-infiltrating T lymphocytes to peptide-MHC levels elicits strong antitumor reactivity.** *J Immunol* 2005, **174:**6888–6897.
15. Stamou P, de Jersey J, Carmignac D, Mamalaki C, Kioussis D, Stockinger B: **Chronic exposure to low levels of antigen in the periphery causes reversible functional impairment correlating with changes in CD5 levels in monoclonal CD8 T cells.** *J Immunol* 2003, **171:**1278–1284.
16. Kassiotis G, Zamoyska R, Stockinger B: **Involvement of avidity for major histocompatibility complex in homeostasis of naive and memory T cells.** *J Exp Med* 2003, **197:**1007–1016.
17. Hawiger D, Masilamani RF, Bettelli E, Kuchroo VK, Nussenzweig MC: **Immunological unresponsiveness characterized by increased expression of CD5 on peripheral T cells induced by dendritic cells in vivo.** *Immunity* 2004, **20:**695–705.
18. Indraccolo S, Mion M, Zamarchi R, Coppola V, Calderazzo F, Amadori A, Chieco-Bianchi L: **A CD3 + CD8+ T cell population lacking CD5 antigen expression is expanded in peripheral blood of human immunodeficiency virus-infected patients.** *Clin Immunol Immunopathol* 1995, **77:**253–261.
19. Acierno PM, Newton DA, Brown EA, Maes LA, Baatz JE, Gattoni-Celli S: **Cross-reactivity between HLA-A2-restricted FLU-M1:58–66 and HIV p17 GAG:77–85 epitopes in HIV-infected and uninfected individuals.** *J Transl Med* 2003, **1:**3.
20. Mason RD, Bowmer MI, Howley CM, Gallant M, Myers JC, Grant MD: **Antiretroviral drug resistance mutations sustain or enhance CTL recognition of common HIV-1 Pol epitopes.** *J Immunol* 2004, **172:**7212–7219.
21. Mason RD, Bowmer MI, Howley CM, Grant MD: **Cross-reactive cytotoxic T lymphocytes against human immunodeficiency virus type 1 protease and gamma interferon-inducible protein 30.** *J Virol* 2005, **79:**5529–5536.
22. Lin MT, Chang HM, Huang CJ, Chen WL, Lin CY, Chuang SS: **Massive expansion of EBV + monoclonal T cells with CD5 down regulation in EBV-associated haemophagocytic lymphohistiocytosis.** *J Clin Pathol* 2007, **60:**101–103.
23. Toga A, Wada T, Sakakibara Y, Mase S, Araki R, Tone Y, Toma T, Kurokawa T, Yanagisawa R, Tamura K, Nishida N, Taneichi H, Kanegane H, Yachie A, Nishida N, Nishida N, Taneichi H, Taneichi H, Kanegane H, Yachie A: **Clinical significance of cloned expansion and CD5 down-regulation in Epstein-Barr Virus (EBV)-infected CD8+ T lymphocytes in EBV-associated hemophagocytic lymphohistiocytosis.** *J Infect Dis* 2010, **201:**1923–1932.
24. Friedlein G, El Hage F, Vergnon I, Richon C, Saulnier P, Lecluse Y, Caignard A, Boumsell L, Bismuth G, Chouaib S, Mami-Chouaib F: **Human CD5 protects circulating tumor antigen-specific CTL from tumor-mediated activation-induced cell death.** *J Immunol* 2007, **178:**6821–6827.
25. Dasu T, Qualls JE, Tuna H, Raman C, Cohen DA, Bondada S: **CD5 plays an inhibitory role in the suppressive function of murine CD4(+) CD25(+) T (reg) cells.** *Immunol Lett* 2008, **119:**103–113.
26. Yang Y, Contag CH, Felsher D, Shachaf CM, Cao Y, Herzenberg LA, Tung JW: **The E47 transcription factor negatively regulates CD5 expression during thymocyte development.** *Proc Natl Acad Sci U S A* 2004, **101:**3898–3902.
27. Arman M, Calvo J, Trojanowska ME, Cockerill PN, Santana M, Lopez-Cabrera M, Vives J, Lozano F: **Transcriptional regulation of human CD5: important role of Ets transcription factors in CD5 expression in T cells.** *J Immunol* 2004, **172:**7519–7529.
28. Terasaki PI, Bernoco D, Park MS, Ozturk G, Iwaki Y: **Microdroplet testing for HLA-A, –B, –C, and -D antigens. The Phillip Levine Award Lecture.** *Am J Clin Pathol* 1978, **69:**103–120.

18

HIV related pulmonary arterial hypertension: epidemiology in Africa, physiopathology, and role of antiretroviral treatment

Jean Joel R. Bigna[1*], Paule Sandra D. Sime[2] and Sinata Koulla-Shiro[2,3]

Abstract

The development of HIV related pulmonary arterial hypertension (PAH) reduces the probability of survival by half as compared with HIV-infected individuals without HIV related PAH. HIV infected patients have a greater incidence of PAH compared to general population and have a 2500-fold increased risk of developing PAH. It is therefore important to have a recent overview of the problem in Africa, the most HIV affected part of the world (70 % of all HIV infection in the world). First, we discussed the epidemiology of HIV-related PAH in Africa. Second, the current understanding of the HIV-related PAH pathogenesis has been covered. Third, role of highly active antiretroviral therapy on HIV-related PAH has been revisited. There are few data concerning epidemiology of HIV related pulmonary hypertension in Africa leading to necessity to conduct further prospective large studies. The prevalence of PAH among HIV infected people in Africa varies from 5 to 13 %. The prevalence of HIV-related PAH in Africa is notably high compared to those in developed countries and in general population. The pathogenesis of PAH is clearly complex, and probably results from the interaction of multiple modulating genes with environmental factors. The physiopathology includes cytokines secretion increase which induces dysregulation of endothelial and vascular smooth muscle cell growth and imbalance of endogenous vasodilators and constrictors; HIV viral proteins which induces vascular oxidative stress, smooth myocyte proliferation and migration, and endothelial injury and genetic predisposition due to some major histocompatibility complex alleles, particularly HDL-DR6 and HLA-DR5. Histologically, HIV related PAH has the same characteristics with other types PAH. Antiretroviral therapy have a beneficial effect on the outcome of HIV related pulmonary hypertension, but it lacks evidence from large prospective studies.

Keywords: HIV, AIDS, Pulmonary hypertension, Pulmonary arterial hypertension, Africa, Antiretroviral therapy

Background

Pulmonary hypertension (PH) is defined as mean pulmonary arterial pressure (mPAP) ≥25 mmHg on right heart catheterization at rest [1]. The classification of PH involves five groups: pulmonary arterial hypertension (PAH) which includes human immunodeficiency virus (HIV) related PH, PH due to left heart diseases, PH due to respiratory diseases and/or hypoxemia, PH due to chronic embolic disease, and PH having unclear multifactorial mechanism [1]. PAH is defined by a mPAP ≥25 mmHg, pulmonary capillary wedge pressure ≤15 mmHg and pulmonary vascular resistance >3 Wood units at the time of right heart catheterization [1].

Symptoms result from right ventricular dysfunction. The first clinical manifestation is effort intolerance and exertional dyspnea that will progress to the point of breathlessness at rest. These symptoms are nonspecific, of course, and overlap with those of many other diseases, including pulmonary and cardiac conditions. Echocardiography is an extremely useful tool for the diagnosis of

*Correspondence: bignarimjj@yahoo.fr
[1] Department of Epidemiology and Public Health, Pasteur Center of Cameroon Member of International Network of the Pasteur Institutes, Yaoundé, Cameroon

HIV related PAH, and Doppler echocardiography can be used to estimate systolic pulmonary artery pressure. Assessment of hemodynamic measures by catheterization remains, however, the best test for evaluating the response to therapy. Cardiac catheterization is mandatory to definitively diagnose the disease and exclude any underlying cardiac shunt as the etiology [2].

About two-thirds of the deaths in patients with HIV-related PAH were due to the consequences of PAH, such as right heart failure, cardiogenic shock, and sudden death [3]. HIV infected patients have a greater incidence of PH compared to general population [4]. In comparison with the incidence of idiopathic PAH in the general population (1–2 per million), HIV-infected patients have a 2500-fold increased risk of developing PAH [5]. The development of HIV related PAH reduces the probability of survival by half as compared with HIV infected individuals without HIV related PAH. It therefore is important to have a recent overview of the problem in sub-Saharan Africa, the most HIV affected part of the world with 24.7 million people living with HIV (70 % of all the world) [6], and to summarize current knowledge on HIV-related PAH.

First, we discussed the epidemiology of HIV-related PAH in Africa. Second, the current understanding of the HIV-related PAH pathogenesis has been covered. Third, role of highly active antiretroviral therapy on HIV-related PAH has been revisited.

Epidemiology of HIV related pulmonary arterial hypertension in Africa

There are few data concerning epidemiology of HIV related pulmonary hypertension in Africa which come all from cross-sectional studies (Table 1). A study conducted in 2012 including 116 vertically HIV-infected adolescents (10–19 years) in Zimbabwe revealed a prevalence of 7 % for PAH [7]. In another study including 102 HIV infected patients in Tanzania, pulmonary hypertension was present among 13 % of patients [8]. In a retrospective cross-sectional study conducted in Burkina-Faso among 79 HIV-infected patients, the prevalence was 5 % [9]. In a cross sectional study in South Africa including 518 HIV-infected patients, the prevalence was 8 % [10].

The prevalence of PH among HIV infected people in Africa varies from 5 to 13 %. With around 24.7 million of HIV infected people in sub-Saharan Africa [6], between 1.2 and 3.2 million might have PAH. There is no difference between the prevalence in male (6–19 %) and the prevalence in female (around 10 %). The prevalence in sub-Saharan Africa is notably high compared to those in developed countries where the prevalence is close to 0.5 % [4, 11–13]. The possible explanation is that, the diagnosis and the management of HIV infection were made at an advanced stage of HIV disease. And also, in most developed countries, antiretroviral therapy is initiated regardless CD4 count and HIV infection clinical stage compared to developing countries which take in account these parameters.

There is need for large prospective studies to better estimate burden of HIV related PAH in Africa. In all of the studies mentioned above, the diagnostic tool was echocardiography, therefore there is need studies using cardiac catheterization which gold standard [2] to better estimate epidemiology. As demonstrated by a study, echocardiographic assessment of pulmonary arterial pressure was inaccurate in 19.7 % of patients compared to right heart catheterization [14].

Physiopathology of HIV related pulmonary hypertension

The pathogenesis of PAH is clearly complex, and probably results from the interaction of multiple modulating genes with environmental factors. The mechanism is unclear and to date not completely understood. Several key aspects involved in the pathophysiological process of HIV related PAH. HIV infection itself plays a major role in the development of PAH. The mechanism is not directly due to the action of the virus because attempts to localize the virus in the vascular lesions or endothelial cells of affected patients have been unsuccessful [15], suggesting that a direct role of the virus is unlikely, and indicating that the underlying mechanism in pulmonary arterial hypertension associated with HIV is related to the indirect action of infection, possibly through the action of viral proteins and chronic inflammation cytokines mediated due to HIV infection. Three main mechanisms are responsible for the HIV PAH: the HIV viral proteins found in the pulmonary vascular endothelium, cytokines due to the presence of HIV and increase the genetic predisposition due to HIV (Fig. 1). The pathogenesis of PAH is characterized by three major processes including vasoconstriction, vascular remodeling and microthrombotic events [16].

Role of cytokines and inflammation

HIV infection induces high secretion of some cytokines by monocytes, macrophages and lymphocytes including interleukin (IL)-1, IL-6, IL8, IL-13, tumor necrosis factor (TNF) α and platelet-derived growth factors which can exacerbates a patent PAH or induces inflammation of vascular endothelium leading to PAH [16–23]. The activation of platelet derived growth factor [24] and vascular endothelial pathway [25] can result to aberrant pulmonary vascular activity. These growth factors and cytokines can lead to dysregulation of endothelial and vascular smooth muscle cell growth and imbalance of endogenous

Table 1 Characteristics of studies reporting epidemiology of pulmonary hypertension among HIV infected people in Africa

First author name, Publication year	Study design	Patients characteristics	Prevalence	Diagnostic	Setting	Factors associated with PH
Ferrand, 2012 [7]	Cross sectional	N = 116 Mean age = 14 years (10–19) Women = 69 %	7 %	Mean pulmonary artery pressure >25 mmHg with Doppler echocardiography	Zimbabwe	Not researched
Chillo, 2012 [8]	Cross sectional	N = 102 Mean age = 42 years (18–72) Women = 69 %	Overall: 13 % Men: 19 % (6/32) Women: 10 % (7/70)	Pulmonary arterial pressure >35 mmHg with Doppler echocardiography	Tanzania	None (researched: SBP, DBP, duration of HIV infection, cholesterol level, age, gender and use of HAART)
Sliwa, 2012 [10]	Cross sectional	N = 518 Mean age = 42 years (18–72) Women = 62 %	Overall: 8 % Men : 6 % (11/197) Women: 10 % (31/321)	Pulmonary artery pressure >25 mmHg with Doppler echocardiography	South Africa	Not researched
Niakara, 2002 [9]	Retrospective cross sectional	N = 79 Mean age = 46 years Women = 44 %	5 %	Echocardiography	Burkina Faso	Not researched

SBP systolic blood pressure, *DBP* diastolic blood pressure, *HAART* highly active antiretroviral treatment

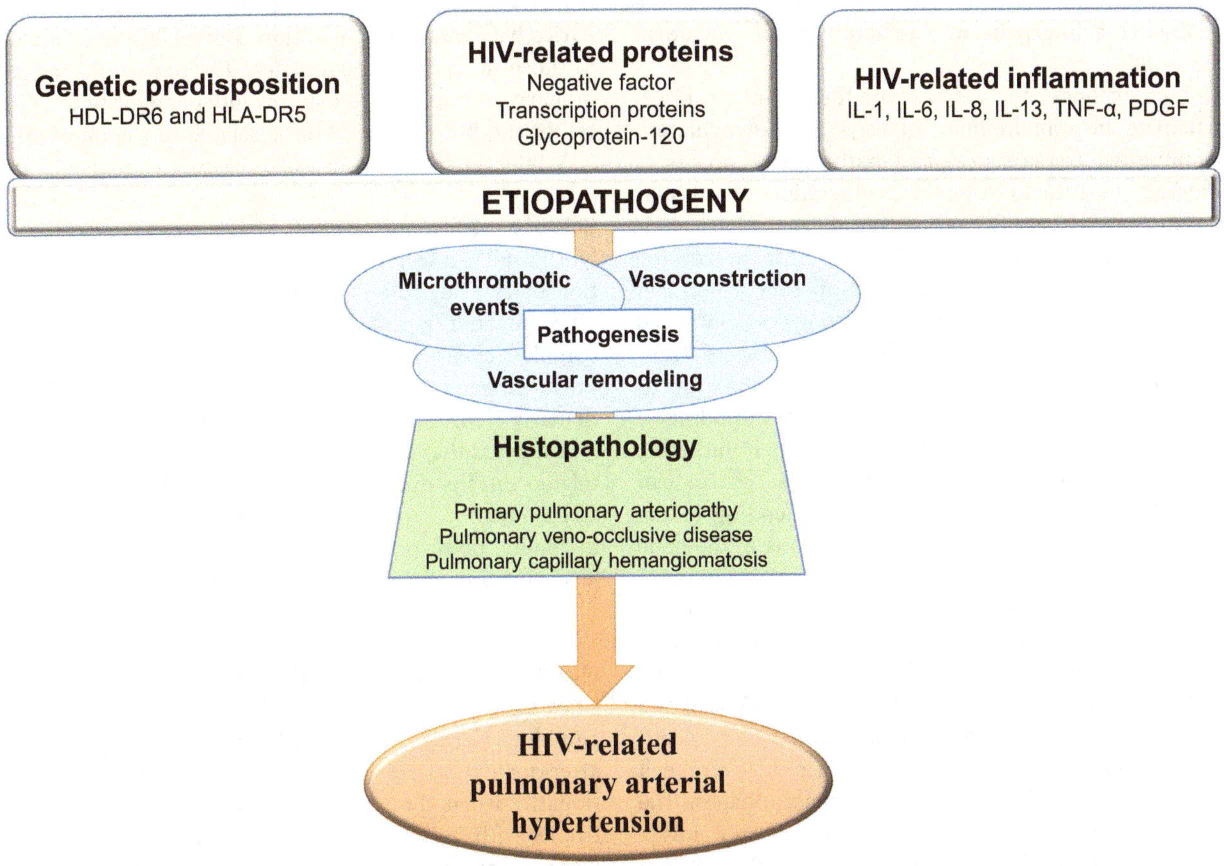

Fig. 1 Physiopathology of HIV-related pulmonary hypertension

vasodilators and constrictors (in favor of constrictors). IL-1 appears to have deleterious effects for the development and progression of pulmonary hypertension. The exact mechanisms, however, remain unclear [16]. It was shown that elevated levels of IL-6 resulted in an upregulation of vascular endothelial growth factor receptor II and matrix metalloproteinase-9, an endopeptidase that promotes angiogenesis through regulation of cell attachment, proliferation, and migration [16, 26]. IL-8 is thought to play an important role in the development of PAH, especially in early phases of vascular remodeling. IL-8 is known to have proangiogenic and antiapoptotic activities and acts as a growth factor for endothelial cells [27]. IL-13 acts as an important mediator of cell proliferation and tissue remodeling in lungs [28]. This is explain by imbalance of NO homeostasis and increased muscularization of pulmonary arteries [16]. Similarly to other inflammatory cytokines, elevated serum levels of TNF-α were described in PAH patients. TNF-α might play an important role in the development of pulmonary hypertension, even though the concrete mechanisms remain unknown [29]. Interestingly some studies show that TNF-α blockers ameliorate pulmonary pressure, while other studies found no significant effects [16].

Role of HIV viral proteins

These HIV viral proteins include negative factor (Nef), transcription proteins (Tat) and glycoprotein 120 (gp-120) [30–35]. These proteins probably induce vascular oxidative stress, smooth myocyte proliferation and migration, and endothelial injury leading to HIV related PAH.

Nef induces complex plexiform lesion in the pulmonary vasculature, this has been demonstrated in a study comparing macaque Nef-positive simian immunodeficiency virus (SIV) and macaque Nef-negative SIV [30]. The involvement of Nef in the occurrence of HIV-related PAH has been also demonstrated in porcine model study and among HIV infected persons [31, 33], because Nef is present in the endothelial cells of HIV infected patients with PAH. Nef can enter into the pulmonary endothelial cells via the CXCR 4 receptor and therefore induce proliferation and apoptosis of endothelial cells in lung [36, 37]. Thus, localization of Nef to the lipid rafts may be sufficient to trigger the changes associated with the endothelial cell expansion characteristic of plexiform lesions [38].

Bone morphogenetic protein type II receptor (BMPR2) participate in a multiplicity of ways in the regulation of numerous physiological and pathological processes including the inhibition of the proliferation of vascular smooth muscle tissue by promoting the survival of pulmonary arterial endothelial cells, therefore preventing arterial damage and adverse inflammatory responses [39]. Its wide-ranging biological functions is controlled by several mechanisms, including regulation of transcription, complex formation among the signaling receptors (oligomerization) and with co-receptors, binding of the receptors to scaffolding proteins or their targeting to specific membrane domains [39]. This control can be breakdown by a mutation the gene encoding to the BMPR2. A heterozygous germline mutations in the gene encoding the BMPR2), can lead to heritable PAH in more than 70 % of cases [40–42]. Tat represses transcription of gene encoding to BMPR2 in monocytes, suggesting that Tat-mediated reduction of BMPR2 may be linked to the development of HIV related PAH [43]. The BMPR2 is a member of the transforming growth factor-beta receptor family and is expressed on the surface of several cell types including endothelial cells and macrophages. The modulation of host gene transcription by HIV infection might genetically alter expression of BMPR2. As the HIV Tat protein is the major transcriptional regulator of host gene expression during HIV infection, Tat downregulates BMPR2 expression and signaling by half. This level of decreased BMPR2 expression can lead to abnormal pulmonary vascular function with exuberant cellular proliferation [43]. Tat enhance the activity of vascular endothelial cells via interleukin-6 [44].

Secreted HIV gp120 proteins induce lung endothelial cell injury and could contribute to the development of HIV-related PAH. The mechanism is by apoptosis and smooth cell proliferation due to exposure of HIV-1 gp120 proteins to primary human lung microvascular endothelial cells [32]. Gp120 also significantly increases secretion of the potent vasoconstrictor endothelin-1 by human lung endothelial cells [45].

Nevertheless, it is essential to state that only a small proportion of infected patients with HIV will develop HIV related PAH. Other factors, including stage of immune depression, likely play a role in the occurrence of the HIV related PAH. It is possible that, the implication of HIV viral proteins be related with high level HIV-RNA, because detectable plasma HIV-RNA is associated with the risk to develop PAH, as demonstrated in a cross-sectional study [11, 46]. This can also explain why the prevalence of HIV-related PAH is high in Africa compared to developed countries, because HIV-infected patients in Africa have more HIV infection control failure compared to those in developed countries. The occurrence of pulmonary arterial hypertension is independent of the CD4 cell count, but it appears to be related to the duration of HIV infection [47].

Role of genetic predisposition

Not all HIV infected develop PAH. Genetic predisposition plays a key role in the development of PAH among HIV infected people. Some major histocompatibility complex alleles have been incriminated by their high prevalence among HIV infected people with PAH, particularly HDL-DR6 and HLA-DR5 [48, 49].

It appears that the mechanism mainly specific to HIV-related PAH is due to viral proteins. Other mechanisms of HIV-related PAH are associated to either an increase in genetic predisposition or to an increase in the serum level of cytokines involved in the PAH.

Histopathology

Histologically, HIV related PAH has the same characteristics with other types PAH [50]. There are three histopathological presentation including primary pulmonary arteriopathy (plexiform arteriopathy, thrombotic arteriopathy, isolated medial hypertrophy, and medial hypertrophy with intimal fibrosis), pulmonary veno-occlusive disease, and pulmonary capillary hemangiomatosis [51]. Concerning the importance of form, the most common histological form of HIV related PAH is the plexogenic pulmonary arteriopathy followed by thrombotic pulmonary arteriopathy, pulmonary medial hypertrophy with intimal fibrosis, and pulmonary veno-occlusive disease [50].

Role of antiretroviral therapy in the treatment of HIV related pulmonary hypertension

There is no cure for pulmonary arterial hypertension [47]. It is essential to note that the treatment of HIV-related PAH is similar to the treatment of other forms of PAH. Several medications may be adjunctively (non-specific therapies) used in the management of PAH depending on the clinical presentation of PAH. These include: (1) anticoagulants because PAH patients are at risk for small intrapulmonary thrombus due to prothrombotic state, sedentary lifestyle, and cardiac dilation [22, 52]; (2) supplemental oxygen because patients with PAH often develop hypoxemia which can further exacerbate pulmonary arterial vasoconstriction [22, 52]; (3) diuretic agents which can be used in the case of volume overloaded; Digoxin in the case right sided heart failure [22, 52]; (4) Calcium channel blocker among PAH patients who develop decrease in mPAP between 10 mmHg and

40 mmHg. This reduction in mPAP must be accompanied by improved or at least unchanged cardiac output and unchanged or minimally reduced systemic blood pressure [22, 52, 53].

Several medicines are available in the specific management of PAH, the same both for non HIV-related PAH and HIV-related PAH, such as endothelin receptor antagonists, prostaglandin analogs, and phosphodiesterase 5 inhibitors [52].

There have been no large prospective studies of the effects of antiretroviral treatment on HIV related PAH. Most of the studies demonstrated the beneficial effect of the use of highly active antiretroviral therapy (HAART) among HIV infected patients with PAH on their outcome. As demonstrated in a cross sectional study, detectable plasma HIV-RNA was associated with the risk to develop PAH [11]. This suggests that the use of HAART, whose aim is to prevent the multiplication of HIV and thus make undetectable viral load; could reduce the risk of developing PAH in patients infected with HIV. In a prospective cohort study [54], highly active antiretroviral therapy (HAART) improved pulmonary artery pressure in HIV/AIDS patients if instituted at early stages (WHO classes I and II). However, at more advanced stages of pulmonary artery hypertension, it does not have any significant effect on reduction of the same. In the view of these results, early detection of PAH in HIV/AIDS patients is essential and prompt institution of HAART should be considered in them even when those patients do not fulfill the conventional criteria for initiation of this treatment. Further studies was needed to investigate these possibility. HAART should not be used as a sole therapy for HIV-related PAH, and the initiation of PAH-specific therapy is of paramount importance. HAART only ameliorate the outcome of patients with HIV-related PAH. In a cross-sectional study including 400 HIV infected patients, a current use of Tenofovir was associated with lower PAH prevalence [55]. Several other studies also show the beneficial effect of the use of HAART in the treatment of PAH [56, 57]. HAART also reduce mortality [58] and cardiac involvement [59] among HIV infected patients with PAH. Therefore, it is necessary that all patients with HIV-related PAH start HAART regardless HIV disease clinical stage and CD4 count. However, it is necessary to conduct large prospective studies to better estimate the effect of HAART on PAH.

Conclusions

There is a high prevalence of PAH in patients infected with HIV in Africa, although there are very few studies, hence the need for further studies including research also risk factors. This prevalence is very high compared to that in the developed countries and compared with that in the general population. The pathophysiologic mechanism responsible for PAH in subjects infected with HIV remains to be explored. One notes nevertheless the involvement of HIV viral proteins, cytokines and genetic predisposition in the pathophysiologic mechanism. Although the pathophysiological mechanism of HIV-related PAH is different from other PAH, histological presentation is the same. The beneficial role of antiretroviral drugs in the treatment of PAH associated with HIV is not yet established, which requires large prospective studies to clarify.

Abbreviations

BMPR2: bone morphogenic protein receptor 2; Gp120: glycoprotein 120; HAART: highly active antiretroviral therapy; HIV: human immunodeficiency virus; Nef: negative factor; PAH: pulmonary arterial hypertension; PH: pulmonary hypertension; SIV: simian immunodeficiency virus; Tat: transcription proteins.

Authors' contributions

JJRB conceived and designed the study, and drafted manuscript. PSDS and SK-S conceived and designed the study, and revised manuscript for important intellectual content. All authors read and approved the final manuscript.

Author details

[1] Department of Epidemiology and Public Health, Pasteur Center of Cameroon Member of International Network of the Pasteur Institutes, Yaoundé, Cameroon. [2] Faculty of Medicine and Biomedical Sciences, University of Yaoundé 1, Yaoundé, Cameroon. [3] Infectious Diseases Unit, Yaoundé Central Hospital, Yaoundé, Cameroon.

Acknowledgements

This paper needed no particular funding.

Competing interests

The authors declare that they have no competing interests.

References

1. Simonneau G, Gatzoulis MA, Adatia I, Celermajer D, Denton C, Ghofrani A, GomezSanchez MA, KrishnaKumar R, Landzberg M, Machado RF, et al. Updated clinical classification of pulmonary hypertension. J Am Col Cardiol. 2013;62(25 Suppl):D34–41.
2. Cicalini S, Almodovar S, Grilli E, Flores S. Pulmonary hypertension and human immunodeficiency virus infection: epidemiology, pathogenesis, and clinical approach. Clin microbiol Infect Off Publ Eur Soc Clin Microbiol Infect Dis. 2011;17(1):25–33.
3. Opravil M, Pechere M, Speich R, Joller-Jemelka HI, Jenni R, Russi EW, Hirschel B, Luthy R. HIV-associated primary pulmonary hypertension. A case control study. Swiss HIV Cohort Study. Am J Respir Crit Care Med. 1997;155(3):990–5.
4. Crothers K, Huang L, Goulet JL, Goetz MB, Brown ST, Rodriguez-Barradas MC, Oursler KK, Rimland D, Gibert CL, Butt AA, et al. HIV infection and risk for incident pulmonary diseases in the combination antiretroviral therapy era. Am J Respir Crit Care Med. 2011;183(3):388–95.
5. Correale M, Palmiotti GA, Lo Storto MM, Montrone D, Foschino Barbaro MP, Di Biase M, Lacedonia D. HIV-associated pulmonary arterial hypertension: from bedside to the future. Eur J Clin Invest. 2015;45(5):515–28.
6. Global statistics [http://www.unaids.org/sites/default/files/media_asset/20140716_FactSheet_en.pdf].
7. Ferrand RA, Desai SR, Hopkins C, Elston CM, Copley SJ, Nathoo K, Ndhlovu CE, Munyati S, Barker RD, Miller RF, et al. Chronic lung disease in adolescents with delayed diagnosis of vertically acquired HIV infection. Clin Infect Dis Off Publ Infect Dis Soc Am. 2012;55(1):145–52.

8. Chillo P, Bakari M, Lwakatare J. Echocardiographic diagnoses in HIV-infected patients presenting with cardiac symptoms at Muhimbili National Hospital in Dar es Salaam, Tanzania. Cardiovas J Africa. 2012;23(2):90–7.
9. Niakara A, Drabo YJ, Kambire Y, Nebie LVA, Kabore NJP, Simon F. Cardiovascular diseases and HIV infection: a study of 79 cases in the national hospital of Ouagadougou (Burkina Faso). Bull Soc Pathol Exot. 2002;95(1):23–6.
10. Sliwa K, Carrington MJ, Becker A, Thienemann F, Ntsekhe M, Stewart S. Contribution of the human immunodeficiency virus/acquired immunodeficiency syndrome epidemic to de novo presentations of heart disease in the Heart of Soweto Study cohort. Eur Heart J. 2012;33(7):866–74.
11. Quezada M, Martin-Carbonero L, Soriano V, Vispo E, Valencia E, Moreno V, de Isla LP, Lennie V, Almeria C, Zamorano JL. Prevalence and risk factors associated with pulmonary hypertension in HIV-infected patients on regular follow-up. AIDS. 2012;26(11):1387–92.
12. Speich R, Jenni R, Opravil M, Pfab M, Russi EW. Primary pulmonary hypertension in HIV infection. Chest. 1991;100(5):1268–71.
13. Sitbon O, Lascoux-Combe C, Delfraissy JF, Yeni PG, Raffi F, De Zuttere D, Gressin V, Clerson P, Sereni D, Simonneau G. Prevalence of HIV-related pulmonary arterial hypertension in the current antiretroviral therapy era. Am J Respir Crit Care Med. 2008;177(1):108–13.
14. Selby VN, Scherzer R, Barnett CF, MacGregor JS, Morelli J, Donovan C, Deeks SG, Martin JN, Hsue PY. Doppler echocardiography does not accurately estimate pulmonary artery systolic pressure in HIV-infected patients. AIDS. 2012;26(15):1967–9.
15. Mette SA, Palevsky HI, Pietra GG, Williams TM, Bruder E, Prestipino AJ, Patrick AM, Wirth JA. Primary pulmonary hypertension in association with human immunodeficiency virus infection. A possible viral etiology for some forms of hypertensive pulmonary arteriopathy. Am Rev Respir Dis. 1992;145(5):1196–200.
16. Groth A, Vrugt B, Brock M, Speich R, Ulrich S, Huber LC. Inflammatory cytokines in pulmonary hypertension. Respir Res. 2014;15:47.
17. Pellicelli AM, Palmieri F, Cicalini S, Petrosillo N. Pathogenesis of HIV-related pulmonary hypertension. Ann N Y Acad Sci. 2001;946:82–94.
18. Aliyu ZY, Kato GJ, Taylor Jt, Babadoko A, Mamman AI, Gordeuk VR, Gladwin MT. Sickle cell disease and pulmonary hypertension in Africa: a global perspective and review of epidemiology, pathophysiology, and management. Am J Hematol. 2008;83(1):63–70.
19. Olivetta E, Percario Z, Fiorucci G, Mattia G, Schiavoni I, Dennis C, Jager J, Harris M, Romeo G, Affabris E, et al. HIV-1 Nef induces the release of inflammatory factors from human monocyte/macrophages: involvement of Nef endocytotic signals and NF-kappa B activation. J Immunol. 2003;170(4):1716–27.
20. Dai HL, Zhang M, Xiao ZC, Guang XF, Yin XL. Pulmonary arterial hypertension in HIV infection: a concise review. Heart, Lung Circ. 2014;23(4):299–302.
21. Pellicelli AM, D'Ambrosio C, Vizza CD, Borgia MC, Tanzi P, Pino P, Zachara E, Soccorsi F. HIV-related pulmonary hypertension. From pathogenesis to clinical aspects. Acta Cardiol. 2004;59(3):323–30.
22. Mirrakhimov AE, Ali AM, Barbaryan A, Prueksaritanond S. Human immunodeficiency virus and pulmonary arterial hypertension. ISRN cardiology. 2013;2013:903454.
23. Tcherakian C, Couderc LJ, Humbert M, Godot V, Sitbon O, Devillier P. Inflammatory mechanisms in HIV-associated pulmonary arterial hypertension. Sem Resp Critic Care Med. 2013;34(5):645–53.
24. Petitpretz P, Brenot F, Azarian R, Parent F, Rain B, Herve P, Simonneau G. Pulmonary hypertension in patients with human immunodeficiency virus infection. Comparison with primary pulmonary hypertension. Circulation. 1994;89(6):2722–7.
25. Ascherl G, Hohenadl C, Schatz O, Shumay E, Bogner J, Eckhart L, Tschachler E, Monini P, Ensoli B, Sturzl M. Infection with human immunodeficiency virus-1 increases expression of vascular endothelial cell growth factor in T cells: implications for acquired immunodeficiency syndrome-associated vasculopathy. Blood. 1999;93(12):4232–41.
26. Steiner MK, Syrkina OL, Kolliputi N, Mark EJ, Hales CA, Waxman AB. Interleukin-6 overexpression induces pulmonary hypertension. Circ Res. 2009;104(2):236–44 **(228p following 244)**.
27. Li A, Varney ML, Valasek J, Godfrey M, Dave BJ, Singh RK. Autocrine role of interleukin-8 in induction of endothelial cell proliferation, survival, migration and MMP-2 production and angiogenesis. Angiogenesis. 2005;8(1):63–71.
28. Wynn TA. Fibrotic disease and the T(H)1/T(H)2 paradigm. Nat Rev Immunol. 2004;4(8):583–94.
29. Soon E, Holmes AM, Treacy CM, Doughty NJ, Southgate L, Machado RD, Trembath RC, Jennings S, Barker L, Nicklin P, et al. Elevated levels of inflammatory cytokines predict survival in idiopathic and familial pulmonary arterial hypertension. Circulation. 2010;122(9):920–7.
30. Marecki JC, Cool CD, Parr JE, Beckey VE, Luciw PA, Tarantal AF, Carville A, Shannon RP, Cota-Gomez A, Tuder RM, et al. HIV-1 Nef is associated with complex pulmonary vascular lesions in SHIV-nef-infected macaques. Am J Respir Crit Care Med. 2006;174(4):437–45.
31. Voelkel NF, Cool CD, Flores S. From viral infection to pulmonary arterial hypertension: a role for viral proteins? AIDS. 2008;22(Suppl 3):S49–53.
32. Kanmogne GD, Primeaux C, Grammas P. Induction of apoptosis and endothelin-1 secretion in primary human lung endothelial cells by HIV-1 gp120 proteins. Biochem Biophys Res Commun. 2005;333(4):1107–15.
33. Duffy P, Wang X, Lin PH, Yao Q, Chen C. HIV Nef protein causes endothelial dysfunction in porcine pulmonary arteries and human pulmonary artery endothelial cells. J Surg Res. 2009;156(2):257–64.
34. Rusnati M, Presta M. HIV-1 Tat protein and endothelium: from protein/cell interaction to AIDS-associated pathologies. Angiogenesis. 2002;5(3):141–51.
35. Mermis J, Gu H, Xue B, Li F, Tawfik O, Buch S, Bartolome S, O'Brien-Ladner A, Dhillon NK. Hypoxia-inducible factor-1 alpha/platelet derived growth factor axis in HIV-associated pulmonary vascular remodeling. Respir Res. 2011;12:103.
36. James CO, Huang MB, Khan M, Garcia-Barrio M, Powell MD, Bond VC. Extracellular Nef protein targets CD4+ T cells for apoptosis by interacting with CXCR4 surface receptors. J Virol. 2004;78(6):3099–109.
37. Choi HJ, Smithgall TE. HIV-1 Nef promotes survival of TF-1 macrophages by inducing Bcl-XL expression in an extracellular signal-regulated kinase-dependent manner. J Biol Chem. 2004;279(49):51688–96.
38. Tuder RM, Marecki JC, Richter A, Fijalkowska I, Flores S. Pathology of pulmonary hypertension. Clin Chest Med. 2007;28(1):23–42.
39. Ehrlich M, Gutman O, Knaus P, Henis YI. Oligomeric interactions of TGF-beta and BMP receptors. FEBS Lett. 2012;586(14):1885–96.
40. Soubrier F, Chung WK, Machado R, Grunig E, Aldred M, Geraci M, Loyd JE, Elliott CG, Trembath RC, Newman JH, et al. Genetics and genomics of pulmonary arterial hypertension. J Am Coll Cardiol. 2013;62(25 Suppl):D13–21.
41. Li W, Dunmore BJ, Morrell NW. Bone morphogenetic protein type II receptor mutations causing protein misfolding in heritable pulmonary arterial hypertension. Proc Am Thorac Soc. 2010;7(6):395–8.
42. Austin ED, Loyd JE, Phillips JA 3rd. Genetics of pulmonary arterial hypertension. Sem Resp Critic Care Med. 2009;30(4):386–98.
43. Caldwell RL, Gadipatti R, Lane KB, Shepherd VL. HIV-1 TAT represses transcription of the bone morphogenic protein receptor-2 in U937 monocytic cells. J Leukoc Biol. 2006;79(1):192–201.
44. Hofman FM, Wright AD, Dohadwala MM, Wong-Staal F, Walker SM. Exogenous tat protein activates human endothelial cells. Blood. 1993;82(9):2774–80.
45. Ehrenreich H, Rieckmann P, Sinowatz F, Weih KA, Arthur LO, Goebel FD, Burd PR, Coligan JE, Clouse KA. Potent stimulation of monocytic endothelin-1 production by HIV-1 glycoprotein 120. J Immunol. 1993;150(10):4601–9.
46. Degano B, Guillaume M, Savale L, Montani D, Jais X, Yaici A, Le Pavec J, Humbert M, Simonneau G, Sitbon O. HIV-associated pulmonary arterial hypertension: survival and prognostic factors in the modern therapeutic era. AIDS. 2010;24(1):67–75.
47. Farber HW, Loscalzo J. Pulmonary arterial hypertension. N Engl J Med. 2004;351(16):1655–65.
48. Morse JH, Barst RJ, Itescu S, Flaster ER, Sinha G, Zhang Y, Fotino M. Primary pulmonary hypertension in HIV infection: an outcome determined by particular HLA class II alleles. Am J Respir Crit Care Med. 1996;153(4 Pt 1):1299–301.
49. Itescu S, Rose S, Dwyer E, Winchester R. Certain HLA-DR5 and -DR6 major histocompatibility complex class II alleles are associated with a CD8 lymphocytic host response to human immunodeficiency virus type 1 characterized by low lymphocyte viral strain heterogeneity and slow disease progression. Proc Natl Acad Sci USA. 1994;91(24):11472–6.
50. Mehta NJ, Khan IA, Mehta RN, Sepkowitz DA. HIV-Related pulmonary hypertension: analytic review of 131 cases. Chest. 2000;118(4):1133–41.

51. Pietra GG, Edwards WD, Kay JM, Rich S, Kernis J, Schloo B, Ayres SM, Bergofsky EH, Brundage BH, Detre KM, et al. Histopathology of primary pulmonary hypertension. A qualitative and quantitative study of pulmonary blood vessels from 58 patients in the National Heart, Lung, and Blood Institute, Primary Pulmonary Hypertension Registry. Circulation. 1989;80(5):1198–206.
52. McLaughlin VV, Archer SL, Badesch DB, Barst RJ, Farber HW, Lindner JR, Mathier MA, McGoon MD, Park MH, Rosenson RS, et al. ACCF/AHA 2009 expert consensus document on pulmonary hypertension a report of the American College of Cardiology Foundation Task Force on Expert Consensus Documents and the American Heart Association developed in collaboration with the American College of Chest Physicians; American Thoracic Society, Inc.; and the Pulmonary Hypertension Association. J Am Coll Cardiol. 2009;53(17):1573–619.
53. Fuso L, Baldi F, Di Perna A. Therapeutic strategies in pulmonary hypertension. Front Pharmacol. 2011;2:21.
54. Pal J, Sen K, Sarkar G, Mandal A, Chakraborty S, Deb A. Effect of antiretroviral therapy on pulmonary hypertension in HIV patients. J Indian Med Assoc. 2013;111(12):845–6.
55. Olalla J, Urdiales D, Pombo M, del Arco A, de la Torre J, Prada JL. Pulmonary hypertension in human immunodeficiency virus-infected patients: the role of antiretroviral therapy. Med Clin. 2014;142(6):248–52.
56. Cicalini S, Chinello P, Grilli E, Petrosillo N. Treatment and outcome of pulmonary arterial hypertension in HIV-infected patients: a review of the literature. Curr HIV Res. 2009;7(6):589–96.
57. Reinsch N, Buhr C, Krings P, Kaelsch H, Kahlert P, Konorza T, Neumann T, Erbel R. Effect of gender and highly active antiretroviral therapy on HIV-related pulmonary arterial hypertension: results of the HIV-HEART Study. HIV medicine. 2008;9(7):550–6.
58. Zuber JP, Calmy A, Evison JM, Hasse B, Schiffer V, Wagels T, Nuesch R, Magenta L, Ledergerber B, Jenni R, et al. Pulmonary arterial hypertension related to HIV infection: improved hemodynamics and survival associated with antiretroviral therapy. Clin Infect Dis Off Publ Infect Dis Soc Am. 2004;38(8):1178–85.
59. Pugliese A, Isnardi D, Saini A, Scarabelli T, Raddino R, Torre D. Impact of highly active antiretroviral therapy in HIV-positive patients with cardiac involvement. J Infect. 2000;40(3):282–4.

19

HIV-1 protease inhibitor drug resistance in Kenyan antiretroviral treatment-naive and -experienced injection drug users and non-drug users

Valentine Budambula[1], Francis O. Musumba[2,3], Mark K. Webale[2], Titus M. Kahiga[4], Francisca Ongecha-Owuor[5], James N. Kiarie[6], George A. Sowayi[7], Aabid A. Ahmed[8], Collins Ouma[2,9] and Tom Were[10*]

Abstract

Background: Although injection drug use drives antiretroviral drug resistance, the prevalence of protease inhibitor (PI) resistance among Kenyan IDUs remains undetermined. We, therefore, explored PI resistance mutations and their association with viral load and CD4+ T cell counts in HIV-1 infected IDUs (ART-naive, n = 32; and -experienced, n = 47) and non-drug users (ART-naive, n = 21; and -experienced, n = 32) naive for PI treatment from coastal Kenya.

Results: Only IDUs harboured major PI resistance mutations consisting of L90M, M46I and D30 N among 3 (6.4 %) ART-experienced and 1 (3.1 %) -naive individuals. Minor PI mutations including A71T, G48E, G48R, I13V, K20I, K20R, L10I, L10V, L33F, L63P, T74S, V11I, and V32L were detected among the ART-experienced (36.2 vs. 46.9 %) and -naive (43.8 vs. 66.7 %) IDUs and non-drug users, respectively. All the four IDUs possessing major mutations had high viral load while three presented with CD4+ T cell counts of <500 cells/ml. Among the ART-naive non-drug users, CD4+ T cell counts were significantly lower in carriers of minor mutations compared to non-carriers ($P < 0.05$).

Conclusion: Transmitted drug resistance may occur in IDUs underscoring the need for genotyping resistance before initiating PI treatment.

Keywords: HIV-1, Protease inhibitor, Drug resistance, Antiretroviral, Treatment-naive, Treatment-experienced, Injection drug users, Non-drug users, Coastal Kenya

Background

Despite up-scaling of antiretroviral drugs for treatment and prevention, HIV-1 remains an important cause of infectious disease burden in the world. In the year 2013, an estimated 35 million people globally were infected with HIV of whom 24.7 million reside in Sub-Saharan Africa [1]. Substance consumption including injection drug use is an emerging epidemic that is driving the high HIV burden on the continent [2]. Among the 243 million people using substances in the world, 12.7 million are injection drug users (IDUs) of whom 13.1 % are living with HIV [1]. Africa is home to nearly 1.02 million IDUs of which 12.1 % are harbouring HIV infections [1]. In Kenya, about 18.3 % of the 49,000 IDUs, mainly concentrated in Nairobi and Coastal regions, are living with HIV [3]. Non-drug users are individuals not consuming illicit drugs classified by the United Nations Office on Drug and Crime (UNODC) [1]. However, non-drug users are also at increased risk of acquiring HIV infection, largely through engaging in unprotected and high risk sexual activities with IDUs [4–6]. As such, effective interventions are urgently required to reduce the high burden of HIV in these most-at-risk-populations.

The current standard regimen for first-line HIV treatment in Kenya consists of two nucleoside reverse transcriptase inhibitors (NRTI) mainly tenofovir disoproxil

*Correspondence: mugogwe@yahoo.com
[10] Department of Medical Laboratory Sciences, Masinde Muliro University of Science and Technology, P. O. Box 190, Kakamega 50100, Kenya

fumarate (TDF) or azidovudine (AZT), lamuvudine (3TC) and one non-nucleoside reverse transcriptase inhibitor (NNRTI) efevirenz (EFV) or nevirapine (NVP) [7]. Protease inhibitor (PI) drugs serve as HIV-1 pre- and post-exposure prophylaxis and substitute treatment in cases of first line antiretroviral treatment failures and/or intolerance [8]. Protease inhibitors are recommended in cases of virological failure, defined as a viral load >1000 copies/ml after 12 months of therapy or an increase in the viral load after initial viral suppression [7]. Consequently, PIs have been effective in further lowering HIV-associated morbidity and mortality [9, 10]. However, continued use of PIs as effective salvage treatment is hindered by emergence of drug resistance, largely due to poor accessibility and adherence to treatment [11]. Two classes of point mutations in the protease gene, designated major and minor mutations, mediate resistance to PIs [12]. Major mutations decrease susceptibility to PI drugs leading to poor virologic response and treatment failure, while minor mutations only enhance viral replication in the presence of major mutations [12]. In addition, previous studies reporting higher rates of major and minor PI resistance (24 vs. 8 %) among ART-experienced PI-naive IDUs compared to non-drug users [10], suggest spontaneous emergence of PI resistance in PI-naive individuals. To our knowledge, no study has concurrently determined rates of PI resistance in ART-naive and -experienced IDUs and non-drug users among PI treatment-naive individuals.

Several studies across Kenya show widespread resistance to NRTIs and non-NNRTIs in ART-naive and -experienced adults and children, breastfeeding infants and IDUs [13–31]. More importantly, previous studies showing 13.8 % resistance rates to first line (NRTIs and NNRTIs) ART regimens among IDUs from Mombasa, coastal Kenya, suggest existence of resistance to these drugs that are commonly used in combination with PIs [27]. In such cases of suspected drug resistance, the NNRTIs (NVP or EFV) or NRTIs (ABC) are often substituted with PIs (either LPV/r or ATV/r) as second-line treatment [7]. In addition, resistance to integrase inhibitors has also been detected in the country [32]. While a number of studies in the country show existence of resistance to PIs in ART-naive and -experienced individuals in adults and children from the general population, and treatment-naive female sex workers [16, 18, 29, 33, 34] no studies to date have established PI resistance in Kenyan IDUs. Since, high drug injection intensity particularly under the selection pressure of antiretroviral therapy accelerates emergence of resistance [35], this cross-sectional study, examined PI resistance in ART-naive and -experienced IDUs from Mombasa, a coastal city in Kenya.

Methods

Study design and population

This cross-sectional study was conducted in HIV-1 infected IDUs and non-drug using controls at Bomu Hospital, a social enterprise facility in Mombasa City, coastal Kenya. Injection drug users were recruited via respondent-driven, snowball and makeshift-outreach sampling methods. In the context of the current study, IDUs comprised of individuals exhibiting injection needle-stick scars and reporting a history of injecting any illicit drug classified by UNODC at least once in the previous month [1] while non-drug users were individuals reporting having never used any of the substances and drugs in the UNODC registry [1]. HIV-1 infection status of consenting IDUs and non-drug users was confirmed using Determine™ (Abbott Laboratories, Tokyo, Japan) and Unigold™ (Trinity Biotech Plc, Bray, Ireland) in accordance with the Kenya's guidelines for adult HIV testing [36]. Those yielding positive results on both tests were subsequently recruited into the study. In addition, ART-naive study participants had not been initiated on ART. The ART-experienced study participants were on first-line ART (NRTIs and NNRTIs) consisting of TDF or AZT + 3TC + NVP or EFV [37]. None of the participants were on PIs.

Clinical evaluations

In brief, about, 3.0 ml venous blood was collected from study participants in ethylenediaminetetraacetic acid vacutainer tubes (Becton–Dickinson, Franklin Lakes, USA) and used for enumerating CD4+ T cells, and plasma harvesting for HIV-1 viral load quantification. A drop of whole blood was applied on Whatman-FTA® 903 cards (Schleicher & Schuell BioScience, Dassel, Germany) for preparing dry blood spots (DBS) that were stored at −20 °C until used for pro-viral DNA extraction. For enumerating CD4+ T cell counts, 5.0 µl of blood were stained with CD3/CD4/CD45 monoclonal antibody reagent (BD Tritest) and analysed on BD FACSCalibur™ according to the manufacturer's protocols. HIV-1 viral load was determined in 0.2 ml plasma samples using the Abbott Molecular m2000sp sample preparation and m2000rt real-time amplification and detection systems (Abbott Molecular Inc., Illinois, USA) according to the manufacturer's methods.

HIV-1 DNA extraction and amplification

HIV-1 pro-viral DNA was extracted from DBS using QIAamp™ DNA blood mini kit (QIAGEN, Valencia, USA) according to the manufacturer's recommendations. HIV-1 pro-viral DNA encoding protease gene was amplified by nested PCR with primers; Nyupol_7 (5′-GGGAATTTTCTTCAGAGCAG-3′)

HXB2 nucleotide position 2125–2144, and Nyupol_8 (5′-TCTTCTGTCAATGGCCATTGT-3′) HXB2 nucleotide position 2635–2615 in the first round. Nyupol_9 (5′-TCCTTAACTTCCCTCAAATCACT-3′) HXB2 nucleotide position 2241–2264 and Nyupol_10 (5′-CTGGCACGGTTTCAATAG GACT-3′) HXB2 nucleotide position 2577–2556 were used in the second round. First and second round PCR was conducted in a 25 μl volume containing 5 μL DNA, 1× PCR buffer, 1.5 mM $MgCl_2$, 1 U/μL *Taq* polymerase (KemTaq®), 200 μM of each dNTP (Invitrogen™, Carlsbad, USA), and 0.5 μM of each first or second round primers. Amplification consisted of initial denaturation at 94 °C for 4 min, followed by 40 cycles of 94 °C for 15 s, 50 °C for 30 s, and 72 °C for 1 min, with a final extension of 72 °C for 5 min. PCR products were electrophoresed in 1 % ethidium bromide-stained agarose gel, and visualized under ultraviolet light. PCR product sizes of approximately 330 bp were diagnostic for HIV-1 pro-viral DNA.

HIV-1 protease inhibitor drug resistance mutations

PCR amplicons were purified with QIAquick™ PCR purification kit (Qiagen, Valencia, USA) according to the manufacturer's protocol. Direct sequencing was performed using BigDye™ sequencing chemistry (Applied Biosystems®, Foster City, USA) on an ABI PRISM® 3100 Genetic Analyzer (Applied Biosystems®, Foster City, USA) as per the manufacturer's protocols. Primer pair Nyupol_9 and Nyupol_10 was used for forward and reverse sequencing reactions, respectively. Forward and reverse chromatograms were visually inspected and edited for base mis-calls using MEGA version 6.0 [38]. Pair-wise alignment and contiguous sequences were generated using DNA Baser Sequence Assembler version 4.20.0 (Heracle BioSoft, http://www.DnaBaser.com). Protease inhibitor drug resistance mutations were identified and interpreted using Stanford web-based HIV drug resistance database [39, 40] and the International AIDS Society-USA (IAS-USA) drug resistance panel [12].

Data analysis

Data analysis was conducted using IBM® SPSS 20.0 (IBM® SPSS Statistics for Windows, Version 20.0. Armonk, NY: IBM Corp.). Age and CD4+ T cell counts and viral load were compared across study groups using Kruskal–Wallis test and Dunn's post hoc correction for multiple comparisons. Differences in distribution of gender were compared across the study groups using Chi-square test. Rates of resistance mutations in each study group were summarised as numbers and proportions. Statistical significance was set at $P < 0.05$.

Ethical considerations

This study was conducted following ethical approval obtained from Kenyatta University Ethical Review Committee, approval number PKU019/116 of 2012 in accordance with Helsinki declaration [41]. Written informed consent was obtained from all participants prior to enrolment into the study. Confidentiality was maintained throughout the study.

Results

Baseline characteristics of the study participants

Baseline characteristics of the study participants are presented in Table 1. Recruitment was within HIV-infected cohort thus sero-conversion rate is unknown. A total of 132 HIV-1 sero-positive study participants were successfully sequenced for protease inhibitor drug resistance. The study participants consisted of IDUs (ART-naive, n = 32 and -experienced, n = 47) and non-drug users (ART-naive, n = 21 and -experienced, n = 32). Gender distribution was similar among the study groups ($P = 0.531$). Age was significantly different across the groups ($P = 0.009$) with ART-naive IDUs (median, 30.1; IQR, 7.2) having younger individuals relative to ART-naive non-drug users (median, 36.0; IQR, 13.8; $P < 0.05$). In addition, 20 (42.5 %), 24 (51.1 %) and 3 (6.4 %) ART-experienced IDUs while 3 (9.3 %), 7 (21.9 %) and 22 (68.8 %) ART-experienced non-drug users were on antiretroviral therapy for <1, 1–3, and >3 years, respectively. The CD4+ T cell counts were similar across the study groups ($P = 0.379$). The HIV-1 viral load was significantly different across the study groups ($P = 0.004$) with ART-naive (median, 3.4; IQR, 2.7; $P < 0.05$) and -experienced (median, 3.5; IQR, 2.7; $P < 0.01$) IDUs presenting with lower levels compared to ART-naive non-drug users (median, 4.5; IQR, 2.8).

Protease inhibitor drug resistance

Major and minor HIV-1 protease drug resistance mutations detected in the study participants are shown in Table 2. Although major PI resistance mutations was not detected in the non-drug users, three major PI resistance mutations including L90M, M46I and D30N were detected in 4 (5.1 %) IDUs. Interestingly, mutation L90M co-existed with K20R minor mutation in 1 (2.1 %) ART-experienced IDU, while D30N co-existed with T74S+K20R minor mutations in 1 (3.1 %) ART-naive IDU. In addition, D30N+M46I co-existed with G48E and K20I minor mutations, respectively, in 2 (4.2 %) ART-experienced IDUs. Fourteen (29.8 %) ART-experienced IDUs harboured only minor mutations comprising of 1(2.1 %) K20I, 7 (8.5 %) K20R, 3 (6.4 %) L10I, 1 (2.1 %) V32L and 2 (12.5 %) L10V+K20R. In addition, 13 (40.6 %) ART-naive IDUs had only minor mutations including 1

Table 1 Baseline characteristics of the study participants

Characteristic	Non-drug users		Injection drug users		*P*
	ART (−), *n* = 21	ART (+), *n* = 32	ART (−), *n* = 32	ART (+), *n* = 47	
Female, n (%)	16 (76.2)	20 (62.5)	18 (56.3)	30 (63.8)	0.531
Age, years	36.0 (13.8)	35.2 (10.6)	30.1 (7.2)[a]	31.6 (7.4)	*0.009*
Duration (years) on ART, n (%)					
<1	0 (0.0)	3 (9.3)	0 (0.0)	20 (42.5)	
1–3	0 (0.0)	7 (21.9)	0 (0.0)	24 (51.1)	–
>3	0 (0.0)	22 (68.8)	0 (0.0)	3 (6.4)	
CD4+ T cell counts/ml	568 (673)	412 (554)	532 (472)	426 (423)	0.379
Log_{10} HIV-1 RNA, copies/ml	4.5 (2.8)	4.3 (1.6)	3.4 (2.7)[a]	3.5 (2.7)[b]	*0.004*

Data are presented as medians (IQR, interquartile range) or indicated as number (n) and proportion (%) of subjects

ART (−) anti-retroviral treatment-naive, *ART (+)* antiretroviral treatment-experienced, *HIV-1* human immunodeficiency virus-1

[a] $P < 0.05$ vs. ART (−) non-drug users

[b] $P < 0.01$ vs. ART (−) non-drug users

Significant *P* values are shown in italic

Table 2 Protease inhibitor drug resistance mutations

Mutation	Non-drug users		Injection drug users	
	ART (−), *n* = 21	ART (+), *n* = 32	ART (−), *n* = 32	ART (+), *n* = 47
L90**M** + K20R	0 (0.0)	0 (0.0)	0 (0.0)	1 (2.1)
D30**N** + T74S + K20R	0 (0.0)	0 (0.0)	1 (3.1)	0 (0.0)
D30**N** + **M**46**I** + G48E	0 (0.0)	0 (0.0)	0 (0.0)	1 (2.1)
D30**N** + **M**46**I** + K20I	0 (0.0)	0 (0.0)	0 (0.0)	1 (2.1)
G48E	0 (0.0)	0 (0.0)	1 (3.1)	0 (0.0)
G48R	0 (0.0)	0 (0.0)	1 (3.1)	0 (0.0)
K20I	1 (7.1)	0 (0.0)	0 (0.0)	1 (2.1)
K20R	8 (38.1)	5 (15.6)	5 (15.6)	7 (8.5)
L10I	2 (9.5)	0 (0.0)	2 (6.3)	3 (6.4)
L10V	0 (0.0)	2 (6.3)	1 (3.1)	0 (0.0)
L33F	0 (0.0)	2 (6.3)	0 (0.0)	0 (0.0)
V32L	0 (0.0)	0 (0.0)	0 (0.0)	1 (2.1)
I13V + L63P	0 (0.0)	1 (3.1)	0 (0.0)	0 (0.0)
L10I + K20R	1 (7.1)	0 (0.0)	1 (3.1)	0 (0.0)
L10V + K20R	0 (0.0)	1 (3.1)	2 (6.3)	2 (4.3)
L10V + T74S	0 (0.0)	3 (9.4)	0 (0.0)	0 (0.0)
L10V + V11I	2 (9.5)	0 (0.0)	0 (0.0)	0 (0.0)
L33F + A71T	0 (0.0)	1 (3.1)	0 (0.0)	0 (0.0)

Data presented are number and proportion of subjects. Mutations are denoted based on Stanford drug resistance database and International Antiviral Society-USA drug resistance mutations panel [12, 39, 40], where number shows amino acid position in the protease gene, and letter before position is wild type amino acid and after the position mutant amino acid

Major mutations are shown in bold

A alanine, *D* aspartic acid, *E* glutamic acid, *F* phenylalanine, *G* glycine, *I* isoleucine, *K* lysine, *L* leucine, *M* methionine, *N* asparagine, *P* proline, *R* arginine, *S* serine, *T* threonine, *V* valine, *ART (−)* antiretroviral treatment-naive, *ART (+)* antiretroviral treatment-experienced, *HIV-1* human immunodeficiency virus type-1

(3.1 %) G48E, 1 (3.1 %) G48R, 5 (15.6 %) K20R, 2 (6.3 %) L10I, 1 (3.1 %) L10V, 1 (3.1 %) L101+K20R and 2 (6.3 %) L10V + K20R.

In non-drug users, 15 (46.9 %) ART-experienced individuals had minor mutations consisting of 5 (15.6 %) K20R, 2 (6.3 %) L10V, 2 (6.3 %) L33F, 1 (3.1 %) I13V + L63P, 1 (3.1 %) L10V + K20R, 3 (9.4 %) L10V + T74S and 1 (3.1 %) L33F + A71T. In addition, 14 (66.7 %) ART-naive non-drug users harboured minor mutations comprising of 1 (7.1 %) K20I, 8 (38.1 %) K20R,

2 (9.5 %) L10I, 1 (7.1 %) L101 + K20R, and 2 (9.5 %) L10V + V11I.

Association of protease inhibitor resistance with viral load and CD4+ T cell counts

Viral load and CD4+ T cell counts of individuals with major and minor mutations are presented in Tables 3 and 4, respectively. All the four individuals harbouring major mutations presented with high viral load of 4624, 291,124, 141,341 and 209,871 copies/ml, which was greater than 1000 copies/ml viral load threshold required for viral suppression in the community [42]. In addition, three of the individuals with major mutations presented with CD4+ T cell counts of 473, 39, and 162 cells/μl which were <500 cells/μl. Carriage of minor mutations was not associated with viral load in all the study groups ($P > 0.05$), but among ART-naive non-drug users, CD4+ T cell counts were significantly lower in carriers of minor mutations compared to non-carriers (median, 455; IQR , 599 vs. 989, 507; $P = 0.005$).

Discussion

Effective use of protease inhibitors in HIV-1 treatment and prevention is largely impeded by the increasing development and spread of acquired and transmitted resistance [43]. Antiretroviral treatment-naive and -experienced IDUs are at an increased risk of acquiring antiretroviral drug resistance as a consequence of high risk sexual and injection practices [44]. In addition, increased selection of protease drug resistance in ART-experienced IDUs is linked to high drug injection intensity and poor adherence to treatment [35, 44]. Thus, continuous surveillance of drug resistance is important in planning for effective and successful treatment programs in IDUs. This study, determined PI resistance in ART-naive and -experienced IDUs in Mombasa City, in the coastal region in Kenya.

In the current study, major PI mutations were detected only in IDUs with the antiretroviral treatment-experienced (L90M, D30N and M46I) individuals having higher rates than -naive (D30N) individuals. Most importantly,

Table 3 HIV-1 viral load and CD4+ T cell counts of individuals with major protease inhibitor drug resistance mutations

ID	Mutation	Age, years	Gender	ART duration, years	HIV-1 RNA (log_{10} HIV-1 RNA), copies/ml	CD4+ T cells/ml
#1	**D30N** + **M46I** + G48E	36.4	M	<0.5	4624 (3.7)	473
#2	**L90M** + K20R	34.6	M	1–3	291,124 (5.5)	637
#3	**D30N** + **M46I** + K20I	30.1	F	1–3	141,341 (5.2)	39
#4	**D30N** + T74S + K20R	33.3	M	Naive	209,871 (5.3)	162

Mutations are denoted according to Stanford drug resistance database and International Antiviral Society-USA drug resistance mutations panel [12, 39, 40]

Major mutations are shown in bold

D aspartic acid, *E* glutamic acid, *G* glycine, *I* isoleucine, *K* lysine, *L* leucine, *M* methionine, *N* asparagine, *S* serine; *T* threonine, *ART* antiretroviral therapy, *HIV-1* human immunodeficiency virus type-1

Table 4 Association between minor protease inhibitor resistance mutations, viral load and CD4+ T cell count

	Injection drug users					
	ART (−)			ART (+)		
	Mutation (−), $n = 18$	Mutation (+), $n = 13$	*P*	Mutation (−), $n = 30$	Mutation (+), $n = 14$	*P*
CD4+ T cell count/μl	529 (276)	568 (597)	0.708	412 (415)	424 (648)	0.762
Log_{10} HIV-1 RNA, copies/ml	4.4 (2.7)	2.2 (1.9)	0.183	3.6 (2.7)	2.2 (1.7)	0.142
	Non-drug users					
	ART (−)			ART (+)		
	Mutation (-), $n = 7$	Mutation (+), n = 14	*P*	Mutation (−), $n = 17$	Mutation (+), $n = 15$	*P*
CD4+ T cell count/μl	989 (507)	455 (599)	*0.005*	351 (526)	554 (461)	0.350
Log_{10} HIV-1 RNA, copies/ml	3.6 (1.9)	4.8 (2.5)	0.313	4.3 (1.3)	4.3 (2.0)	0.852

Data presented are medians (IQR, interquartile range) in carriers and non-carriers of only minor protease resistance mutations. Statistical analysis was performed using Mann–Whitney test

Significant *P*-values are shown in italic

ART (−) anti-retroviral treatment-naive, *ART (+)* anti-retroviral treatment-experienced, *Mutation (+)* minor protease resistance mutation carrier, *Mutation (−)* minor protease resistance mutation non-carrier, *HIV-1* human immunodeficiency virus type

major mutations, D30N and M46I co-existed with minor mutations, G48E, K20I and T74S, suggesting that these mutations mediate evolution of major drug resistance [45]. Our findings of L90M, D30N, and M46I mutations, are partly consistent with previous studies reporting on the presence of major PI mutations D30N and M46I in ART-naive sex workers, a most-at-risk-population from Nairobi, Kenya [34]. Our results are also, in part, consistent with previous studies in Canada showing D30N, M46I, and L90M PI resistance mutations among individuals reporting a history of injection drug use [46]. Likewise, our results are similar to previous studies showing presence of L90M, D30N, and M46I mutations among antiretroviral-naive IDUs in Rio de Janeiro, Brazil [47]. Importantly, phenotypic and/or clinical evidence indicate that D30N mutation confers high-level resistance to nelfinavir; L90M imparts resistance to nelfinavir, sequinavir, indinavir, and lopinavir; while M46I confers resistance to indinavir, lopinavir, fosamprenavir and nelfinavir [12, 39, 40]. In this study, most of the ART-experienced IDUs and non-drug users had been receiving first-line antiretroviral treatment (NRTIs and NNRTIs) for at least a year, eliminating the possibility of cross-resistance to PIs [12]. Although not determined in the current study, it is possible that development of major PI resistance in ART-experienced IDUs is attributable to PI transmitted drug resistance, increased drug-injection frequency, particularly under the selection pressure of antiretroviral therapy [35]. Therefore, tipranavir/ritonavir and darunavir/ritonavir to which the above mutations have no effect [12] may be adopted as drugs of choice for second line treatment in Kenyan IDUs. Altogether, screening prior to initiating highly active antiretroviral therapy (HAART), monitoring of treatment and routine surveillance are important in achieving effective clinical care and preventing emergence and spread of resistance in this most-at-risk-population.

Overall, higher rates of minor mutations were found in IDUs relative to non-drug users, suggesting heterogeneity of HIV-1 strains in IDUs. The detection of A71T, G48E/R, I13V, K20I/R, L10I/V, L33F, L63P, T74S, V11I, and V32L minor mutations in this study is, in part, consistent with previous studies that reported K20R, L10I/V, L33F/I, and L63P minor mutations among HIV-positive women attending antenatal clinics in a large HIV treatment study in western Kenya [33]. In addition, our results corroborate previous studies showing K20I/M/R, L10I/V, I13V, and L63P minor mutations among HIV infected treatment-naive individuals in Morocco [48]. Of note are the higher rates of minor PI mutations in antiretroviral treatment-naive individuals in both the IDUs and non-drug users supporting a mechanism(s) of spontaneous emergence [49]. However, it is also possible that drug-related selective pressure enhances development of minor resistance in IDUs [35].

The high viral load among individuals carrying major PI mutations is consistent with phenotypic and clinical studies showing absence or low virologic response in patients having these major mutations [50]. It is important to emphasize that three of the individuals with major mutations concurrently harboured G48E, K20I, K20R and T74S minor mutations. This is not surprising because G48E inhibits as K20I, K20R and T74S enhance viral replication [12, 51]. In addition, CD4+ T cell counts were <500 cells/μl in three of the patients, indicating progression to immunodeficiency. Although minor PI mutations do not directly cause reduced phenotypic and/or clinical response to PI resistance [12], the lower CD4+ T cell counts observed in ART-naive users possibly suggests that minor mutations may contribute to viral fitness and infectivity in treatment-naive individuals [52]. This hypothesis is underscored by previous studies reporting that polymorphic compensatory mutations in the protease gene, may improve the replicative capacity of HIV-1 even in the absence of drug selective pressure or major resistance mutations [52]. Interestingly, previous studies have also reported low CD4+ T cell counts in anti-retroviral treatment naive IDUs harbouring minor PI mutations [53]. Therefore, our findings suggest that appearance of minor PI mutations may indicate disease progression among newly-infected individuals.

While a prospective design would have been important in examining the emergence of PI resistance in treatment-naive and -experienced IDUs, this cross-sectional study provides the first baseline evidence of occurrence of PI resistance in IDUs from Kenya. Although specific antiretroviral regimens used by the ART-experienced individuals were not evaluated in this study, poor adherence to ART by injection drug users, generate suboptimal antiretroviral drug levels that exert selective pressure on the viral genome leading to resistance [44]. Since interactions of substances consumed and antiretroviral drugs in IDUs cause hepatic hyper-inflammation and derangements in metabolic functions [54, 55], toxicological analysis and monitoring of response to ART in a prospective approach will provide insights into the mechanisms underlying development of resistance. In addition, analysis of mutations outside the protease gene, such as *env* [56] that confer resistance to PI will identify additional mutants mediating resistance.

Conclusion

Protease inhibitor transmitted drug resistance is likely to occur among Kenyan IDUs. Therefore, performing HIV-1 drug resistance analyses prior to initiating PI treatment in HIV patients from high-risk population groups is critical in achieving better treatment outcomes and prolonging the effectiveness of these drugs in the country.

Sequence data

The 125 sequences described in this study were submitted to the GenBank under accession numbers: KP791995, KP791996, KP791997, KP791998, KP791999, KP792000, KP792001, KP792002, KP792003, KP792004, KP792005, KP792006, KP792007, KP792008, KP792009, KP792010, KP792011, KP792012, KP792013, KP792014, KP792015, KP792016, KP792017, KP792018, KP792019, KP792020, KP792021, KP792022, KP792023, KP792024, KP792025, KP792026, KP792027, KP792028, KP792029, KP792030, KP792031, KP792032, KP792033, KP792034, KP792035, KP792036, KP792037, KP792038, KP792039, KP792040, KP792041, KP792042, KP792043, KP792044, KP792045, KP792046, KP792047, KP792048, KP792049, KP792050, KP792051, KP792052, KP792053, KP792054, KP792055, KP792056, KP792057, KP792058, KP792059, KP792060, KP792061, KP792062, KP792063, KP792064, KP792065, KP792066, KP792067, KP792068, KP792069, KP792070, KP792071, KP792072, KP792073, KP792074, KP792075, KP792076, KP792077, KP792078, KP792079, KP792080, KP792081, KP792082, KP792083, KP792084, KP792085, KP792086, KP792087, KP792088, KP792089, KP792090, KP792091, KP792092, KP792093, KP792094, KP792095, KP792096, KP792097, KP792098, KP792099, KP792100, KP792101, KP792102, KP792103, KP792104, KP792105, KP792106, KP792107, KP792108, KP792109, KP792110, KP792111, KP792112, KP792113, KP792114, KP792115, KP792116, KP792117, KP792118, KP792119, KT033003, KT033004, KT033005, KT033006, KT033007, KT033008, and KT033009.

Authors' contributions

TW and VB conceived and designed the study. TW, FOM and MWK performed laboratory, statistical and bioinformatics analyses. TW, FOM, MWK co-drafted the manuscript. AA was involved in study design, and clinical analyses. TMK, FOO, JNK, GA, and CO critically revised the manuscript. VB and FOM contributed equally to the writing of this manuscript. All authors read and approved the final manuscript.

Author details

[1] Department of Environment and Health Sciences, Technical University of Mombasa, Mombasa, Kenya. [2] Department of Biomedical Science and Technology, Maseno University, Maseno, Kenya. [3] Centre for Virus Research, Kenya Medical Research Institute, Nairobi, Kenya. [4] Department of Pharmacy and Complementary Medicine, Kenyatta University, Nairobi, Kenya. [5] Department of Medicine, Therapeutics, Dermatology and Psychiatry, Kenyatta University, Nairobi, Kenya. [6] Department of Obstetrics and Gynecology, University of Nairobi, Nairobi, Kenya. [7] Department of Medical Laboratory Sciences, Masinde Muliro University of Science and Technology, Kakamega, Kenya. [8] Bomu Hospital, Mombasa, Kenya. [9] Health Challenges and Systems Program, African Population and Health Research Centre, Nairobi, Kenya. [10] Department of Medical Laboratory Sciences, Masinde Muliro University of Science and Technology, P. O. Box 190, Kakamega 50100, Kenya.

Acknowledgements

We thank the study participants for participating in the study. We are also grateful to staff and management of Bomu Hospital for their support during the study. We thank Raphael Lihana for technical advice on laboratory, bioinformatic analyses and critical review of this manuscript. This research was partly funded by National Commission on Science, Technology and Innovation (NCST/5/003/065) and Partnership for Innovative Medical Education in Kenya (NIH IR24TW008889) awards to TW and VB.

Competing interests

The authors declare that they have no competing interests.

References

1. UNODC (2014) World drug report 2014
2. Reid SR (2009) Injection drug use, unsafe medical injections, and HIV in Africa: a systematic review. Harm Reduct J 6:24
3. NASCOP, MOH (2012) MARPs surveillance report 2012. NASCOP, Nairobi
4. Hacker MA, Leite I, Friedman SR, Carrijo RG, Bastos FI (2009) Poverty, bridging between injecting drug users and the general population, and "interiorization" may explain the spread of HIV in southern Brazil. Health Place 15:514–519
5. Masur H, Michelis MA, Wormser GP, Lewin S, Gold J, Tapper ML, Giron J, Lerner CW, Armstrong D, Setia U et al (1982) Opportunistic infection in previously healthy women. Initial manifestations of a community-acquired cellular immunodeficiency. Ann Intern Med 97:533–539
6. Panda S, Chatterjee A, Bhattacharya SK, Manna B, Singh PN, Sarkar S, Naik TN, Chakrabarti S, Detels R (2000) Transmission of HIV from injecting drug users to their wives in India. Int J STD AIDS 11:468–473
7. NASCOP, MOH (2014) Guidelines on use use of antiretroviral drugs for treating and preventing HIV infection: a rapid advice. NASCOP, Nairobi
8. WHO (2014) March 2014 supplement to the 2013 consolidated guidelines on the use of antiretroviral drugs for treating and preventing HIV infection. Recommendations for a public health approach
9. Floridia M, Fragola V, Galluzzo CM, Giannini G, Pirillo MF, Andreotti M, Tomino C, Vella S (2002) HIV-related morbidity and mortality in patients starting protease inhibitors in very advanced HIV disease (CD4 count of <50 cells/microL): an analysis of 338 clinical events from a randomized clinical trial. HIV Med 3:75–84
10. Kowalski J, Gange SJ, Schneider MF, Tsai HL, Templeton A, Shao Q, Zhang GW, Yeh MF, Young M, Markham RB (2009) Relationship of injection drug use, antiretroviral therapy resistance, and genetic diversity in the HIV-1 pol gene. J Acquir Immune Defic Syndr 50:381–389
11. Ajose O, Mookerjee S, Mills EJ, Boulle A, Ford N (2012) Treatment outcomes of patients on second-line antiretroviral therapy in resource-limited settings: a systematic review and meta-analysis. AIDS 26:929–938
12. Wensing AM, Calvez V, Gunthard HF, Johnson VA, Paredes R, Pillay D, Shafer RW, Richman DD (2014) 2014 Update of the drug resistance mutations in HIV-1. Top Antivir Med 22:642–650
13. Beck IA, Deng W, Payant R, Hall R, Bumgarner RE, Mullins JI, Frenkel LM (2014) Validation of an oligonucleotide ligation assay for quantification of human immunodeficiency virus type 1 drug-resistant mutants by use of massively parallel sequencing. J Clin Microbiol 52:2320–2327
14. Chung MH, Beck IA, Dross S, Tapia K, Kiarie JN, Richardson BA, Overbaugh J, Sakr SR, John-Stewart GC, Frenkel LM (2014) Oligonucleotide ligation assay detects HIV drug resistance associated with virologic failure among antiretroviral-naive adults in Kenya. J Acquir Immune Defic Syndr 67:246–253
15. Graham SM, Masese L, Gitau R, Jalalian-Lechak Z, Richardson BA, Peshu N, Mandaliya K, Kiarie JN, Jaoko W, Ndinya-Achola J et al (2010) Antiretroviral adherence and development of drug resistance are the strongest predictors of genital HIV-1 shedding among women initiating treatment. J Infect Dis 202:1538–1542
16. Hassan AS, Mwaringa SM, Obonyo CA, Nabwera HM, Sanders EJ, Rinke de Wit TF, Cane PA, Berkley JA (2013) Low prevalence of transmitted HIV type 1 drug resistance among antiretroviral-naive adults in a rural HIV clinic in Kenya. AIDS Res Hum Retroviruses 29:129–135

17. Hassan AS, Nabwera HM, Mwaringa SM, Obonyo CA, Sanders EJ, Rinke de Wit TF, Cane PA, Berkley JA (2014) HIV-1 virologic failure and acquired drug resistance among first-line antiretroviral experienced adults at a rural HIV clinic in coastal Kenya: a cross-sectional study. AIDS Res Ther 11:9
18. Kiptoo M, Brooks J, Lihana RW, Sandstrom P, Ng'ang'a Z, Kinyua J, Lagat N, Okoth F, Songok EM (2013) HIV-1 drug resistance-associated mutations among HIV-1 infected drug-naive antenatal clinic attendees in rural Kenya. BMC Infect Dis 13:517. doi:10.1186/1471-2334-13-517
19. Kiptoo M, Ichimura H, Wembe RL, Ng'Ang'a Z, Mueke J, Kinyua J, Lagat N, Okoth F, Songok EM (2008) Prevalence of nevirapine-associated resistance mutations after single dose prophylactic treatment among antenatal clinic attendees in north rift Kenya. AIDS Res Hum Retroviruses 24:1555–1559
20. Koigi P, Ngayo MO, Khamadi S, Ngugi C, Nyamache AK (2014) HIV type 1 drug resistance patterns among patients failing first and second line antiretroviral therapy in Nairobi, Kenya. BMC Res Notes 7:890
21. Lehman DA, Chung MH, Mabuka JM, John-Stewart GC, Kiarie J, Kinuthia J, Overbaugh J (2009) Lower risk of resistance after short-course HAART compared with zidovudine/single-dose nevirapine used for prevention of HIV-1 mother-to-child transmission. J Acquir Immune Defic Syndr 51:522–529
22. Lehman DA, Wamalwa DC, McCoy CO, Matsen FA, Langat A, Chohan BH, Benki-Nugent S, Custers-Allen R, Bushman FD, John-Stewart GC, Overbaugh J (2012) Low-frequency nevirapine resistance at multiple sites may predict treatment failure in infants on nevirapine-based treatment. J Acquir Immune Defic Syndr 60:225–233
23. Lihana RW, Khamadi SA, Lubano K, Lwembe R, Kiptoo MK, Lagat N, Kinyua JG, Okoth FA, Songok EM, Makokha EP, Ichimura H (2009) HIV type 1 subtype diversity and drug resistance among HIV type 1-infected Kenyan patients initiating antiretroviral therapy. AIDS Res Hum Retroviruses 25:1211–1217
24. Lihana RW, Khamadi SA, Lubano K, Mwangi J, Kinyua JG, Okoth VO, Lagat NJ, Okoth FA, Songok EM, Makokha EP (2010) Genetic characterization of HIV type 1 among patients with suspected immune reconstitution inflammatory syndrome after initiation of antiretroviral therapy in Kenya. AIDS Res Hum Retroviruses 26:833–838
25. Lwembe R, Ochieng W, Panikulam A, Mongoina CO, Palakudy T, Koizumi Y, Kageyama S, Yamamoto N, Shioda T, Musoke R et al (2007) Anti-retroviral drug resistance-associated mutations among non-subtype B HIV-1-infected Kenyan children with treatment failure. J Med Virol 79:865–872
26. Nyamache AK, Waihenya R, Ng'ang'a ZW, Muigai AW, Khamadi SA (2011) Reverse transcriptase inhibitors drug resistance mutations in drug-naive HIV type 1 positive Kenyans. East Afr Med J 88:4–8
27. Osman S, Lihana RW, Kibaya RM, Ishizaki A, Bi X, Okoth FA, Ichimura H, Lwembe RM (2013) Diversity of HIV type 1 and drug resistance mutations among injecting drug users in Kenya. AIDS Res Hum Retroviruses 29:187–190
28. Sigaloff KC, Mandaliya K, Hamers RL, Otieno F, Jao IM, Lyagoba F, Magambo B, Kapaata A, Ndembi N (2012) Rinke de Wit TF: Short communication: High prevalence of transmitted antiretroviral drug resistance among newly HIV type 1 diagnosed adults in Mombasa, Kenya. AIDS Res Hum Retroviruses 28:1033–1037
29. Steegen K, Luchters S, Dauwe K, Reynaerts J, Mandaliya K, Jaoko W, Plum J, Temmerman M, Verhofstede C (2009) Effectiveness of antiretroviral therapy and development of drug resistance in HIV-1 infected patients in Mombasa, Kenya. AIDS Res Ther 6:12
30. Wamalwa DC, Lehman DA, Benki-Nugent S, Gasper MA, Gichohi R, Maleche-Obimbo E, Farquhar C, John-Stewart GC, Overbaugh J (2013) Long-term virologic response and genotypic resistance mutations in HIV-1 infected Kenyan children on combination antiretroviral therapy. J Acquir Immune Defic Syndr 62:267–274
31. Zeh C, Weidle PJ, Nafisa L, Lwamba HM, Okonji J, Anyango E, Bondo P, Masaba R, Fowler MG, Nkengasong JN et al (2011) HIV-1 drug resistance emergence among breastfeeding infants born to HIV-infected mothers during a single-arm trial of triple-antiretroviral prophylaxis for prevention of mother-to-child transmission: a secondary analysis. PLoS Med 8:e1000430
32. Nyamache AK, Muigai AW, Nganga Z, Khamadi SA (2011) HIV Type 1 genetic diversity and naturally occurring polymorphisms in HIV type 1 Kenyan isolates: implications for integrase inhibitors. AIDS Res Hum Retroviruses 28:933–936
33. Kantor R, DeLong A, Balamane M, Schreier L, Lloyd RM Jr, Injera W, Kamle L, Mambo F, Muyonga S, Katzenstein D et al (2014) HIV diversity and drug resistance from plasma and non-plasma analytes in a large treatment programme in western Kenya. J Int AIDS Soc 17:19262
34. Sampathkumar R, Shadabi E, La D, Ho J, Liang B, Kimani J, Ball T, Francis A Plummer FA, Luo M (2014) Naturally occurring protease inhibitor resistance mutations and their frequencies in HIV proviral sequences of drug-naïve sex workers in Nairobi, Kenya. In: 16th International Conference on Human Retroviruses:HTLV and Related Viruses. Montreal, Canada. BMC retrovirology
35. Carneiro M, Yu XF, Lyles C, Templeton A, Weisstein AE, Safaeian M, Farzadegan H, Vlahov D, Markham RB (1999) The effect of drug-injection behavior on genetic evolution of HIV-1. J Infect Dis 180:1025–1032
36. NASCOP (2010) National Guidelines for HIV Testing and Counselling in Kenya, 2nd edn. MOPHS, Nairobi
37. NASCOP (2012) Guidelines for antiretroviral therapy in Kenya 2011, 4th edn. Ministry of Medical Services, Kenya, Nairobi
38. Tamura K, Stecher G, Peterson D, Filipski A, Kumar S (2013) MEGA6: molecular evolutionary genetics analysis version 6.0. Mol Biol Evol 30:2725–2729
39. Rhee SY, Taylor J, Fessel WJ, Kaufman D, Towner W, Troia P, Ruane P, Hellinger J, Shirvani V, Zolopa A, Shafer RW (2010) HIV-1 protease mutations and protease inhibitor cross-resistance. Antimicrob Agents Chemother 54:4253–4261
40. Shafer RW, Schapiro JM (2008) HIV-1 drug resistance mutations: an updated framework for the second decade of HAART. AIDS Rev 10:67–84
41. Parsa-Parsi RW, Ellis R, Wiesing U (2014) Fifty years at the forefront of ethical guidance: the world medical association declaration of Helsinki. South Med J 107:405–406
42. Jordan MR, Bennett DE, Bertagnolio S, Gilks CF, Sutherland D (2008) World Health Organization surveys to monitor HIV drug resistance prevention and associated factors in sentinel antiretroviral treatment sites. Antivir Ther 13(Suppl 2):15–23
43. Ssemwanga D, Lihana RW, Ugoji C, Abimiku A, Nkengasong J, Dakum P, Ndembi N (2015) Update on HIV-1 Acquired and Transmitted Drug Resistance in Africa. AIDS Rev 17:3–20
44. Vlahov D, Celentano DD (2006) Access to highly active antiretroviral therapy for injection drug users: adherence, resistance, and death. Cad Saude Publica 22:705–718
45. Wainberg MA, Brenner BG (2012) The impact of HIV genetic polymorphisms and subtype differences on the occurrence of resistance to antiretroviral drugs. Mol Biol Int 2012:256982
46. Wood E, Hogg RS, Yip B, Dong WW, Wynhoven B, Mo T, Brumme CJ, Montaner JS, Harrigan PR (2005) Rates of antiretroviral resistance among HIV-infected patients with and without a history of injection drug use. AIDS 19:1189–1195
47. Maia Teixeira SL, Bastos FI, Hacker MA, Guimaraes ML, Morgado MG (2006) Trends in drug resistance mutations in antiretroviral-naive intravenous drug users of Rio de Janeiro. J Med Virol 78:764–769
48. Bakhouch K, Oulad-Lahcen A, Bensghir R, Blaghen M, Elfilali KM, Ezzikouri S, Abidi O, Hassar M, Wakrim L (2009) The prevalence of resistance-associated mutations to protease and reverse transcriptase inhibitors in treatment-naive (HIV1)-infected individuals in Casablanca, Morocco. J Infect Dev Ctries 3:380–391
49. Pires IL, Soares MA, Speranza FA, Ishii SK, Vieira MC, Gouvea MI, Guimaraes MA, de Oliveira FE, Magnanini MM, Brindeiro RM, Tanuri A (2004) Prevalence of human immunodeficiency virus drug resistance mutations and subtypes in drug-naive, infected individuals in the army health service of Rio de Janeiro, Brazil. J Clin Microbiol 42:426–430
50. Paolucci S, Baldanti F, Zavattoni M, Comolli G, Labo N, Menzo S, Clementi M, Gerna G (2003) Comparison of levels of HIV-1 resistance to protease inhibitors by recombinant versus conventional virus phenotypic assay and two genotypic interpretation procedures in treatment-naive and HAART-experienced HIV-infected patients. J Antimicrob Chemother 51:135–139
51. Zimmer JM, Roman F, Lambert C, Jonckheer A, Vazquez A, Plesseria JM, Servais JY, Covens K, Weber J, Van Laethem K et al (2008) Impact on replicative fitness of the G48E substitution in the protease of HIV-1: an in vitro and in silico evaluation. J Acquir Immune Defic Syndr 48:255–262

52. Theys K, Deforche K, Vercauteren J, Libin P, van de Vijver DA, Albert J, Asjo B, Balotta C, Bruckova M, Camacho RJ et al (2012) Treatment-associated polymorphisms in protease are significantly associated with higher viral load and lower CD4 count in newly diagnosed drug-naive HIV-1 infected patients. Retrovirology 9:81
53. Tossonian HK, Raffa JD, Grebely J, Viljoen M, Mead A, Khara M, McLean M, Krishnamurthy A, DeVlaming S, Conway B (2009) Primary drug resistance in antiretroviral-naive injection drug users. Int J Infect Dis 13:577–583
54. Valente MJ, Carvalho F, Bastos M, de Pinho PG, Carvalho M (2012) Contribution of oxidative metabolism to cocaine-induced liver and kidney damage. Curr Med Chem 19:5601–5606
55. Were T, Wesongah JO, Munde E, Ouma C, Kahiga TM, Ongecha-Owuor F, Kiarie JN, Ahmed AA, Makokha EP, Budambula V (2014) Clinical chemistry profiles in injection heroin users from Coastal Region, Kenya. BMC Clin Pathol 14:32
56. Rabi SA, Laird GM, Durand CM, Laskey S, Shan L, Bailey JR, Chioma S, Moore RD, Siliciano RF (2013) Multi-step inhibition explains HIV-1 protease inhibitor pharmacodynamics and resistance. J Clin Invest 123:3848–3860

20

Rates and risk factors associated with the progression of HIV to AIDS among HIV patients

Lin Chen[1*], Jiezhe Yang[1], Renjie Zhang[1], Yun Xu[1], Jinlei Zheng[1], Jianmin Jiang[1], Jun Jiang[1], Lin He[1], Ning Wang[2], Philip Chun Yeung[3] and Xiaohong Pan[4]

Abstract

Objectives: The objective of this study was to determine the rate of acquired immune deficiency syndrome (AIDS) in Zhejiang province and to identify specific factors associated with progression of this disease.

Methods: This study utilized a retrospective cohort to identify the specific factors involved in the progression of human immunodeficiency virus (HIV) to AIDS. We collected data of patients existing in care between 2008 and 2012 from the national surveillance system databases. We performed our analyses using a multivariate Cox proportional hazards model.

Results: This study included 9216 HIV-positive patients (75.6 % male), which yielded 12,452 person-years (py) of follow-up-data. The AIDS progression rates were 33.9 % (2008), 33.6 % (2009), 38.1 % (2010), 30.6 % (2011) and 25.9 % (2012). We observed a significant reduction in the rate of progression Of HIV to AIDS post-2010 (Pearson $\chi^2 = 4341.9$, $P < 0.001$). The cumulative AIDS progression incidence rates were 33.4, 35.4, 36.4, 37.0 and 37.04 per 100 py in 1 each of the 5 years of follow-up. This study found that age was an independent risk factor for the progression of HIV to AIDS. Compared with patients infected with HIV by homosexual transmission, patients infected with HIV by heterosexuals transmission or blood transfusion had a reduced hazard ratio (*HR*) for progression to AIDS (heterosexual transmission: $HR = 0.695, 0.524, P = 0.007$; blood transfusion: HR = 0.524, $P = 0.015$). Diagnosed with HIV from 2011 to 2012 and having a higher CD4+ cell count (350–500 cells/mm^3; or >500 cells/mm^3) at baseline were independently associated with lower rates of HIV progression to AIDS [HR = 0.382, 0.380, 0.187, $P < 0.001$]. Patients with a CD+ T-cell count of 200–350 cells/mm^3 or greater than 350 cells/mm^3 were less likely to develop AIDS following HIV diagnosis than were those patients without HAART treatment.

Conclusion: This study found a high progression rate from HIV to AIDS in HIV patients residing within Zhejiang province from 2008 to 2010. This rate decreased after 2010, which coincided with the new criteria for HAART treatment, which likely contributed to the observed reduction in the rate of progression. Initiation of HAART with higher CD4+ T-cell count may reduce rate of AIDS progression. Based on our results, we conclude that efficient strategies for HIV screening, as well as early diagnosis and treatment are necessary to reduce the progression of HIV to AIDS.

Keywords: HIV, AIDS, HAART

Background

Human immunodeficiency virus (HIV), the causative agent of acquired immune deficiency syndrome (AIDS), has posed a major global threat since its discovery in 1983 [1]. Today, approximately 40 million people globally are infected with HIV. Specifically, in China, there is a steadily increasing rate in the prevalence of HIV and subsequent progression to AIDS [2, 3]. In 2009, AIDS became the leading cause of death due to infectious agents in China [4]. Prior to 2009, the People's Republic of China

*Correspondence: lchen@cdc.zj.cn
[1] Zhejiang Provincial Center for Diseases Control and Prevention, Hangzhou, China

(PRC) launched the Four Frees and One Care' (FFOC) policy in 2003 to reduce the transmission of HIV. 'Four Frees' represent free antiretroviral treatment, prevention of mother-to-child transmission, voluntary counselling and testing, schooling for Children orphaned by AIDS' [5]. 'One care' represents care and economic assistance to the households of people living with HIV/AIDS. In 2010, the criteria for highly active antiretroviral therapy (HAART) was broadened from standards that included patients with a CD4+ T-cell count $\leq$200 cells/mm^3 to those that included patients with a CD4+ T-cell count $\leq$350 cells/mm^3. This modification allowed a greater number of people living with HIV (PLHIV) receive free treatment at an earlier stage of the infection. Zhejiang province, located on the southern coast of China, is one of the most developed areas in China. In 2012, there were a total of 8144 HIV/AIDS patients in Zhejiang. Interestingly, Zhejiang has a higher rate of HIV/AIDS patients than other Chinese provinces with similar populations and economic levels [6, 7]. Although 57.0 % of the total patients in Zhejiang have been treated with HAART.

The number of newly diagnosed HIV cases has steadily increased between 2008 and 2012 (from 1066 to 2744 patients). Despite HAART treatment, the number of HIV/AIDs patients in Zhejiang has increased. Therefore, it is essential that we understand the efficacy of current HIV/AIDS management strategies so that we can develop supplementary measures that will delay or prevent the progression of AIDS and, ultimately, reduce the rate of mortality.

Previous studies involving mathematical prediction models suggest that HIV-infected patients to in developing countries are more likely to acquire AIDS and subsequently die compared with those in developed countries [8–10]. In this study, we retrospectively analyzed data from HIV-infected patients in Zhejiang collected from 2008 to 2012. The goal of this study was to utilize patient data to identify risk factors associated with AIDS progression. Because China is the largest developing country in the world, this study examined whether the risk factors identified in developed countries might also be responsible for AIDS progression in developing countries.

Methods

Data source

A retrospective cohort study was conducted to evaluate the progression of HIV to AIDS in HIV-infected patients from Zhejiang, China. We utilized patient data from the Chinese National Case Reporting System collected from January 1, 2008 to December 31, 2012. After patients had been positively confirmed as HIV-positive, a uniform questionnaire designed by the Chinese Centers for Disease Control was used to collect patient information. The data were then uploaded to the National Surveillance System Database and the National Treatment Database. Patient information is confidential and could not be released without permission. Information retrieved from these databases included the following: demographic characteristics, disease progression (HIV or AIDS), year of confirmed diagnosis, method of diagnosis, transmission mode, dates, as well as details regarding AIDS progression and treatment [e.g., date of AIDS onset, HAART treatment dates, death (if applicable) CD4+ T-cell count]. After diagnosis, patients were followed until they died, were lost from the database, or until December 31, 2012. Observation stops once AIDS were developed.

Sampling method

Between January 1, 2008 and December 31, 2012, a total of 9216 HIV-positive patients were enrolled in Group One. All participants had to meet the following criteria: diagnosed as HIV-positive before 2008 and alive on December 31, 2007 or newly diagnosed with HIV during 2008 to 2012; HIV-positive status was defined as testing positive for an HIV-1 on ELISA and Western blot analysis. During the 5 years study observation, 441 (4.8 %) subjects died or dropped out of the database.

Our analysis also focused on the role of potential risk factors in HIV progression to AIDS. Therefore, Group Two consisted of patients with the following characteristics: newly diagnosed as HIV-positive from 2008 to 2012, had CD4+ T-cell count tested within 3 months after diagnosis, no immediate progression to AIDS. Of the 9216 patients, 4121 had AIDS at the time of HIV-positive diagnosis to AIDS. Patients who developed AIDS within 6 months after HIV diagnosis, or patients without a CD4 test within 3 month after diagnosis were excluded in the study to reduce bias. Thus, 3898 patients were enrolled in group two.

Diagnosis of AIDS

In 2006, the World Health Organization (WHO) stated the progression of HIV to AIDS has occurred when an individual has a CD4+ T-cell count less than or equal to 200 cells/mm^3, or WHO stage 3 or 4 [11].

Statistical analysis

The survival time of those patients diagnosed with AIDS was estimated by the number of years from their first visit to the midpoint between the last visit with AIDS-free and the first visit with AIDS. Individuals who remained AIDS-free were monitored until their last follow-up visit. All statistical analyses for this report were conducted using SPSS 17.0 statistical analysis software package (SPSS, Chicago, IL, USA). Data from Group One were analyzed using an abridged life table method, which described the incidence of AIDS from 2008 to 2012; and estimate the effect of HAART treatment on patient outcomes. For Group Two, Cox proportional hazards models were fitted to examine the effects of region, gender, age, education, marriage, occupation, CD4+ T-cell count and HAART treatment on the time to between HIV diagnosis and AIDS diagnosis. Results with p values of less than 0.05 were considered statistically significant. We excluded patients with missing data from the analysis.

Results

Patient characteristics

The mean age of the 9216 HIV-positive patients enrolled in Group One was 35 years (range = 1–88 years). In this study, the majority of patients were men (75.6 %) and 45.3 % were married. In terms of educational level, approximately 69.0 % patients did not proceed beyond junior high school. Additionally, 47.4 % patients were migrants from other provinces and most patients held one of the following jobs:worker, famer and commercial servant (64.3 %). Patients demographic characteristics are presented in Table 1.

Table 1 Selected characteristics of patients with HIV infection in Zhejiang province

Characteristic	Number (total = 9216)	%
Sex		
Male	6961	75.6
Female	2242	24.4
Occupation		
Farmer	1788	19.4
Worker	2365	25.7
Unemployed	994	10.8
Commercial service	1764	19.2
Doctor, teacher, retired people, government officials	526	5.7
Others	1766	19.2
Marriage		
Unmarried	3396	36.9
Married	4166	45.3
Divorced or widowed	1588	17.3
Unknown	53	0.6
Ethnic group		
Han	8548	92.9
Other	651	7.1
Unknown	4	0.0
Education		
Primary school or under	2461	26.7
Junior high school	3879	42.1
Senior high school	1634	17.8
College or above	1226	13.3
Unknown	3	0.0
Age (years)		
0–24	1964	21.3
25–34	3196	34.7
35–44	2215	24.1
45–54	993	10.8
55 or above	835	9.1
Census register		
Zhejiang Province	4837	52.6
Other Province	4366	47.4

AIDS development from 2008 to 2012

A total of 9216 patients in Group One were followed up for 12,452 person-years (py). By December 31, 2012, 3868 patients progressed from HIV to AIDS in Group one. There were 441 patients who returned to their home country or died (ranging from 0.30 to 4.70 person-years following HIV diagnosis). Following HIV diagnosis, the mean CD4+ T-cell count was 437 cells/mm^3. No significant differences between the demographic characteristics of patients who stopped being monitored during the time of our study compared with those patients whose information was available throughout the study time frame (data not shown) (Table 2).

During the entire observation period (2008–2012), HIV-positive patients progressed to AIDS (Group one) at the following rates: 33.9 % (2008), 33.6 % (2009), 38.1 % (2010), 30.6 % (2011) and 25.9 % (2012) (Table 2). The cumulative AIDS incidence probability were 33.43, 35.37, 36.38, 36.96 and 37.04 % in 1–5 years of follow-up, respectively (Table 3).

AIDS progression in patients treated with HAART

The prevalence of AIDS in Zhejiang from 2008 to 2010 was 35.7 %, and it decreased to 27.9 % between 2011 and 2012 (Table 2). To initially qualify for treatment with HAART (2008–2010), patients needed a CD4+ T-cell count of less than or equal to 200 cells/mm^3; however, the eligibility for HAART treatment was broadened to include patients with a CD4+ T-cell count of less than 350 cells/mm^3 (2011–2012) (Table 2). Figure 1 show that AIDS progression rates decreased in all CD4 level groups except the unknown one. The largest reduction in the rate of AIDS progression was observed in patients with a baseline CD4+ T-cell count of 200–350 cells/mm^3 (25.8/100 py of the patients in 2008–2010 and 17.7/100 py of the patients in 2011–2012, $P < 0.001$). Figure 2 indicates that the progression rates for all modes of transmission decreased after the eligibility criteria for HAART were broadened to include patients with a CD4+ T-cell count of less than 350 cells/mm^3. In particular, patients who were infected by HIV through homosexual transmission showed the most dramatic

Table 2 AIDS progression rates by time period

Time period	Person-years of observation (py)	Incidence observed (n)	AIDS progression rate (/100 py)	Male		Female	
				AIDS, n (py)	AIDS progression rate (/100 py)	AIDS, n (py)	AIDS progression rate (/100 py)
2008	1093	370	33.9	243 (714)	34.0	127 (379)	33.6
2009	1626	546	33.6	395 (1112)	35.5	151 (514)	29.4
2010	2296	874	38.1	676 (1618)	41.8	198 (678)	29.2
2008–2010	5015	1790	35.7*	1314 (3444)	38.2*	476 (1571)	30.3*
2011	3163	969	30.6	726 (2317)	31.3	243 (846)	28.7
2012	4274	1109	25.9	869 (3232)	26.9	240 (1042)	23.0
2011–2012	7437	2078	27.9*	1595 (5549)*	28.8*	483 (1888)	25.6*

* Pearson χ^2 test, P value for AIDS progression rates 2008–2010 vs. 2011–2012 of whole group, male and female are 0.000, 0.000, 0.002, respectively

Table 3 Cumulative AIDS incidence between 2008 and 2012

Time to AIDS onset (year)	AIDS (n)	Incidence probability (%)	Cumulative incidence probability (%)
0–	2763	33.43	33.43
1–	335	5.81	35.37
2–	151	2.84	36.38
3–	81	1.59	36.96
4–	12	0.24	37.04
Total	3342	–	–

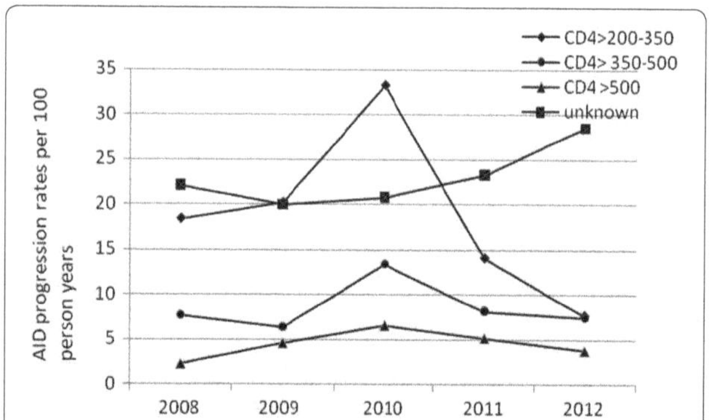

Fig. 1 AIDS progression rates by baseline CD4+ cell count among 2008–2012: this *figure* demonstrated the progression of HIV to AIDS among patients with different CD4+ T-cell count

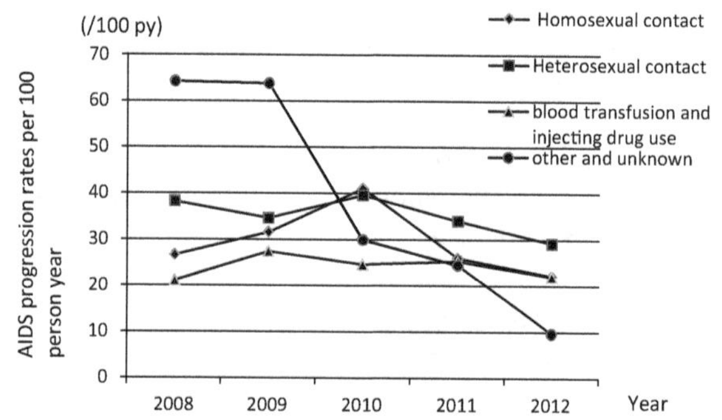

Fig. 2 AIDS progression rates by mode of transmission among 2008–2012: this *figure* demonstrated the progression of HIV to AIDS among patients with different transmission routes

reduction in the rates of AIDS (36.2/100 py in 2008–2010 to 23.6/100 py in 2011–2012, $P < 0.001$).

Changes over calendar time

The demographic characteristics of patients changed over the course of this study, from 2008 to 2012. In 2012, patients with first positive HIV test had a higher median age (39.8 years) compared with that of the comparable group of patients in 2008 (37.9 years old) ($P < 0.05$); HIV infection from homosexual transmission occurred more frequently in patients in 2012 (36.4 %) compared with in 2008 (18.8 %) ($P < 0.001$); However, baseline CD4 T-cell count counts were similar in 2008 and 2012 (median: 319 and 328 cell/μl, respectively; $P > 0.05$); The rate of HAART treatment during the first year of diagnosed with HIV was significantly higher (27.5 %) in 2012 than in 2008 (3.1 %) ($P < 0.001$).

Risk factors involved in the progression of HIV to AIDS

Patients in Group Two (3989 patients) were followed up for 12,452 py. As of December 31, 2012, it was known that 611 patients had progressed to AIDS. Cox proportional hazards regression was performed to determine the relative contribution of each factor (i.e., demographic characteristics, mobility, transmission routes, year of diagnosis, treatment with HAART and CD4+ T-cell count at baseline) to the progression of HIV of AIDS (Table 4). Cox regression analysis revealed that several factors, including age at diagnosis, transmission routes, census register, year of diagnosis, baseline CD4+ T-cell count and CD4+ T-cell count

Table 4 Cox proportional hazards model of risk factors for development of AIDS

Risk factor	Unadjusted relative hazard *HR* (95 % *CI*)	*P*	Adjusted relative hazard *HR* (95 % *CI*)	*P*
Sex				
Male	1 (reference)		–	–
Female	0.996 (0.827–1.200)	0.966	–	–
Age (year)				
0~	1 (reference)		1 (reference)	
25~	1.176 (0.949–1.457)	0.139	1.221 (0.982–1.518)	0.072
35~	1.310 (1.031–1.666)	0.027	1.364 (1.065–1.746)	0.014
45~	1.556 (1.167–2.075)	0.003	1.692 (1.247–2.297)	0.001
55~	1.950 (1.412–2.694)	0.000	1.915 (1.357–2.703)	0.000
Education				
Primary school and under	1 (reference)		–	–
Junior high school	0.981 (0.798–1.206)	0.856	–	–
Senior high school	0.943 (0.739–1.205)	0.641	–	–
College and above	0.874 (0.673–1.135)	0.312	–	–
Marital status				
Single	1 (reference)		–	–
Married	1.198 (1.007–1.425)	0.042	–	–
Divorced or widowed	1.094 (0.863–1.386)	0.457	–	–
Unknown	1.313 (0.486–3.526)	0.590	–	–
Mode of transmission				
Homosexual contact	1 (reference)		1 (reference)	
Heterosexual contact	1.019 (0.862–1.205)	0.824	0.695 (0.571–0.844)	0.000
Blood	0.789 (0.514–1.212)	0.279	0.524 (0.336–0.816)	0.004
Other and unknown	0.951 (0.470–1.927)	0.890	0.689 (0.336–1.415)	0.311
Testing mode				
VCT consultant	1 (reference)			–
Health checkup	1.027 (0.807–1.306)	0.831	–	–
Seeing doctor for other disease	1.261 (1.006–1.579)	0.044	–	–
Spouse and children of patient, blood donors	1.380 (1.007–1.891)	0.045	–	–
Others	1.112 (0.720–1.718)	0.633	–	–
Census register				
Zhejiang Province	1 (reference)		1 (reference)	
Other Province	0.765 (0.651–0.898)	0.001	0.670 (0.562–0.799)	0.000
Mobility				
Between Provinces	1 (reference)		–	–
Between Cites	0.905 (0.636–1.287)	0.579	–	–
Between County	0.977 (0.777–1.228)	0.840	–	–
Immobility	0.970 (0.795–1.182)	0.761	–	–
Reported time (year)				
2008–2010	1 (reference)		1 (reference)	
2011–2012	0.346 (0.274–0.437)	0.000	0.382 (0.302–0.483)	0.000
Baseline CD4+ T-cell count				
200–350	1 (reference)	0.000	1 (reference)	
350–500	0.464 (0.388–0.556)	0.000	0.380 (0.316–0.458)	0.000
>500	0.262 (0.206–0.332)	0.000	0.187 (0.147–0.239)	0.000
CD4+ T-cell count of initial HAART				
No HAART	1 (reference)		1 (reference)	
≤200	2.166 (1.273–3.685)	0.004	1.165 (0.679–1.999)	0.580

Table 4 continued

Risk factor	Unadjusted relative hazard *HR* (95 % *CI*)	*P*	Adjusted relative hazard *HR* (95 % *CI*)	*P*
200–350	0.402 (0.320–0.504)	0.000	0.225 (0.178–0.285)	0.000
>350	0.295 (0.110–0.789)	0.015	0.168 (0.063–0.451)	0.000

VCT voluntary counselling test

of initial HAART played significant influence roles in the progression of HIV to AIDS. HIV patients older than 55 years showed a higher risk of progressing to AIDS than patients who were younger than 25 years old ($HR = 1.915$, 95 % CI: 1.357–2.703, $P < 0.001$). The rate of AIDS progression was significantly higher among those infected by homosexual transmission than among patients infected by heterosexuals transmission ($HR = 0.695$, 95 % CI: 0.571–0.844, $P < 0.05$) or by blood borne transmission ($HR = 0.524$, 95 % CI: 0.336–0.816, $P < 0.05$). Patients diagnosed with HIV between 2011 and 2012 were at a lower risk of acquiring AIDS than were those patients diagnosed between 2008 and 2010 ($HR = 0.382$, 95 % CI: 0.302–0.483, $P < 0.001$). Our results also indicate that a higher CD4+ T-cell count was associated with a lower rate of AIDS progression ($HR = 0.380$, 0.187, $P < 0.001$). Patients with a CD4+ T-cell count of 200–350 cells/mm^3 or greater than 350 cells/mm^3 were less likely to develop AIDS following HIV diagnosis than were those patients without HAART treatment ($HR = 0.225$, 0.168, $P < 0.001$) (Table 4).

Discussion

The rate at which HIV progressed to AIDS decreased from 33.9 % in 2008 to 25.9 % in 2012. These rates were greater than those observed in developed countries, such as British Columbia (7 % in 2013), Brazil (6.2 % between 2000 and 2008), but they were similar to the rates in Africa and Asia countries [12–16]. In this study, AIDS was diagnosed within 1 year of HIV diagnosis, which is similar to the diagnostic process in developed countries. The rates at which patients diagnosed with HIV progressed to AIDS within 12 months in developed countries were as follows: Australia: 65.0 %, Canada: 64.0 % and France: 64.8 % [17]. Our study found late diagnosis of HIV in Zhejiang and other Chinese provinces, which probably affects the survival of patients.

Several studies in developed countries have demonstrated that non-HAART treatment, hepatitis B coinfection, tuberculosis coinfection, being older than 50 years of age, having black or brown skin, intravenous drug abuse, lack of schooling as well as a baseline CD4+ T-cell count lower than 500 cells/mm^3 were predictors of higher rate of AIDS progression [18–20].

The results from our study suggest that increasing the CD4+ T-cell count necessary to begin HAART treatment is an effective way to delay AIDS progression among PLHIV. The overall AIDS progression rate underwent a steady reduction after 2010 (from 38.1 to 25.9 %) as the treatment was available to patients with a CD4+ T-cell count of 350 cells/mm^3 [21]. Our analysis also indicated that patients with a CD4+ T-cell count greater than 200–350 cells/mm^3 benefit the most from early HAART treatment. The progression rate for patients with unknown CD4+ T-cell counts increased over time, with 33.5 % of these patients being diagnosed at the time of death. We hypothesize that these phenomena relate to the fact that these specific individuals did not seek care in time. Furthermore, most of these patients were migrants, had lower lever of education, and older. HAART plays an important role in delaying the progression of HIV to AIDS because it can reduce the HIV–RNA concentration and restoring the immune system [22–24]. In recent years, increasing number of researches encouraged early treatment with CD4+ T-cell count less than 500 cells/mm^3 or more [25–27]. Although the beneficial effects of HAART have been already observed in patients with a CD4+ T-cell count greater than 200 cells/mm^3, or greater than or equal to 350 cells/mm^3, developing counties, including Asia and Africa, need to understand other important factors [e.g. economic factors, side effects or serious non AIDS events (ANAEs) like cancer and cardiovascular disease].

Several factors, including mode of transmission, region, age and CD4+ T-cell count at baseline were related to the rate of AIDS progression in HIV-positive patients. A study performed by Hongjing Yan found a higher rate of disease progression from HIV to AIDS among homosexuals compared with among heterosexuals, intravenous drug users (IDUs) or blood donors [8]. Similar results were observed in this study; however, the proportion of late diagnosis in male who have sex with male (MSM) patients was 19.1 %, which was lower than that of heterosexuals (30.9 %) and others (29.7 %) in Zhejiang (data not published). The high rate of AIDS progression among homosexual patients might be a result of other important factors including stigma, psychological characteristics, genetic or molecular characteristics, as well as coinfection with other disease, such as hepatitis; or tuberculosis

[28]. Although this information was not collected in our particular patient database, further investigations are warranted. In Zhejiang, the central regions have the highest rate of AIDS development, which might be related to the fact that these regions contain the highest proportions of homosexuals. A study in Hangzhou conducted between 2006 and 2008 indicated that the infection rates of homosexuals from pubs, bathrooms and clubhouses were 3.5, 12.8 and 2.8 %, respectively, all of which were higher than those observed in any other cities in Zhejiang [29, 30]. The results of our study also suggest that age and baseline CD4+ T-cell count were critical factors that determine the rate of progression of HIV to AIDS. Patients who have lower baseline CD4+ T-cell count and were of an older age tended to have a higher %consistent with previously published works [31].

This retrospective cohort study of patients from Zhejiang, provides information on the rate and contributors to the progression of HIV to AIDS. Our observations highlight the impact of late HIV testing and delayed diagnosis of HIV/AIDS in Zhejiang. Previous studies have suggested that an undamaged immune system predicts delayed progression to AIDS [32] and late diagnosis leads to exhaustion of the immune system. Therefore, the use of additional strategies, such as VCT and provider-initiated HIV testing and counseling (PITC), for HIV screening is necessary to delay the progression of HIV to AIDS.

Limitations

This has a few limitations. As the cohort was not strictly designed, inaccurate follow-up was inevitable. First, the amount of time between HIV diagnosis to AIDS diagnosis might have been exaggerated or underestimated. Second, CD4+ T-cell count, which is an important diagnostic tool for AIDS, was not available for all patients. A large number subjects are excluded in group two for their AIDS status as diagnosis and without CD4+ T-cell count in first 3 month following diagnosis were excluded for confounding variables, which may have introduced selection bias. Although we recommend early HAART treatment, data on side effect or additional information regarding earlier treatment have not been reported. The role of early HAART treatment in patient health will need to be assessed in the future.

Conclusions

In conclusion, HIV progression to AIDS was affected by the patient's age at diagnosis, transmission routes and baseline CD4+ T-cell counts. Early HAART treatment in patients with a higher CD4+ T-cell count significantly delayed progression to AIDS in these patients. Thus effective interventions, such as PITC or VCT, should be utilized to target those at high risk. Our results support use of early HAART treatment, an approach that is already recommended by the current WHO treatment guidelines for HIV infection.

Authors' contributions

LC carried out study design as well as data collection, data analysis, and write manuscript. XHP designed the study, reviewed the manuscript and approved the final version. RJZ and PCY revised the manuscript. JMJ and NW reviewed the manuscript. JZY, YX, JLZ, JJ, LH helped to collect and manage data. All authors read and approved the final manuscript.

Author details

[1] Zhejiang Provincial Center for Diseases Control and Prevention, Hangzhou, China. [2] National Center for AIDS/STD Control and Prevention, China CDC, Beijing, China. [3] Department of Surgery, Faculty of Medicine, The Chinese University of Hong Kong, Shatin, Hong Kong. [4] Department of HIV/AIDS Prevention and Control, Zhejiang Provincial Center for Diseases Control and Prevention, 3399 Binsheng Road, Hangzhou, Zhejiang, People's Republic of China.

Acknowledgements

The authors thank the staff of local Health Bureaus and local CDCs in Zhejiang province for their assistance in the fieldwork.

Grant support

Our funding was provided by The National Science and Technology Pillar Program (Grant No. 2012ZX10001001).

Sources of support

Key Projects in the National Science and Technology Pillar Program during the Twelfth five-year plan period (Grant No. 2012ZX10001001).

Competing interests

The authors declare that they have no competing interests.

References

1. Barré-Sinoussi F, Chermann JC, Rey F, et al. Isolation of a T-lymphotropic retrovirus from a patient at risk for AIDS. Science. 1983;220:868–71.
2. UNAIDS epidemic update 2007. http://www.who.int/hiv/pub/epidemiology/epiupdate2007/en/. Accessed 10 May 2013.
3. Wang L, Wang L, Ding ZW, et al. HIV prevalence among populations at risk, using sentinel surveillance data from 1995 to 2009 in China. Chin J Epidemiol. 2011;32:20–4.
4. BBC News. Aids take deathly toll in China. February 18, 2009. http://news.bbc.co.uk/2/hi/asia-pacific/7896133.stm/. Accessed 2 May 2012.
5. Shen J, Yu D. Governmental policies on HIV infection in China. Cell Res. 2005;15:903–7.
6. Wang ZY, Zheng YF, Liu L, et al. High prevalence of HIV-associated neurocognitive disorder in HIV-infected patients with a baseline CD4 count ≤350 cells/μL in Shanghai, China. Biosci Trends. 2013;7:284–9.
7. Wu JR, Wang B, Zhou LJ, et al. Mycoplasmas infection in male HIV/AIDS patients in Jiangsu, China. Microb Pathog. 2013;63:54–8.
8. Yan HJ, Yang HT, Li JJ, et al. Emerging disparity in HIV/AIDS disease progression and mortality for men who have sex with men, Jiangsu Province, China. AIDS Behav. 2014;S1:5–10.
9. Yoichi C, Kavita V. Adverse psychosocial factors predict poorer prognosis in HIV disease: a meta-analytic review of prospective investigations. Brain Behav Immun. 2009;23:434–45.
10. Steele KT, Steenhoff AP, Newcomb CW, et al. Early mortality and AIDS progression despite high initial antiretroviral therapy adherence and virologic suppression in Botswana. PLoS One. 2011;6(6):e20010.
11. World Health Organization (WHO). HIV/AIDS Programme. WHO case definitions of HIV for surveillance and revised clinical staging and immunological classification of HIV-related disease in adults and children.

2006. http://www.who.int/hiv/pub/guidelines/hivstaging/en/. Accessed 13 May 2014.

12. Nicola L, Katie P, Rebecca C, et al. AIDS survival and progression in black Africans living in south London, 1986–1994. Genitourin Med. 1996;72:12–6.
13. Lima VD, Lourenço L, Yip B, et al. Trends in AIDS incidence and AIDS-related mortality in British Columbia between 1981 and 2013. Lancet HIV. 2015;2(3):e92–7.
14. Luz PM, Bruyand M, Ribeiro S. AIDS and non-AIDS severe morbidity associated with hospitalizations among HIV-infected patients in two regions with universal access to care and antiretroviral therapy, France and Brazil, 2000–2008: hospital-based cohort studies. BMC Infect Dis. 2014;21(14):278.
15. Gabillard D, Lewden C, Ndoye I. Mortality, AIDS-morbidity, and loss to follow-up by current CD4 cell count among HIV-1-infected adults receiving antiretroviral therapy in Africa and Asia: data from the ANRS 12222 collaboration. J Acquir Immune Defic Syndr. 2013;62(5):555–61.
16. Jiang HB, Xie NH, Cao BB. Determinants of progression to AIDS and death following HIV diagnosis: a retrospective cohort study in Wuhan, China. PLoS One. 2013;8(12):e83078.
17. Hall HI, Halverson J, Wilson DP. Late diagnosis and entry to care after diagnosis of human immunodeficiency virus infection: a country comparison. PLoS One. 2013;8(11):e77763.
18. Tancredi MV, Waldman EA. Predictors of progression to AIDS after HIV infection diagnosis in the pre- and post-HAART eras in a BrazilianAIDS-free cohort. Trans R Soc Trop Med Hyg. 2014;108(7):408–14.
19. Edelman EJ, Cheng DM, Krupitsky EM. Heroin use and HIV disease progression: results from a Pilot Study of a Russian Cohort. AIDS Behav. 2015;19(6):1089–97.
20. Kawado M, Hashimoto S, Yamaguchi T. Difference of progression to AIDS according to CD4 cell count, plasma HIV RNA level and the use of antiretroviral therapy among HIV patients infected through blood products in Japan. J Epidemiol. 2006;16(3):101–6.
21. WHO. Rapid advice: antiretroviral therapy for HIV infection in adults and adolescents. http://www.who.int/hiv/pub/arv/rapid_advice_art.pdf. Accessed 15 May 2013.
22. Li X, Xu Y, Nie S, et al. The effect evaluation of highly active antiretroviral therapy to patients with AIDS in Hubei province of China. J Huazhong Univ Sci Technol Med Sci. 2009;29:580–4.
23. Wong KH, Chan KCW, Lee SS, et al. Delayed progression to death and to AIDS in a Hong Kong cohort of patients with advanced HIV type 1 disease during the era of highly active antiretroviral therapy. Clin Infect Dis. 2004;39:853–60.
24. Pezzotti P, Dorrucci M, Donisi A, et al. Survival, progression to AIDS and immunosuppression in HIV-positive individuals before and after the introduction of the highly active antiretroviral therapy (HAART). Epidemiol Prev. 2003;27:348–55.
25. Drechsler H, Zhang S, Holodniy M, et al. CD4 counts and mortality in virologically suppressed US veterans. J Int Assoc Provid AIDS Care. 2014;13(2):120–6.
26. Cagigi A, Rinaldi S, Cotugno N, et al. Early highly-active antiretroviral therapy enhances B-cell longevity: a 5 year follow-up. Pediatr Infect Dis J. 2014;33(5):e126–31.
27. Mills FP, Ford N, Nachega JB, et al. Earlier initialization of highly active antiretroviral therapy is associated with long-term survival and is cost-effective: findings from a deterministic model of a 10-year Ugandan cohort. J Acquir Immune Defic Syndr. 2012;61(3):364–9.
28. Lim HJ, Okwera A, Mayanja-Kizza H. Effect of tuberculosis preventive therapy on HIV disease progression and survival in HIV-infected adults. HIV Clin Trials. 2006;7(4):172–83.
29. Shao B, Li Y, Yu L, et al. The HIV/AIDS epidemic characteristics in a northeast province of China—men who have sex with men have made a tremendous contribution to the growth of the HIV epidemic. J Infect. 2014;68(3):273–80.
30. Wraivg LH, Xu YY, Weivg J, et al. Cross-sectional investigation on HIV prevalence and HIV related risk behavior among men who have sex with men in Taizhou, Zhejiang. Dis Surveill. 2013;1:362–5.
31. Symeon M, Olga T, Lemonia S, et al. Older HIV-infected patients—an underestimated population in northern Greece: epidemiology, risk of disease progression and death. Int J Infect Dis. 2013;17:e883–91.
32. Maloy KJ, Burkhart C, Junt TM, et al. CD4pT cell subsets during virus infection. Protective capacity depends on effector cytokine secretion and on migratory capability. J Exp Med. 2000;191:2159–70.

21

Community-based ART distribution system can effectively facilitate long-term program retention and low-rates of death and virologic failure

Stephen Okoboi[1*], Erin Ding[2], Steven Persuad[3], Jonathan Wangisi[1], Josephine Birungi[1], Susan Shurgold[2], Darius Kato[1], Maureen Nyonyintono[1], Aggrey Egessa[1], Celestin Bakanda[1], Paula Munderi[4], Pontiano Kaleebu[4] and David M. Moore[2,3]

Abstract

Background: Community-drug distribution point is a care model for stable patients in the community designed to make ART delivery more efficient for the health system and provide appropriate support to encourage long-term retention of patients. We examined program retention among ART program participants in rural Uganda, which has used a community-based distribution model of ART delivery since 2004.

Methods: We analyzed data of all patients >18 years who initiated ART in Jinja, Ugandan site of The AIDS Support Organization between January 1, 2004 and July 31, 2009. Participants attended clinic or outreach visits every 2–3 months and had CD4 cell counts measured every 6 months. Retention to care was defined as any patient with at least one visit in the 6 months before June 1, 2013. We then identified participants with at least one visit in the 6 months before June 1, 2013 and examined associations with mortality and lost-to-follow-up (LTFU). Participants with >4 years of follow up during August, 2012 to May, 2013 had viral load conducted, since no routine viral load testing was available.

Results: A total of 3345 participants began ART during 2004–2009. The median time on ART in June 2013 was 5.69 years. A total of 1335 (40 %) were residents of Jinja district and 2005 (60 %) resided in outlying districts. Of these, 2322 (69 %) were retained in care, 577 (17 %) died, 161 (5 %) transferred out and 285 (9 %) were LTFU. Factors associated with mortality or LTFU included male gender, [Adjusted Hazard Ratio (AHR) = 1.56; 95 % CI 1.28–1.9], CD4 cell count <50 cells/μL (AHR = 4.09; 95 % CI 3.13–5.36) or 50–199 cells/μL (AHR = 1.86; 95 % CI 1.46–2.37); ART initiation and WHO stages 3 (AHR = 1.35; 95 % CI 1.1–1.66) or 4 (AHR = 1.74; 95 % CI 1.23–2.45). Residence outside of Jinja district was not associated with mortality/LTFU (p value = 0.562). Of 870 participants who had VL tests, 756 (87 %) had VLs <50 copies/mL.

Conclusion: Community-based ART distribution systems can effectively mitigate the barriers to program retention and result in good rates of virologic suppression.

Keywords: Antiretroviral therapy, Virologic failure, Lost-to-follow-up; mortality, Retention, Sub-Saharan Africa, Uganda

*Correspondence: stephenokoboi@yahoo.co.uk; okobois@tasouganda.org

[1] Mulago Hospital Complex, The AIDS Support Organization (TASO), P.O BOX 10443, Kampala, Uganda

Background

Large-scale antiretroviral treatment (ART) programs for HIV and AIDS were launched in sub-Saharan Africa in 2003–2004 with the increases in funding made available through the Global Fund Against AIDS, Tuberculosis and Malaria and the President's Emergency Plan for AIDS Relief (PEPFAR) [1–3]. From their inception, much attention was then focused on patients' day-to-day adherence to ART which have generally shown very good results [1, 3–5].

However, long-term retention of patients in treatment programs, a prerequisite for achieving any adherence at all has gained more attention in recent years [4]. Most large-scale treatment providers have few resources available to track missing patients; and patient attrition is often not prioritized as a primary outcome and clinical studies often focus solely on describing those patients who are retained in care. In a study conducted in 17 facilities in Uganda, Tanzania and Zambia, loss to follow up ranged from an average of 25.9 % at 1 year to 41.9 % at 4 years [8]. Other studies have shown that transportation costs, absence of treatment partner or lack of family support as significant barrier to program retention [6, 7, 12, 16, 24].

In studies with follow-up beyond the first 4 years of treatment, LTFU has been shown to vary between 7 % in a program in Malawi [6, 10] to 56 % for one program in Uganda [7]. In a recent systematic review of participant retention in ART programs in Africa, researchers found an estimated median retention of care of 64.4 % (range 57.5–72.1 %) after 3 years after ART initiation among 39 cohorts with over 225,000 patients in total [8]. LTFU was the most common factor for not been retained [13, 18]. Possible explanations for these variations in patient retention include patients having to pay for their medication, patients accessing care at another facility and unreported mortality [6, 10 16]. Additionally, lack of transportation and distance from the clinic, financial strain, work or child care responsibilities, social issues, and feeling that their health was too poor or too good to warrant continuing have all been identified as barriers to being retained in care [6, 10, 16]. When investigated, the proportion of patients LTFU who were then discovered to have died ranged from 25 to 50 % [1, 10, 17, 19].

We undertook an analysis of program data at one of the TASO centers in Jinja, Uganda to examine program retention, LTFU and mortality among clients enrolled in the first 5 years of the ART program. Our primary interest was in examining whether clients from districts which were distant from the TASO centre had the same likelihood of being retained in care, as those who resided close to the TASO clinic. In a sample of those retained in care after 5 years of treatment, we also conducted VL testing to measure the prevalence of virologically defined treatment failure in a program without access to routine VL testing.

Results

A total of 3340 participants began ART during 2004–2009 and the median time on ART for these individuals in June 2013 was 5.7 years (IQR = 4.1–7.2). Of these individuals, 2379 (71 %) were females, the median age at ART initiation was 40 years (IQR = 34–46), and 1618 (55 %) of the participants had some primary education as their highest level attained. The median CD4 cell count at initiation was 184 cells/μL (IQR = 95–298). A total of 1335 (40 %) were residents of Jinja district and 2005 (60 %) resided in outlying districts. A total of, 1361 (44 %) of the participants began treatment on Nevirapine, Zidovudine and Lamivudine, 950 (31 %) began with Niverapine, Stavudine and Lamivudine and 323 (11 %) began with Efavirenz, Zidovudine and Lamivudine.

A total of 2317 (69 %) participants had at least one recorded clinic or outreach visit recorded between November 1, 2012–May 31, 2013. For participants not retained in care, 577 (17 %) were known to have died, 161 (5 %) had transferred out and 285 (9 %) were classified as LTFU. The mortality rate was 3.22/100 and the rate LTFU was 1.59/100 person years. Table 1 shows the bivariate analysis of factors associated with mortality or LTFU. Male participants represented a higher proportion of those who died or LTFU than those who were retained in care 37 vs 25 %, respectively; ($p < 0.001$). We also found that WHO stage at treatment initiation ($p < 0.001$), CD4 cell count at initiation ($p < 0.001$) hemoglobin values at ART initiation ($p < 0.001$) and occupation ($p = 0.045$) were higher in those who died or were LTFU. District of residence at ART initiation was also unequally distributed across the four vital status categories ($p < 0.001$). However, when expressed as row percentages (rather than column percentages as in Table 1) the proportion retained in care had a fairly narrow range from a low 67 % in Jinja to a high 73 % in surrounding districts (data not shown). Mortality ranged from 14 % in Buikwe to 20 % in Mayuge and LTFU ranged from 4 % in Mayuge to 10 % in "other districts".

In the multivariate Cox proportional hazards analysis of factors associated with time to death or LTFU as in Table 1, male gender [adjusted hazard ratio (AHR) = 1.56; 95 % CI 1.28–1.9] was significantly associated with LTFU or mortality. CD4 cell count <50 (AHR = 4.09; 95 % CI. 3.13–5.36) or 50–199 cells/μL (AHR = 1.86; 95 % CI 1.46–2.37) at ART initiation and WHO stages 3 (AHR = 1.35; 95 % CI 1.1–1.66) or 4 (AHR = 1.74; 95 % CI 1.23–2.45) were also associated with the outcome. Participants who received Stavudine, Lamivudine and Nevirapine, (AHR = 1.38; 95 %

Table 1 Cox proportional hazards analysis of factors associated with time to mortality or loss to follow up

List of clinical factors	Univariate		Multivariate	
	HR (95 % CI)	p value	HR (95 % CI)	p value
Age at ART initiation	0.99 (0.98, 1.00)	0.065	1.00 (0.99, 1.01)	0.720
First ARV regimen				
Nevirapine/zidovudine/lamivudine	1.00 (–)	0.018	1.00 (–)	0.003
Efavirenz/stavudine/lamivudine	0.64 (0.39, 1.03)		0.87 (0.53, 1.44)	
Efavirenz/zidovudine/lamivudine	0.61 (0.42, 0.89)		0.74 (0.51, 1.09)	
Nevirapine/stavudine/lamivudine	0.91 (0.74, 1.14)		1.38 (1.08, 1.76)	
Other ARV regimen	1.21 (0.86, 1.71)		1.41 (1.00, 1.99)	
WHO stage				
Stages 1 and 2	1.00 (–)	<0.001	1.00 (–)	0.002
Stage 3	1.52 (1.24, 1.85)		1.36 (1.1, 1.67)	
Stage 4	1.82 (1.3, 2.56)		1.72 (1.21, 2.43)	
CD4 at ART initiation				
≥200	1.00 (–)	<0.001	1.00 (–)	<0.001
50–199	2.21 (1.75, 2.8)		1.86 (1.46, 2.37)	
<50	5.25 (4.07, 6.78)		4.11 (3.13, 5.4)	
District of residence at ART initiation				
Jinja	1.00 (–)	0.879	1.00 (–)	0.562
Buikwe	0.87 (0.65, 1.15)		0.92 (0.69, 1.22)	
Iganga	0.87 (0.65, 1.15)		0.77 (0.58, 1.03)	
Kamuli	0.92 (0.66, 1.28)		0.92 (0.66, 1.28)	
Mayuge	0.95 (0.7, 1.27)		0.95 (0.7, 1.28)	
Other	0.85 (0.55, 1.31)		0.77 (0.5, 1.19)	
Education level				
None/preprimary/other	1.00 (–)	0.587	1.00 (–)	0.400
Higher education	0.89 (0.5, 1.58)		0.73 (0.39, 1.38)	
Some secondary	0.91 (0.67, 1.25)		0.81 (0.58, 1.12)	
Some primary	1.07 (0.82, 1.39)		0.97 (0.74, 1.28)	
Gender				
Female	1.00 (–)	<0.001	1.00 (–)	<0.001
Male	1.62 (1.34, 1.96)		1.6 (1.3, 1.97)	
Occupation				
Peasant	1.00 (–)	0.136	1.00 (–)	0.065
Casual laborer	1.24 (0.9, 1.72)		1.13 (0.81, 1.58)	
None	1.32 (1.02, 1.71)		1.34 (1.02, 1.74)	
Other	1.15 (0.83, 1.6)		1.13 (0.8, 1.58)	
Paid employee	1.01 (0.7, 1.45)		0.92 (0.61, 1.39)	
Vendor/business person	0.86 (0.63, 1.17)		0.79 (0.57, 1.08)	
Year of ART initiation	1.39 (1.29, 1.51)	<0.001	1.32 (1.2, 1.46)	<0.001

CI 1.08–1.76) or atypical ARV regimens (AHR = 1.41; 95 % CI 1.00–1.99) also had an increased hazard of mortality/LTFU in comparison to those who began therapy with Nevirapine, Zidovudine and Lamivudine. As well, the year of ART initiation (AHR = 1.32 per year; 95 % CI 1.20–1.46) was significantly associated with mortality/LTFU. Notably, residence in any of the areas outside of Jinja district, again was not associated with mortality/LTFU in this analysis (p value = 0.562) in comparison to those who resided in Jinja.

We conducted HIV viral load testing on 870 clients of TASO Jinja who had been on ART for more than 4 years and presented for care between June 2012 and August 2013. Of these, we could link 805 (92.5 %) to the electronic database records. These individuals had been receiving ART for a median of 7.0 (IQR 5.0–8.0) years.

The similarities and differences in this sample in comparison to the entire TASO-Jinja cohort are presented in Table 2. Note that this sample included six participants who were identified as having transferred out and two who were considered LTFU. The sample had more female participants (77 vs. 69.2 %; $p < 0.001$) had higher CD4 cell counts at enrollment (97 vs. 69 %; $p < 0.001$) (74.7 % female vs 69.4 %; $p < 0.001$) (Table 3).

Of these individuals, 753 (87 %) of the patients had > 90 % adherence to therapy based on self-report of missed doses. A total of 756 (87 %) participants had VLs < 50 copies/mL and 809 (93 %) had VLs <1000 copies/ml. Table 4 shows the bivariate analysis of factors associated with virologic failure, defined as a VL ≥1000 copies/mL. Patients with VLs ≥1000 copies/mL were likely to be older than those with VLs <1000 copies/mL (median 45 Vs 42 years; $p < 0.003$). A lower proportion of women had virologic failure (67 vs 77 %), but this was only marginally significant ($p = 0.083$). Those with VLs ≥1000 copies/mL had lower CD4 cell counts at the time of VL testing (median 253 cells/μL) than those with VLs <1000 copies/mL (575 cells/μL; $p < 0.001$). We found a significant association between virologic failure meeting the CD4 cell count criteria treatment failure as defined by WHO ($p < 0.001$). Those with virologic failure were also younger than those without (median age 42 vs. 45 years; $p < 0.001$). There were no significant associations between virologic failure with regimen type, education level, or occupation in the bivariate analysis. Logistic regression analysis revealed that the most recent CD4 cell count [adjusted odds ratio (AOR) = 0.51 per 100 cells/μl; 95 % CI 0.43–0.60] and age (AOR = 0.96 per year; 95 % CI 0.92–0.99) were significantly associated with virologic failure as shown in Table 4. We also found that participants whose initial ART regimen was Nevirapine/Stavudine/Lamivudine had an increased odds of virologic failure (AOR = 1.38; 95 % CI 1.08–1.76) in comparison to those who started with Nevirapine/Zidovudine/Lamivudine (reference category).

Discussion

This study of over 3000 participants in the TASO ART Program in Jinja, Uganda demonstrated that more than 69 % of patients who initiated ART from 2004 to 2009 were retained in care after more than 5 years of treatment. This finding demonstrates that high retention rates are possible even in rural, resource-limited settings, particularly when programs are designed to be client-centered. Not only was retention in care quite high only 9 % of participants became LTFU and mortality was relatively low at 17 % and among those retained in care 93 %, had a VL result of <1000 copies/mL, even without access to VL testing for ART monitoring. While some programs have reported similar rates of retention [3, 17, 21, 23, 25, 26, 27, 28], they most often have been reported with study populations with shorter duration of follow-up (17, 21 22, 23, 25, 26] often in the range of 2 years after ART initiation [1, 16, 20], as opposed to the median of 5 years of follow-up in our study. For example, Assefa et al., in the study of outcomes of the ART services in the 55 health facilities in Ethiopia, reported an average 68 % (95 % CI 51–85) of patients retained in care after 2 years of follow-up [1]. The program at TASO, therefore, has retention figures which are among the better performing programs in the region even over longer follow-up periods.

We also found that, the risk for mortality and LTFU did not differ based on the geographic residence of program participants. This suggests that community-based distribution systems in use at TASO has effectively mitigated the time and cost constraints associated with transportation to ART clinic sites which have been demonstrated as barrier to retaining ART patients in care [3, 7, 31].

Among those retained in care and receiving first-line ART, we found a very low prevalence of virologic failure and very few with detectable VL measurements (i.e. ≥50 copies/mL) even in the absence of VL monitoring. While the new WHO 2013 guidelines for the use of ART in resource-limited settings recommend the use of VL testing, it is important to note that ART programs with only routine CD4 testing and good adherence strategies can achieve excellent outcomes and high rates of virologic suppression, even in the absence of such testing. However, it also appears that even the use of these clinical tools available at TASO have not been completely optimized since, we found 44 individuals (5 %) in our sub-study of virologic failure who met criteria for immunologic failure and whom had not yet been switched to second-line therapy. The fact that only 19 of the 44 were found to have VLs ≥1000 copies/mL, suggests confirming virologic failure amongst individuals who meet clinical or immunologic criteria for failure may be a more useful role for VL testing than screening large numbers of participants who are clinically well.

While our mortality rate was fairly low (3.22 per 100 person-years), in comparison to other studies in Africa reporting 5.1 per 100 person-years [6–9, 14] previous studies have shown that underreporting of mortality due to LTFU can bias the reporting of mortality, [20, 22]. However, as LTFU in our study was also low, this does not appear to be the explanation for this observation in our study. Of course, since most mortality on ART occurs within the first few months of initiation, it is also expected that studies with longer follow-up time will also yield lower mortality rates [15, 22, 31].

The rate of LTFU of 1.59 per 100 person-years in our cohort is comparable to that observed in the South Africa

Table 2 Comparison of participants in viral load sub-study in 2012 -13 with other participants in Jinja Cohort

Variable	Total N	Participants in VL sub-study				p value
		No (N = 2540)		Yes (N = 805)		
		N	(%)	N	(%)	
Clinical outcomes	3345					<0.001
Survived and retained in care		1525	(60)	797	(99)	
Dead		577	(23)	0	(0)	
Lost to follow-up		283	(11)	2	(0)	
Transferred out		155	(6)	6	(1)	
Gender	3345					<0.001
Female		1757	(69)	623	(77)	
Male		783	(31)	182	(23)	
CD4 at ART initiation	3099					<0.001
<50		429	(18)	55	(7)	
50–199		958	(42)	278	(35)	
≥200		915	(40)	464	(58)	
Hemoglobin count of participant at ARV initiation or clinical visit	2222					0.025
<8		71	(4)	13	(2)	
≥8		1574	(96)	564	(98)	
WHO stage	2829					0.749
Stage 1		40	(2)	10	(1)	
Stage 2		992	(47)	359	(49)	
Stage 3		913	(44)	318	(43)	
Stage 4		147	(7)	50	(7)	
Occupation	2920					0.384
Casual labourer		202	(9)	59	(9)	
Paid employee		187	(8)	48	(7)	
Peasant		940	(41)	268	(41)	
Vendor/business person		321	(14)	98	15)	
Other		246	(11)	61	(9)	
None		401	(17)	89	(14)	
Education level	2920					0.092
None/preprimary/other		382	(17)	100	(16)	
Some primary		1294	(56)	324	(52)	
Some secondary		545	(24)	174	(28)	
Higher education		75	(3)	26	(4)	
First ARV regimen	3076					0.003
Efavirenz/Zidovudine/Lamivudine		233	(10)	90	(11)	
Efavirenz/Stavudine/Lamivudine		136	(10)	64	(8)	
Nevirapine/Stavudine/Lamivudine		688	(30)	262	(33)	
Nevirapine/Zidovudine/Lamivudine		1034	(45)	327	(42)	
Other ARV regimen		198	(7)	44	(6)	
Year of ART initiation	3345	2006	(2006–2008)	2006	(2005–2007)	<0.001

N = 3345 Jinja cohort participants

studies [17], but relatively lower as compared to the rate observed in Western Kenya which found, 5.1 per 100 person-years of observation [31]. The careful design and scale up of ART in TASO may have contributed to the observed LTFU. This program has grown in size dramatically, with our cohort increasing enrolment about 3-fold from 2004 to 2013.

These findings could be limited because death was ascertained by patient record review. Consequently, deaths, which occurred at home, might have not been

Table 3 Bivariate analysis of 870 participants with and without viral load <1000 copies/ml

Variable	Total N	Viral load result (copies/mL)				p value
		<1000 (N = 809)		≥1000 (N = 61)		
		N	(%)	N	(%)	
Gender	870					0.083
Female		623	(77)	41	(67)	
Male		186	(23)	20	(33)	
Most important source of income	870					0.399
Agricultural farming		254	(31)	16	(26)	
Wage or salaried employment		93	(11)	8	(13)	
Crafts and trade work		54	(7)	2	(3)	
Petty trade in kiosks stalls and hawking		198	(24)	22	(36)	
None		77	(10)	5	(8)	
Other		133	(16)	8	(13)	
Education level	869					0.127
No education (including do not know)		173	(21)	8	(13)	
Some/completed primary		357	(44)	25	(41)	
Some/completed high school/higher education		278	(34)	28	(46)	
Current marital status	870					0.186
Single/separated/divorced/widowed		481	(59)	31	(51)	
Legally married/co habiting		328	(41)	30	(49)	
Any evidence of CD4 cell count treatment failure?	867					<0.001
No		781	(97)	42	(69)	
Yes		25	(3)	19	(31)	
Current ARV regimen (first regimen)	870					0.084
Nevirapine		626	(77)	53	(87)	
Efavirenz		183	(23)	8	(13)	
Current ARV regimen (second regimen)	870					0.417
3TC/ZDV		744	(92)	54	(89)	
FTC/TDF		1	(0)	0	(0)	
3TC/TDF		63	(8)	7	(11)	
3TC/ABC		1	(0)	0	(0)	
Frequency taking ARV pills	869					0.826
Never		517	(64)	37	(61)	
Once a week		54	(7)	5	(8)	
More than once a week but less than a month		54	(7)	3	(5)	
More than a month		183	(23)	16	(26)	
Adherence (frequency missing ARV pills)	869					0.956
Never or more than a month		700	(87)	53	(87)	
Once a week or more than once a week but less than a month		108	(13)	8	(13)	
Alcohol within previous month	870					0.903
No		739	(91)	56	(92)	
Yes		70	(9)	5	(8)	
Age at time of VL test	870	45	(40–50)	42	(37–45)	0.003
Most recent CD4 cell count (cells/mm^3)	867	575	(445–757)	253	(118–426)	<0.001
Duration on ART (years)	870	7	(6–8)	7	(5–8)	0.775

N = 870

documented in the patient card. This may underestimate the rate of mortality. For this reason we combined LTFU with mortality as our outcome. As the data we used for this analysis was routinely collected and entered by clinicians as part of providing clinical care, it lacks some accuracy and was not complete. This may underestimate

Table 4 Univariate and multivariate logistic regression analysis of factors associated with virologic failure

	Univariate		Multivariate	
	OR (95 % CI)	p value	OR (95 % CI)	p value
Gender		0.081		
Female	1.00 (–)			
Male	1.65 (0.94, 2.89)			
Education level		0.101		0.132
No education (including do not know)	1.00 (–)		1.00 (–)	
Some/completed Primary	1.47 (0.65, 3.34)		1.51 (0.61, 3.72)	
Some/completed high school/higher education	2.25 (1, 5.04)		2.34 (0.95, 5.76)	
Current marital status		0.265		
Single/separated/divorced/widowed	1.00 (–)			
Legally married/co habiting	1.35 (0.8, 2.28)			
Current ARV regimen (first regimen)		0.091		
Nevirapine	1.00 (–)			
Efavirenz	0.52 (0.24, 1.11)			
Age (in years)	0.95 (0.91, 0.98)	0.003	0.96 (0.92, 0.99)	0.020
Number of child dependents	0.95 (0.88, 1.02)	0.174		
Most recent CD4 cell count (per 100 cells/μl)	0.50 (0.42, 0.59)	<0.001	0.51 (0.43, 0.6)	<0.001

or overestimate some outcome of interest. As well some variables were extensively missing and we could not include them in multivariate analyses. As well, there is some possibility of misclassification as we observed six patients in the virologic failure sub-study who were classified as having transferred out of the program and two other participants in the sub-study met our criteria of LTFU, despite being in care.

Conclusion

Among participants enrolled in an ART program for a median of over 5 years, rates of mortality and LTFU were very low and did not differ based on the geographic residence of program participants. This demonstrates that community-based distribution systems can effectively mitigate the time and cost constraints associated with transportation to ART clinic sites. As well, ART programs which only routine CD4 testing and good adherence strategies can expect good clinical and virologic outcomes.

Methods

Study design

We conducted a retrospective cohort analysis of all patients >18 years old who initiated ART at the TASO service clinic in Jinja. Jinja clinic is one of the eleven TASO ART clinics in Uganda which serves clients within a radius of 75 km. Between January 2004 and July 2009 the CD4 count cut off point for ART eligibility increased from 200 to 250 cell/ml. The AIDS Support Organization (TASO) has the largest non-governmental ART program in the country with more than 80,000 individuals accessing care and over 65,000 individuals receiving ART through 11 service centers, the ART program has been designed to accommodate the needs of clients since its inception. This has been operationalized in terms of providing clients with much more than just clinic visits and medications. Several types of program delivery models have been implemented and revised over the past 10 years at TASO, including home-based care [11, 30] the use of satellite clinics, community drug distribution [29], as well as more conventional clinic-based approaches. In TASO, patients who are initiated on ART after 6 months of ART treatment are evaluated by clinicians and counselors for down referred to Community Drug Distribution Point (CDDP). A CDDP is a small group of 20–50 patients who have been on ART for at least 6 months, are stable clinically, have disclosed their sero-status to a friend or relative and have consented to down referral to the community for continued ART refill, monitoring by lay workers. The patients themselves identify a place within their community where they converge to receive their refills, ART reviews and evaluation by TASO counselors (lay workers) and six monthly reviews by TASO clinical staff. The group elects a leader who is an expert client who then mobilizes and follows up all the patients in his/her group for adherence and other counseling issues, he is also responsible for up referral of the patients to the facility in case of any illness or suspected medication side effect. In the CDDP, Drug refills are conducted every 2 to 3 months, with clinical assessments conducted at the time of drug refills by health professionals and CD4 cell counts performed every 6 months by laboratory technician. No routine VL monitoring is performed as part of this program. For community-based drug distribution, ART is provided at the community by trained lay workers, who are mostly social workers and teachers supervised by Clinical Services Supervisor.

Data collection

In June of 2013, we used the clinical database of TASO Jinja, to extract clinical data at enrollment and subsequent visits, the data collected included WHO stage, baseline CD4, CD4 at subsequent visits, HB, distance to the service centre, ART start date and regimen, as well as basic socio-demographic information. The database also records information on known deaths and patients who have transferred out of the program. When necessary, patient charts in use at TASO Jinja were used to supplement the information found in the clinical database. Individual consent was not obtained from the study participants but the patient records were anonymized and de-identified prior to analysis. Additionally, between August 2012 and May 2013, we obtained funding to conduct viral load (VL) tests for clients who attended the clinic or outreach site and who had been on ART for at least 4 years, while still on a first-line ART regimen. The Participants in this component of the study did provide individual written informed consent. The study protocol and consent forms were approved by the Research Ethics Board of the University of British Columbia, the TASO Research Ethics Committee, the Uganda Virus Research Institute and the Uganda National Council for Science and Technology.

Data analysis

Retention in care was defined by a record of at least one clinic visit in the 6 months before June 1, 2013. We included factors that determined retention and mortality among adults enrolled in HIV service delivery models and conducted bivariate analyse using Kruskal–Wallis and Chi square tests using STATA version 16 to compare clients who remained active program clients throughout the study period, with those who are known to have died or who were LTFU. We used Cox Proportional Hazards Modeling to determine factors associated with the combined outcome of mortality and LTFU, given that the bivariate analysis suggested more similarities between participants in these categories than with those retained in care or transferred out. District of residence was our primary explanatory variables of interest, but we examined other important co-factors, such as CD4 counts at treatment initiation, gender, ethnicity, and other variables for potential inclusion in explanatory models. For the analysis of virologic failure, we calculated the proportion of individuals with virologic failure defined as ≥ 1000 copies/mL. We then conducted a bivariate analysis with participants classified on the basis of presence or absence of viral failure (defined as a VL of ≥ 1000 copies/mL) and examined factors independently associated with virologic failure using multivariate logistic regression.

Abbreviations

TASO: the AIDS Support Organization; CDDP: community drug distribution point; LTFU: lost to follow up.

Authors' contributions

DMM, SP, and SO, designed the study. SO, JW and JB supervised data collection of the study. AE, CB, MN, DK, and, SP collected the data. SS, DE, AE, SO and DMM, conducted or contributed to the data analysis. ED, AE, SS, SO and DMM interpreted the data. SO prepared the original manuscript, PK, PM and DMM contributed to subsequent revisions. All authors read and approved the final manuscript.

Author details

[1] Mulago Hospital Complex, The AIDS Support Organization (TASO), P.O BOX 10443, Kampala, Uganda. [2] The BC Centre for Excellence in HIV/AIDS, Vancouver, Canada. [3] Faculty of Medicine, University of British Columbia, Vancouver, Canada. [4] MRC/UVRI Uganda Research Unit on AIDS, Entebbe, Uganda.

Acknowledgements

We are grateful to The AIDS Support Organization (TASO) for accepting us to access participants' data for this study as per organizational data access policy. We acknowledge the valuable support received from Moore M David inform of mentorship and the Executive Director TASO Dr. Etukoit Bernard for supporting this study including ploughing back the findings into programming. This study was not funded therefore; no body received salary from this study.

Competing interests

The authors declare that they have no competing interests.

References

1. Gill CJ, Hamer D, Simon JL, Thea DM, Sabin L. No room for complacency about adherence to antiretroviral therapy in sub-Saharan Africa. AIDS. 2005;19:1243–9.
2. Lawn SD, Myer L, Orrell C, Bekker LG. Wood R Early mortality among adults accessing a community-based antiretroviral service in South Africa: implications for programme design. AIDS. 2005;19:2141–8.
3. Wester CW, Kim S, Bussmann H, Avalos A, Ndwapi N, et al. Initial response to highly active antiretroviral therapy in HIV-1C-infected adults in a public sector treatment program in Botswana. J Acquir Immune DeficSyndr. 2005;40:336–43.
4. Mills EJ, Nachega JB, Buchan I, Orbinski J, Attaran A, et al. Adherence to antiretroviral therapy in sub-Saharan Africa and North America: a meta-analysis. JAMA. 2006;296:679–90.
5. Akileswaran C, Lurie MN, Flanigan TP. Mayer KH Lessons learned from use of highly active antiretroviral therapy in Africa. Clin Infect Dis. 2005;41:376–85.
6. Rasschaert Freya, Telfer Barbara, Lessitala Faustino, Decroo Tom, Remartinez Daniel, Biot Marc, BaltazarCandrinho Francisco Mbofana, Van Damme Wim. A qualitative assessment of a community antiretroviral-therapy group model in tete. PLOS: Mozambique; 2014.
7. Geng E, Bangsberg D, Musinguzi N, Emenyonu N, Bwana MB, Yiannoutsos C, Glidden D, Deeks SG, Martin J. Understanding reasons for and

outcomes of patients lost to follow-up in antiretroviral therapy programs in africa through a sampling-based approach. JAIDS. 2010;53:405–11.

8. Koole O1, Tsui S, Wabwire-Mangen F, Kwesigabo G, Menten J, Mulenga M, Auld A, et al. Retention and risk factors for attrition among adults in antiretroviral treatment programmes in Tanzania, Uganda and Zambia. Trop Med Int Health. 2014;19(12):1397–1410.
9. Kwong-Leung Yu J, Chih-Cheng S, Kuo-Yang W, Chao-Sung C, Makombe S, Schouten E, Harries A. True Outcomes for patients on antiretroviral therapy who are "lost to follow-up" in Malawi.Bulletin of the World Health Organization. 2007:85:550–554.
10. Dabis Francois, Balestre Eric, Braitstein Paula, Paolo Miotti WG, Brinkhof Martin, Schneider Martin, et al. Cohort Profile: antiretroviral therapy in lower income countries (ART-LINC): international collaboration of treatment cohorts The antiretroviral therapy in lower income countries (ART-LINC) Study Group. Int J Epidemiol. 2005;34:979–86.
11. Amuron B, Levin J, Birunghi J, Namara G, Coutinho A, Grosskurth H, Jaffar S. Mortality in an antiretroviral therapy programme in Jinja, south-east Uganda: a prospective cohort study. AIDS Research and Therapy 2011;8(1):39 **(1186/1742-6405-8-39)**.
12. Hosseinipour MC, Neuhann FH, Kanyama CC, Namarika DC, Weigel R, et al. Lessons learned from a paying antiretroviral therapy service inthe public health sector at kamuzu central hospital, Malawi: 1-year experience. J Int Assoc Physicians AIDS Care. 2006;5:103–8.
13. Stringer JS, Zulu I, Levy J, Stringer EM, Mwango A, et al. Rapid scale up of antiretroviral therapy at primary care sites in Zambia: feasibility and early outcomes. JAMA. 2006;296:782–93.
14. Kwong-Leung Yu J, Chih-Cheng Chen S, Wang K, Chang C, Makombe S, et al. True outcomes for patients on antiretroviral therapy who are "lost to follow-up" in Malawi. Bull World Health Organ. 2007;85:550–554.
15. Tomori C, Kennedy CE, Brahmbhatt H, Wagman JA, Mbwambo JK, Likindikoki S, Kerrigan DL. Barriers and facilitators of retention in HIV care and treatment services in Iringa, Tanzania: the importance of socioeconomic and socio cultural factors. AIDS Care. 2013;26:907–13.
16. Hardon AP, Akurut D, Comoro C, Ekezie C, Irunde HF, et al. Hunger, waiting time and transport costs: time to confront challenges to ART adherence in Africa. AIDS Care. 2007;19:658–65.
17. Grimsrud A, Balkan S, Casas EC, Lujan J, Van Cutsem G, Poulet E, Myer L, Pujades-Rodriguez. Outcomes of antiretroviral therapy over a 10-year period of expansion: a multicohort analysis of African and Asian HIV programmes. Acquir Immune DeficSyndr 2014.
18. Mutasa-Apollo T, Shiraishi RW, Takarinda KC, Dzangare J, Mugurungi O, Murungu J, Abdul-Quader A, Woodfill CJ. Patient retention, clinical outcomes and attrition-associated factors of HIV-infected patients enrolled in Zimbabwe's National Antiretroviral Therapy Programme, 2007–2010. PLoS One. 2014.
19. Lawn SD, Myer L, Harling G, Orrell C, Bekker LG, et al. Determinants of mortality and non death losses from an antiretroviral treatment service in South Africa: implications for program evaluation. Clin Infect Dis. 2006;43:770–6.
20. Morgan D, Mahe C, Mayanja B, Okongo JM, Lubega R, et al. HIV-1 infection in rural Africa: is there a difference in median time to AIDS and survival compared with that in industrialized countries? AIDS. 2002;16:597–603.
21. Lawn SD. Wood R How can earlier entry of patients into antiretroviral programs in low-income countries be promoted? Clin Infect Dis. 2006;42:431–2.
22. Rasschaert F, Decroo T, Remartinez D, Telfer B, Lessitala F, Van Biot M, Damme W. Adapting a community-based ART delivery model to the patients' needs: a mixed methods research in Tete Mozambique. BMC Public Health. 2014;364:1471–2458.
23. Bisson G, Ndwapi N, Rollins C, Avalos A, Gross R, et al. High rates of death among patients lost to follow-up in Botswana's national ART program: implications for monitoring and evaluation, 2007.
24. Bisson GP, Frank I, Gross R, Lo Re V, Strom JB, et al. 3rdOut-of pocket costs of HAART limit HIV treatment responses in Botswana's private sector. AIDS. 2006;20:1333–6.
25. Laurent C, Meilo H, Guiard-Schmid JB, Mapoure Y, Noel JM, et al. Antiretroviral therapy in public and private routine health care clinics in Cameroon: lessons from the Douala antiretroviral (DARVIR) initiative. Clin Infect Dis. 2005;41:108–11.
26. Guiard-Schmid JB, Montagut B, Ribadeau-Dumas F, EdooEdoo G, MakongS, et al. TRICAM: Medico-economic pilot study on HAART for HIV infected-patients in a private company of Cameroon]. 15th International AIDS Conference; 2004 11–16 July; Bangkok, Thailand. 2004: Abstract MoOrD1024.
27. Mosoko JJ, Akam W, Weidle PJ, Brooks J, Aweh A, et al. Survival and adherence to ART in an era of decreasing drug cost in Limbe, Cameroon 14th Conference on Retroviruses and Opportunistic Infections (CROI); Los Angeles, California. 2007: Abstract 536.
28. Kenfak A, Tsague L, Koulla-Shiro S, Tejioken M, Kouanfack C, et al. Challenges in assessing adherence to antiretroviral treatment in low resources settings and impacts on national antiretroviral policy: results of a retrospective multi centric cohort study in Cameroon 16thInternational AIDS Conference; 2007: August 14–18; Toronto, Canada. Abstract CDB0765.
29. Decroo T, Koole O, Remartinez D, dos Santos N, Dezembro S S, Jofrisse M, Rasschaert F, Biot M. Laga. Four-year retention and risk factors for attrition among members of community ART groups in Tete, Mozambique. M. Trop Med Int Health. 2014;19(5):514–21.
30. Jain V, Byonanebye DM, Amanyire G, Kwarisiima D, Black D, Kabami J, Chamie G, etal. Successful antiretroviral therapy delivery and retention in care among asymptomatic individuals with high CD4+ T-cell counts at least 350 cells/μL in Rural Uganda.; the SEARCH Collaboration. AIDS 2014.
31. Ostermann J, Whetten K, Reddy E, Pence B, Weinhold A, Itemba D, Maro V, Mosille E, Thielman N. Treatment retention and care transitions during and after the scale-up of HIV care and treatment in Northern Tanzania. CHAT Research Team. AIDS Care. 2014;11:1352–8.

22

Impact of highly active antiretroviral therapy on hematological indices among HIV-1 infected children

Elizabeth Gathoni Kibaru[1,4*], Ruth Nduati[2], Dalton Wamalwa[2] and Nyambura Kariuki[2,3]

Abstract

Background: HIV infected children experience a range of hematological complications which show marked improvement within 6 months of initiating anti-retroviral therapy. The Objectives of the study was to describe the changes in hematological indices of HIV-1 infected children following 6 months of treatment with first line antiretroviral drugs (ARVs) regimen.

Methods: A retrospective study was conducted between September and November 2008. During this period medical records of children attending Comprehensive Care Clinic at Kenyatta National hospital were reviewed daily. HIV infected children aged 5–144 months were enrolled if they had received antiretroviral drugs for at least 6 months with available and complete laboratory results.

Results: Medical records of 337 children meeting enrollment criteria were included in the study. The median age was 63 months with equal male to female ratio. Following 6 months of HAART, prevalence of anemia (Hemoglobin (Hb) <10 g/dl) declined significantly from 35.9 to 16.6 % a nearly 50 % reduction in the risk of anemia RR = 0.56 [(95 % CI 0.44, 0.70) p < 0.001]. There was significant increase in Hb, mean corpuscular volume (MCV), mean corpuscular hemoglobin (MCH) and platelets above the baseline measurements (p < 0.0001) and a significant decline in total white blood cell counts >11,000 cell/mm^3 but a none significant decrease in red blood cells (RBC). Pre-HAART, World Health Organization (WHO) stage 3 and 4 was associated with a ten-fold increased likelihood of anemia. Chronic malnutrition was associated with anemia but not wasting and immunologic staging of disease.

Conclusion: Hematological abnormalities changed significantly within 6 months of antiretroviral therapy with significant increase in hemoglobin level, MCV, MCH and platelet and decrease in WBC and RBC.

Keywords: Paediatric HIV infection, Hematological abnormalities, Changes of hematological parameters

Background

Hematological complications of human deficiency virus infection (HIV) which include cytopenias of all major cell lines were recognized shortly after the first description of AIDS cases [1]. Unexplained anemia defined as hemoglobin of less than 8 g/dl, neutropenia <1000 cells/mm^3 or thrombocytopenia less than 30,000 platelets/mm^3 persisting for more than one month are currently classified as WHO stage 3 disease [2]. Anemia, the most common abnormality causes chronic fatigue, affects cognitive function and influences the choice of ART and opportunistic infection (OI) medications and has been noted to be the commonest hematological abnormalities in adults in Kenya [3, 4].

In published literature prevalence of anemia among HIV-1 infected children varies from 16 to 94 % and this increases with advancing stage of HIV disease but varies with sex, age and the definition of anemia used [5–10].

*Correspondence: gathonigakinya@yahoo.com
[4] P.O. Box 2275-20100, Nakuru, Kenya

In a meta-analysis of over 2000 HIV infected children, the prevalence of mild [hemoglobin (Hb) 10–12.0] and moderate anemia (Hb 8.0–9.9) was 22–94 % and 3–82 % respectively [10]. The prevalence of mild and moderate anemia in Western settings ranged from 22 to 94 % and 11 to 82 % respectively while in tropical settings it was 50–91 % for mild anemia and 3–38 % for moderate anemia [10]. Neutropenia is present in approximately 10 % of patients with early, asymptomatic HIV infection, and more than half in individuals with more advanced HIV-related immunodeficiency [5, 6, 11]. Thrombocytopenia which is frequently asymptomatic occurs in 20 % to 33 % of paediatric patients with HIV with the prevalence increasing with duration of illness and development of Aids [5, 6, 9, 11, 12].

The most important cause of anemia in HIV infected children is insufficient production of erythrocytes caused by ineffective erythropoiesis, reduced erythropoietin production, associated infections, neoplasia, medications and micronutrient deficiencies. Iron deficiency is the most common cause of nutritional anemia globally. There is significant geographical overlap of areas of the world where iron deficiency anemia (IDA) and paediatric HIV are distributed. The causes of anemia in the community investigated are Multifactorial with iron deficiency prevalence being high due to nutritional deficiency and helminthes. In a study in western Kenya by Footer et al. anemia was found to be prevalent and was present in 71.8 % of children [13]. Factors commonly thought to be associated with anemia were found to be widespread, including malaria parasitemia (32.5 %), iron deficiency (34.6 %), vitamin A deficiency (16.3 %), stunting (29.6 %), wasting (3.3 %), HbS (17.1 %), HbSS (1.6 %), heterozygous α-thalassemia (38.5 %), and homozygous α-thalassemia (9.6 %) [13]. This is similar to WHO finding that Iron deficiency is the most common cause of anemia of micronutrient-related etiology worldwide, affecting about 50 % of women and children in developing countries and about 25 % of men [14]. Another prominent cause of reduced production of all hematological elements in patients with HIV infection is the common use of multiple medications, many of which may cause marrow suppression e.g. Zidovudine (AZT) and other nucleoside analogues can cause a dose-dependent neutropenia [15]. Other medications causing hematological abnormalities include ganciclovir, trimethoprim-sulphamethoxazole, pentamidine and dapsone [9].

Studies have confirmed the ability of HAART to correct or improve the anemia and other hematological parameters of HIV infection. In a study of 6725 HIV-infected patients from across Europe, Microft and colleagues found that the use of Stavudine, zidovudine and Lamivudine was statistically associated with improvement in hemoglobin levels [16]. When used for longer periods of time, HAART was associated with greater likelihood of correcting anemia. Microft et al. found that, 65.5 % of patients were anemic before the use of HAART, 53 % were anemic after 6 months of HAART ($p < 0.0001$), and 46 % were anemic after 12 months of HAART [16]. Huang et al. found an increase in Hb occurring with mean increase from baseline of 13.9 to 14.1 g/dl after 3 months of treatment and this was not statistically significant [17]. After 6 months Hb had increased to 14.6 g/dl ($p < 0.01$), 9 months 14.6 g/dl ($p = 0.001$) and at 12 months mean of 14.3 g/dl ($p < 0.01$) [17]. In a different study in children in Zambia, the mean hemoglobin increased from 10.3 g/dl at baseline to a mean of 11.3 g/dl (CI 95 % 11.2–11.4 g/dl) after 6 months of HAART [18]. In a study in Burkina-Faso hematological changes after 6 months of AZT based HAART showed anemia at 51.4 vs 80.3 % at baseline with $P = 0.0001$ [19]. Other hematological parameter noted to markedly increase after HAART was MCV. Huang et al. found an increase of MCV following treatment from baseline of 5.5 to 98.9 fl $p < 0.1$ at 3 months, 105.5 fl ($p < 0.001$) at 6 months, 106 fl at 9 months ($p < 0.001$) and 102.8 fl $p < 0.001$ at 12 months [17].

The prevalence of hematological abnormalities among children treated with ART in routine care settings in Kenya have not yet been described even though the first line antiretroviral regimen to date includes drugs with significant hematological adverse events such as zidovudine. The objective of the study was to describe the changes in hemoglobin levels, red cell morphology, white blood cells and platelets in HIV-1 infected children aged 5–144 months following 6 months of highly active antiretroviral therapy at the comprehensive care clinic of KNH.

Results

Baseline characteristics of the study participants

A total of 337 children were recruited into the study, among them 53.4 % female and 46.6 % male giving a female to male ratio of 1.1:1, and a median age of 63 months (range of 5–144 months) as shown in the Table 1. Almost all children in the study population received Cotrimoxazole 323 (98.8 %) and the remaining 4 (1.2 %) received dapsone. One eighty nine (56.4 %) presented in WHO clinical stage III at ART initiation while 48 (14.3 %) were in WHO clinical stage IV. The number/proportion of children in stages I and II were 77 (23 %) and 21(6.3 %) respectively. Eighty four children (25 %) were started on iron supplements during the initiation of antiretroviral drugs. Zidovudine-Lamivudine backbone (AZT/3TC) based regimens were the most frequently used first line ART protocol and used by 291 (86.3 %) children in combination with efavirenz (EFV), nevirapine (NVP) or abacavir (ABC).

Table 1 Baseline demographic characteristics of the study participants

Variable	Frequency (n = 337) number, (%), or median
Female	179 (53.4 %)
Male	156 (46.6 %)
Age (months)	
Median	63
IQR	36–97
Weight for age Z score	
SD > −2	130 (39 %)
SD −3 to −2	95 (28 %)
SD < −3	112 (33 %)
Weight for height Z score	
SD > −2	229 (88 %)
SD −3 to −2	22 (6.5 %)
SD < −3	15 (4.4 %)
Height for age Z score	
SD > −2	85 (25 %)
SD −3 to −2	53 (16 %)
SD < −3	198 (59 %)
CD4 count median (1QR)	456 (171.0–753)
CD4 percent median (1QR)	9.9 (5.0–14.0)

Hematological parameters pre and six months post HAART initiation

Hemoglobin level

At baseline 35.9 % study participants had a Hb <10.0 g/dl compared to 16.6 % after 6 months of ART, a statistically significant reduction in risk of anemia RR = 0.56 [(95 % CI 0.44, 077) p < 0.0001] as shown in Table 2. The median Hb at baseline was 10.6 and 11.5 g/dl before and after 6 months of ART, a significant median increase in Hb of 0.9 g/dl (p < 0.0001) as shown in Table 3. The median Hb level of 203 (75 %) children who were not on iron supplements at baseline and after 6 months of ART was 11 g/dl, and 11.8 g/dl respectively a statistical significant change (p < 0.0001). Eighty four children (25 %) who were receiving iron supplements had a baseline median Hb of 9.25 g/dl and increased to 11 g/dl following 6 months of treatment, a significant median increase of Hb 1.75 g/dl (p < 0.0001). Female were reported to have higher hemoglobin levels at the baseline 51.9 % compared to the males 40.3 % although there were more males with moderate anemia (37 %) compared to female 23.1 %. Following 6 months of HAART majority of children of both sexes had hemoglobin levels within the normal ranges with 73.7 % being female and 68.5 % males. Children who initially were reported with severe anemia had reduced to 1.3 % from 4.5 % of female with no male reported to have severe anemia.

Mean corpuscular volume (MCV)

At baseline 31 % of the study participants had a mean corpuscular volume (MCV) below the 70 fl compared to 8.3 % at end of 6 months of ART treatment, a 63 % decline in the risk RR = 0.37 [(95 % CI 0.27,0.52) P < 0.0001] as shown in Table 2. The median corpuscular volume at baseline was 75.9 fl and increased to 89.2 fl after 6 months of HAART, a statistically significant median increase by 13.2 fl of corpuscular volume (p < 0.0001) as show in Table 3.

Table 2 Changes in the prevalence of abnormal haematological parameters

Characteristic N = 337	Baseline no (%)	6 months after initiation of HAART no (%)	Relative risk (95 % CI)	P value
Hb <10 g/dl	121 (35.9)	56 (16.6)	0.56 (0.44, 0.70)	<0.0001
MCV <70 fl	104 (31.0)	28 (8.3)	0.37 (0.27, 0.52)	<0.0001
MCH <24 pg	154 (46.7)	49 (14.6)	0.45 (0.35, 0.59)	<0.0001
Platelets <150,000	67 (20.0)	22 (6.5)	0.46 (0.32, 0.66)	<0.0001
WBC <11,000	33 (10.0)	21 (6.2)	0.76 (0.54, 1.08)	0.09
Granulocytes <1000	22 (6.5)	52 (16)	1.48 (1.25, 1.75)	<0.0001

Table 3 Changes in haemoglobin levels, MCV, MCH and RBC

Characteristic N = 337	Baseline median no (%) or (IQR)	6 months after initiation of HAART no (IQR)	Median change	P value
Hb (g/dl)	10.6 (9.4–11.6)	11.5 (10.5–12.4)	0.9	<0.0001
MCV (fl)	75.9 (68.0–82.3)	89.2 (80.0–97.6)	13.2	<0.0001
MCH (pg)	24.3 (21.5–27.5)	29.1 (25.8–32.1)	4.9	<0.0001
RBC (m/mm^3)	4.3 (3.8–5.0)	4.0 (3.6–4.3)	0.3	0.27

Table 4 Haemoglobin level changes and HAART combination

Drug regimen	Number	Mean Hb at baseline	Mean Hb after 6 months	Mean change	*P* Value
Zidovudine combination	293	10.7	11.4	0.7	0.000
Stavudine combination	38	9.77	11.6	1.83	0.01
Other combinations	6	7.68	11.2	3.52	0.864

Mean corpuscular hemoglobin (MCH)

The prevalence of low mean corpuscular hemoglobin (MCH) before and after 6 months of ARVs was 46.7 and 14.6 % respectively. The relative risk of low MCH was RR = 0.45 [(95 % CI 0.35, 0.59) $p < 0.0001$], a statistically significant reduction. At baseline median MCH was 24.3 pg and increased to 29.0 pg after 6 months of ART a statistically significant median increase of 4.9 pg ($p < 0.0001$) as shown in Table 3.

Red blood cells

At baseline the median number of red cells was 4.3 million/mm^3 and declined to 4.0 million/mm^3 after 6 months of highly active antiretroviral therapy. The median change in RBC was 0.4 million cells/mm^3 and this was not statistically significant ($p = 0.27$) as shown in Table 3.

HAART regimen combination and hemoglobin level

Children with Stavudine combination had higher hemoglobin increments as compared to zidovudine or other combinations as shown in Table 4. There was statistical significant increase in mean Hb level in both zidovudine and Stavudine combinations but the mean hemoglobin change was more with Stavudine combinations at 1.83 g/dl for Stavudine combination and 0.7 g/dl for zidovudine combinations. Indications of choice of regimen to use were based on baseline hemoglobin levels. Majority of children with Hb of above10 g/dl were started on zidovudine combination while Children with low Hb of less than 10 g/dl were started on Stavudine or other combinations.

Platelets

Proportion of children with platelet counts below 150,000/mm3 before and after 6 months of ARV was 20 and 6.5 % respectively, a significant reduction in the risk of thrombocytopenia RR = 0.46 [(95 % CI 0.32, 0.66) $p < 0.0001$] as shown in Table 3. At baseline the median platelets counts were 255 × 10^3/mm^3 (IQR 159 × 10^3/mm^3–352 × 10^3/mm^3), and which increased to a median of 279 × 10^3/mm^3 (IQR 224 × 10^3/mm^3–349 × 10^3/mm^3) following 6 months of ART as shown in Fig. 1.

White blood cells

Before ART initiation 10 % of the children had elevated white blood cell counts above 11,000 cell/mm^3 compared to 6.2 % after 6 months of ARV initiation. The proportion of children with elevated total WBC thus decreased with ART RR = 0.76 [(0.54, 1.08) P = 0.09] a non-significant decline. Overall the median total WBC count at baseline was 9.4 × 10^3/mm^3 which declined significantly to a median of 6.7 × 10^3 cells/mm^3 ($p < 0.0001$). At baseline only 6.5 % of the study participants had granulocyte counts of less than 1000 cells/mm^3 compared to 16 % after 6 months of ARVs, a statistically significant increased likelihood of having low granulocyte counts RR = 1.48 [(1.25, 1.75), $P < 0.0001$]. The total granulocyte count declined significantly following 6 months of ART from a median of 2.8 × 10^3/mm^3–2 × 10^3/mm^3 (IQR 1.4 × 10^3/mm^3–5.1 × 10^3/mm^3) ($p < 0.0001$) as shown in Table 5. The median lymphocyte count was of 5.2 × 10^3 cell/mm^3 before treatment initiation and declined significantly to 4.2 × 10^3 cell/mm^3, ($p < 0.0001$) following 6 months of ART.

Factors associated with low baseline hemoglobin level

In a stratified analysis the 216 (64.1 %) and 121 (35.9 %) children with Hb above and below 10 g/dl respectively were compared to determine demographic and clinical characteristics associated with anemia. Children in WHO stage 3 and 4 were more likely to have Hb of less than or equal to 10 g/dl compared to children in WHO stage 1 and 2 OR = 10.6 (95 % CI 3.64, 36.3) ($P < 0.001$). Children with WAZ greater than −2 SD had significantly reduced likelihood of having Hb of less than 10g/dl OR = 0.62 [(95 % CI 0.38, 1.01) P = 0.04] as shown in Table 6.

Discussion

In this study we report increase in most hematological indices following 6 months of ART in children. Following 6 months of treatment with HAART, hematological reconstitution occurred progressively for all blood lineages except RBC, total WBC, granulocytes and total lymphocytes counts. The positive effect of HAART is probably due to the reduction in viral load, decreased destruction of mature hematopoietic cells of multiple lineages and an improvement in the blunted erythropoietin response [11]. HAART could also have lead to decreased incidences of opportunistic infections [17].

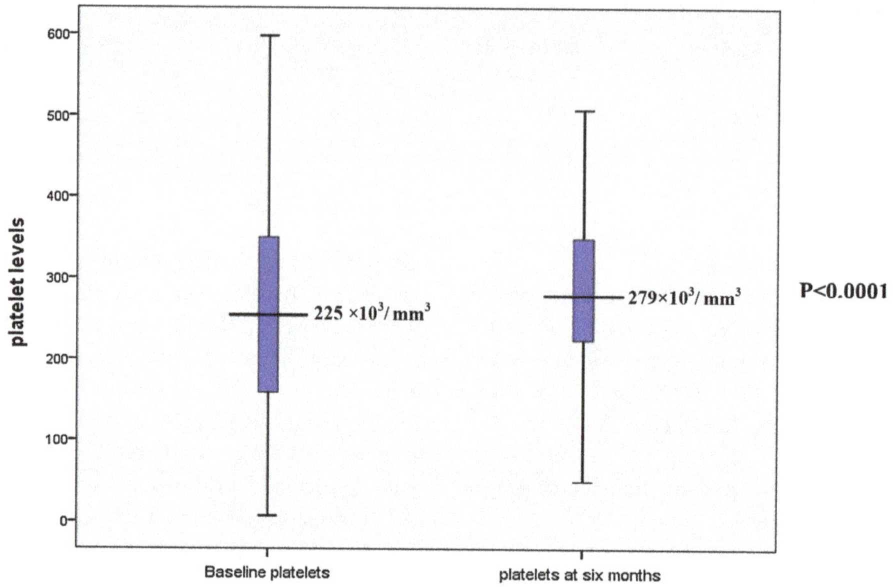

Fig. 1 Comparison of platelet levels at baseline and after 6 months of treatment

Table 5 Changes in WBC, Granulocytes and lymphocytes following six months of HAART

Characteristic N = 337	Baseline Median (IQR)	6 months after of HAART Median (IQR)	Median change	P value
WBC ($\times 10^3/mm^3$)	8.7 (IQR 6.2–11.5)	6.7 (IQR 5.2–8.5)	2.0	<0.0001
Granulocytes $\times 10^3/mm^3$	2.8 (IQR 1.8–4.3)	2.0 (IQR 1.4–2.9)	0.8	<0.0001
Lymphocytes $\times 10^3/mm^3$	4.8 (2.9–6.7)	4.2 (3.0–5.1)	0.6	<0.0001

Table 6 Correlates of low baseline haemoglobin level

	Hb ≥ 10 N = 216 (64.1 %)	Hb ≤10 N = 121 (35.9 %)		P value
CD4 (median)	9.0	10.8		0.2
WHO				<0.0001
Stage 1 and 2	76 (35.2 %)	4 (8.2 %)	1	
Stage 3 and 4	140 (64.8 %)	80 (81.8 %)	10.6 (3.64, 36.3)	
WHZ				0.58
<−2	26 (12.0 %)	17 (14.2 %)	1	
>−2	190 (88.0 %)	103 (85.8 %)	0.83 (0.41, 1.68)	
WAZ				0.04
<−2	124 (57.4 %)	83 (68.6 %)	1	
>−2	92 (42.6 %)	38 (31.4 %)	0.62 (0.38, 1.01)	

The median increase in Hb levels of 0.9 g/dl was well within the range of the 0.8–1.0 g/dl in published studies. Microft et al. in Europe and Huang et al. reported an increase from 13.9 to 14.6 g/dl a statistical association between the level of Hb and duration of use of HAART was also found [16, 17]. In children, Bolton-Moore et al. found that for children with baseline mean Hb of 10.3 g/dl, it had increased to 11.3 g/dl after6 months of HAART almost similar to our study [18]. In another study in Burkina-Faso, Nacoulma et al. found that after 6 months of AZT based HAART anemia prevalence had reduced [19]. Drug regimen was noted to have a big influence on the increments in hemoglobin level with Stavudine combination having a much higher increment as compared to zidovudine combination findings similar to other studies [20].

In this study children who received iron supplements were noted to have higher hemoglobin increments this is similar to the findings in Malawi where iron supplementation in HIV infected children increased hemoglobin levels and reduced the prevalence of anemia by 40 % but iron was noted to increase the risk of malaria [21]. Identification of children to be given iron in this study was based on low baseline hemoglobin levels as recommended by WHO on targeted iron supplementation for children at risk of anemia and iron deficient

[14]. Children who received these drugs had markedly reduced hemoglobin level at baseline. Some of these children were also provided with food supplement and nutritional education and this could have contributed to marked increase. The study was not able to identify whether those given iron supplements had higher risk of sepsis due to retrospective nature of the study.

When we compared the mean corpuscular volume at baseline of 75.9 fl with that after 6 months of treatment of 89.2 fl, we found an increase in median change that was higher than the findings of Huang et al. in adults of 95.5 fl at baseline to 105.5 fl following 6 months of HAART [17]. The increase could have been due to nutritional modification offered, iron supplements or antiretroviral drugs. Macrocytosis was found to have occurred after treatment and this could be attributed to the effect of mainly zidovudine as this has been found in other studies [22]. A striking and discrepant observation was that the circulating RBC counts decreased significantly following six months of HAART despite increase in hemoglobin levels and mean corpuscular volume. This finding is similar to the findings of Huang et al. and may be associated with defect in the production of erythrocytes from erythroid progenitor cells leading to the generation of fewer but larger cells [17].

Total white blood cells were found to decrease significantly from 8.7×10^3 mm^3 to 6.7×10^3 mm^3 in this study probably because at the time of enrollment, the children might have had intercurrent acute or chronic infections causing leucocytosis and following treatment and initiation of HAART the levels were seen to have decreased and this could have been due to the antiretroviral drugs improving immunity leading to less infections. Similar findings were reported by Nacoulma et al. in adults after six months of AZT based HAART of 2.27×10^3 mm^3 at baseline compared to 1.9×10^3 mm^3 after 6 months of HAART [19]. The finding in this study contrast some studies which reported significant increase in WBC following treatment with Huang et al. reporting a mean increase of 0.8 ($p < 0.001$) [17]. In this study, there was a statistical significant increase in platelets levels from 255×10^3 mm^3 to 279×10^3 mm^3 similar to findings by Huang et al. in adults [17].

In this study the first line regimens as recommended by the Ministry of Health of both zidovudine based and Stavudine based were shown to lead to a significant change in hematological parameters similar to the findings in various other studies [17, 18]. Moyle G et al. in their study also assessed the mean decreased in hemoglobin level comparing various regimens after treatment which we were unable to do due the small number of patients that were started on Stavudine based and protease inhibitor based regimens [4].

Conclusion

The findings of this study suggest that Antiretroviral drugs lead to a significant change in hematological parameters with a positive change of hemoglobin levels, MCV, MCH and platelet and decrease in total WBC, granulocytes lymphocytes and RBC. This indicates that zidovudine based regimens may safely be used even in setting with limited laboratory monitoring.

Methods

This retrospective cohort study was carried out at Kenyatta National Hospital comprehensive care centre between September and November 2008. Children were enrolled into the study if they were age 5–144 months, confirmed to be HIV positive by rapid tests for those aged over 18 months and PCR DNA for those aged less than 18 months, attending the Kenyatta National Hospital comprehensive care center. They also had to have received the first line ART according to the Kenyan Ministry of Health guidelines without change of treatment for at least six months with available complete medical records and parents/guardians provided informed consent. Standard study tools were used to abstract data from the medical records of enrolled children and included demographic, clinical and laboratory characteristics. The laboratory data had been analyzed by University of Nairobi Paediatric laboratory which undertakes laboratory procedures relating to the comprehensive care clinic. It uses a semi automated hematology analyzer MS4 and is a GCLP certified (Good Clinical Laboratory Practices) with external quality assurance. There is computerized data for all children attending the clinic who are on HAART and it also details of the regimen the children is on and when started. Using ART number in the data base and patients appointment number we were able to identify the patients' files. Files were retrieved as the clients came for review in their monthly clinic that runs daily from Monday to Friday. Pre and 6-month post ART estimates of, absolute CD4, CD4%, hemoglobin level, total white blood cells count, absolute lymphocyte counts, granulocyte counts, and platelets counts were recorded in an abstract form. In addition information was obtained regarding use of all medications including prophylactic medications, iron supplementation, multivitamins, and HAART regimens. Ethical clearance to conduct the study was obtained from the department of Pediatrics and Child Health and the KNH ethical review Committee.

Statistical methods

Data entry and analysis were done using SPSS version 16.0. The weight for height Z scores (WHZ), height for age Z scores (HAZ) and weight for age Z scores (WAZ) were computed using the nutrition software of Epi Info 3.2 Baseline hematological parameters were compared to those obtained after 6 months of HAART using Pearson Chi square test to compare categorical variables. Wilcoxon paired t-test for non parametric variables was used to determine the difference in baseline hematological parameters and parameters after 6 months of HAART for parameters. Differences in associations and relationships were taken as significant where P was less than 0.05.

Abbreviations

HIV: human immunodeficiency virus; HAART: highly active antiretroviral therapy; ARV: anti retroviral therapy; KNH: Kenyatta National Hospital; Hb: hemoglobin level; RR: relative risk; MCV: mean corpuscular volume; MCH: mean corpuscular hemoglobin; WHO: World Health Organization; WBC: white blood cells; OI: opportunistic infection; ART: anti retroviral therapy; IDA: iron deficiency anemia; AZT: zidovudine; NVP: nevirapine; EFV: efavirenz; RBC: red blood cells; PCR: polymerase chain reaction; ABC: abacavir; 3TC: Stavudine; GCLP certified: good clinical laboratory practices.

Authors' contributions

All authors conceptualized the study and wrote the proposal. EGK carried out the data collection while RN, DW and NK supervised the work and frequently advised during the study. All authors participated in data analysis and wrote the manuscript. All authors read and approved the final manuscript.

Authors' information

EGK is a lecturer and a consultant Paediatrician who received her M.B.ch.B degree from Moi University in Kenya in 2001. She later joined University of Nairobi in Kenya for her Masters degree in Paediatric and child health. She has been working in Egerton University for the last 3 years and she is the Founding Chairperson of the Department of Paediatrics in Egerton University. RN is a Professor of Paediatrics at the School of Medicine, College of Health Sciences, University of Nairobi. She is a Paediatrician and Epidemiologist who has taught at the University of Nairobi for many years. Her major achievement is her contribution to the understanding of the epidemiology and biology of breast milk transmission of HIV and in integration of prevention of mother-to-child transmission (PMTCT) of HIV in resource constrained settings.
DW is an associate Professor in the Department of Paediatrics and Child Health, University of Nairobi and a Consultant Paediatrician. He has experience in conducting research studies in Maternal Newborn and Child Health as well as Paediatric HIV. NK has been in practice for 23 years and she holds an M. B. Ch. B and MMed (Paediatrics) from the University of Nairobi. She has formerly worked at Kenyatta National Hospital, Ministry of Health, Hammersmith Hospital London and the University Of Nairobi School Of Medicine.

Author details

[1] Department of Paediatrics and Child Health, Egerton University, P.O. Box 536-20115, Egerton, Kenya. [2] Department of Paediatrics and Child Health, University of Nairobi, P. O. Box 19676-00202, Nairobi, Kenya. [3] Paediatric Hematology and Oncology, University of London, London, UK. [4] P.O. Box 2275-20100, Nakuru, Kenya.

Acknowledgements

We wish to express our sincere gratitude to the staffs of Kenyatta National Hospital, Comprehensive Care Centre for their support and assistance in provision of medical records, administration of the hospital and the lecturers in the department of paediatric and child health, University of Nairobi for their guidance, patience, commitment and overwhelming support during the period of research. We also wish to acknowledge the Deputy Vice Chancellor Division of Research and Extension, Egerton University for his continued support and encouragement during the preparation of the manuscript.

Competing interests

The authors declare that they have no competing interests.

References

1. Spivak JL, Bender BS, Quinn TC (1984) Hematological abnormalities in the acquired immune deficiency syndrome. Am J Med 77:224
2. Ministry of Health, Government of Kenya (2005) Diagnosis and Staging of HIV in children. In: Ibrahim M, Isaiah T, Sylvia O et al. (eds) Guideline for Antiretroviral therapy in Kenya. p 56
3. Mwanda OW (1997) Hematological changes in human immunodeficiency virus infection. East Afr Med J 1:732–739
4. Moore RD (1999) Human immunodeficiency virus infection, anemia, and survival. Clin. Infect. Dis. 29:44–49 **(Abstract/FREE Full Text)**
5. Consolini R, Benviclli W, Legitimo A, Galli L, Tovo P et al (2007) Pre HAART follow- up study of the hematological manifestation in children with prenatal HIV infection, suggestions for reclassification of clinical disease. Italian register for HIV infection in children. Paediatri. Hematol Oncol 29:376–383
6. Adetifa IM, Temiye EO, Akinsulie AO, Ezeaka VC, Iroha EO (2006) Hematological abnormalities associated with paediatric HIV/AIDS in Lagos. Ann Trop Paediatr 26(2):121–125
7. Totin D, Ndugwa C, Mmiro F et al (2002) Iron deficiency anemia is highly prevalent among HIV infected and uninfected infants in Uganda American Society of nutritional sciences. J Nutri 132:423–429 **(PubMed)**
8. Eley BS, Sive AA, Shuttleworth M, Hussey GD (2002) Prospective cross sectional study of anemia and iron status in HAART naïve HIV infected children in South Africa. BMC Infect Dis 2:3 **(PMC free article, PubMed)**
9. Suarez DA, Rao PR, Miller JS (1994) Prevalence of lymphopenia in children with AIDS. Clin Pediatr 33(4):204–208
10. Calis JC, van Hensbroek MB, de Haan RJ, Moons P, Brabian BJ, Bates I (2008) HIV-associated anemia in children: systemic review from global perspective. AIDS 22(10):1099–1112 **(PubMed)**
11. Ellaurie M, Bernstein LJ, Shah K et al (1986) Thrombocytopenia in Paediatrics AIDS. Blood 68:124a
12. Karpatkin S, Nardi MA, Green D (2002) Platelet and coagulation defect associated with HIV infection. Thromb Haemost 88:389–400
13. Foote EM, Sullivan KM, Ruth LJ, Oremo J, Sadumah I, Williams TN, Suchdev PS (2013) Determinants of Anemia among Preschool Children in Rural, Western Kenya. Am J Trop Med Hyg. 88(4):757–764. doi:10.4269/ajtmh.12-0560
14. WHO (2001) Iron Deficiency Anemia assessment, Prevention, and Control. A guide for programme Managers. http://www.who.int/nutrition/publications/en/ida_assessment_prevention_control.pdf
15. Moyle G, Sawyer W, Law M, Amin J, Hill A (2004) Changes in hematological parameters and efficacy of thymidine analogue based highly active antiretroviral therapy: meta-analysis of six prospective, randomized comparative studies. Clin Ther 26(1):92–97
16. Mocroft A, Kirk O, Barton SE, EuroSIDA Study Group (1999) Anemia is an independent predictive marker for clinical prognosis in HIV infected patients across Europe. AIDS 13:943–950
17. Huang SS, Barbour JD, Deeks SG, Huang SJ, Grant RM et al (2000) Reversal of human immunodeficiency Virus type 1-Associated hematosuppression by effective antiretroviral therapy. Clin Infect Dis 30:504–510
18. Bolton-Moore C, Mubiana-Mbewe M, Cantrell RA, Chintu N, Stringer EM et al (2007) Outcomes and CD4 cell response. Clinical in children receiving Antiretroviral Therapy at Primary health care facilities in Zambia. JAMA 289:1888–1899

19. Nacoulma EW, Some Y, Tieno H, Diallo I, Zoungrana A et al (2007) Hematological parameters evolving during antiretroviral therapy of HIV infected patients in Bukina-faso. Bull Soc Pathol 100(4):271–274
20. Kiragga AN, Castelnuovo B, Nakanjako D, Manabe YC (2010) Baseline severe anemia should not preclude use of zidovudine in antiretroviral-eligible patients in resource-limited settings. J Int AIDS Soc. 13:42. doi:10.1186/1758-2652-13-42 **(PMCID: PMC2991285 Published online 2010 Nov 3)**
21. Esan MO, van Hensbroek MB, Nkhoma E, Musicha C, White SA, Ter Kuile FO, Phiri KS (2013) Iron supplementation in HIV-infected Malawian children with anemia: a double-blind, randomized, controlled trial. Clin Infect Dis 57(11):1626–1634. doi:10.1093/cid/cit528 **(PubMed Abstract Publisher Full Text)**
22. Pryce C, Pierre RB, Steel-Duncan J, Evans-Gilbert T, Palmer P, Moore J, Rodriguez B, Christie CD (2008) Safety of antiretroviral drugs in Jamaican children with HIV. West Indian Med J 57(3):238–245

23

Determinants of late presentation to HIV/AIDS care

Yalemzewod Assefa Gelaw[2*], Goitom Halefom Senbete[1], Akelew Awoke Adane[2] and Kefyalew Addis Alene[2]

Abstract

Background: Late diagnosis and presentation to human immune deficiency virus (HIV)/acquired immune deficiency syndrome care reduce the benefits of antiretroviral therapy and increase the risk of HIV transmission.

Objectives: This study was conducted to identify determinants of late presentation to HIV care among people living with HIV in Southern Tigray, Northern Ethiopia.

Methods: An institution based un-matched case–control (1:2 ratios) supported with qualitative data was conducted in Southern Tigray Zone from March 1 to April 30, 2014. Individuals with HIV enrolled from six randomly selected health facilities were included in the study. Cases were people living with HIV who had cluster of differentiation four count <350 cells/μl or World Health Organization stages 3 or 4. A total of 442 study participants were included by systematic sampling techniques. Bivariable and multivariable binary logistic regression model was used to identify associated factors. Odds ratio with 95 % CI was computed to assess the strength of the associations.

Result: Age categories, 25–29 years [AOR 3, 95 % CI (1.2–8.1)] and 35–39 years [AOR 4.1, 95 % CI (1.4–12.5)], having two [AOR 6, 95 % CI (1.3–28)] and more [AOR 5.2, 95 % CI (1.1–24.8)] lifetime sexual partners, poor social support [AOR 2.3, 95 % CI (1.26–4.30)], second (next to lowest) wealth quintile [AOR 3.3, 95 % CI 91.3–8.5)], fear of stigma [AOR 4.4, 95 % CI (2.2–8.3)], fear of losing job [AOR 6.8, 95 % CI (1.8–24.5)], and reported severe illness [AOR 4.3, 95 % CI (2.26–8)] were identified to be the risk factors for late presentation.

Conclusion: Low socio-economic status and social support, fear of stigma were potential risk factors for late presentation. Efforts towards promoting early care seeking should target on these factors in the study area and other similar settings.

Keywords: Late presentation, HIV/AIDS, Determinants, Case–control, Ethiopia

Background

An estimated of more than 35.3 million adults were living with human immune deficiency virus (HIV) worldwide; and nearly two-third (69 %) of this were found in Sub-Saharan Africa [1]. The European Late Presenter Consensus Working Group (ELPCWG), defines "late presentation" as initial presentation to HIV care with a CD4 cell count of <350 cells/μl, and defines "presentation with advanced HIV disease" as presentation for care with a CD4 count below 200 cells/μl or any acquired immune deficiency syndrome (AIDS)-defining illness or event [2]. Clinically, late presentation limits opportunities to reduce further transmission [1, 2].

Introduction of antiretroviral therapy (ART) has substantially reduced the burden of HIV by decreasing the risk of death and improving treatment response. Late presentation for HIV care is associated with high risk

*Correspondence: yalassefa@gmail.com; pipizewa@gmail.com
[2] Department of Epidemiology and Biostatistics, College of Medicine and Health Sciences, University of Gondar, Gondar, Ethiopia

of death, acquiring opportunistic infection and poor response to treatment [3–5]. Although people on ART have increased risk for non–AIDS illness, early initiations of ART is the option in developing countries including Ethiopia for people with HIV [6].

Previous studies and reports in Sub-Saharan Africa showed that 35–65 % of HIV patients initially present with a CD4 cell counts less than 200 cells/μl or with an AIDS-defining illness [6–9] and 20–40 % start ART with a CD4 counts <100 cells/μl. Such late presentation is associated with lower survival, early mortality and invasive bacterial and fungal infections [4]. It is also a major reason for the decreasing of retention rates in the course of ART [3, 5, 6, 10, 11]. In addition to it, late presentation also poses a higher cumulative risk of HIV transmission to others [6, 12, 13] as well as an economic burden to individuals particularly in the first few months of presentation [12].

Although findings on late presentation are limited, the problem of late ART initiation and its poor outcomes has been reported by some researches in Ethiopia [14–16].

Different scholars from developed [5, 6, 12] and developing countries [3, 5, 6] state various definitions, reasons and determinants of late presentation to HIV care. Studies from Ethiopia are scarce at diversified contextual/ structural, clinical and individual level factors. Identifying the factors associated with late presentation for HIV care seeking is important for the improvement of HIV/ AIDS prevention and control programs. It also helps to early undertakes for decisions makers and program managers on the upcoming revision of country wide HIV testing and care strategies. Therefore, it is important to identify the determinants of late presentation to HIV care.

Methods

Study design and study population

Un-matched case control study design supported with qualitative data was conducted from March 1 to April 20, 2014 (data collection period) in Southern Tigray Zone. The zone is located in the northern part of Ethiopia 645 km away from Addis Ababa, the capital city of Ethiopia. During the study period a total of 20 health facilities (3 general hospitals and 17 health centers) were providing voluntary counseling and testing, prevention of mother to child transmission, ART and treatment of opportunistic infection services.

The study population consisted of people over 18 years of age with HIV who were enrolled in HIV chronic care clinics and had visited the health facilities during the data collection period. Cases were people living with HIV/AIDS who had CD4 count less than 350 cell/mm^3 or World Health Organization (WHO) clinical stage III or IV during their first clinical visit for HIV care. Controls were PLWHA whose CD4 count was ≥350 cell/μl and WHO clinical stage I or II. Focus group discussions (FGD) were conducted with PLWHA who were a member of mother's supporting group.

Sampling techniques and sample size determination

The sample size was calculated using Epi Info version 7.0 by considering the following assumptions: the proportion of HIV status non-disclosure to partners among the cases was 46.2 and 29.4 % among the controls [17], using 95 % CI, 90 % power and case to control ratio of 1 to 2 to detect an odds ratio of 2. Then by adding 10 % non-response rate, the final sample size was 442 (147 cases and 295 controls). Previous studies have indicated that non disclosure of HIV status to partners, alcohol use and perception of stigma increase for late presentation. Non disclosure of HIV status to partner was selected to maximize sample size.

Simple random sampling techniques were applied to select respondents. Two district hospitals and four health centers were selected randomly.

After collecting baseline CD4 count and/or WHO staging using chart reviews, people living with HIV/ AIDS were classified in two groups before data collection began. Cases and controls were then selected using systematic random sampling techniques based on visits that occurred during the data collection period. We divided the sample among the six participating health institutions with a ratio of five cases to two controls. HIV-positive individual's under 18 years of age, those with neither CD4 count data nor WHO HIV/AIDS stage recorded at first visit, and those who were overtly cognitively impaired were excluded from the study.

Data collection and analysis

The data were collected using an interviewer administered technique by 11 trained clinical nurses working in ART clinics and supervised by two health officers. Precoded and structured questionnaires consisted of sociodemographic, socioeconomic, behavioral, psychosocial and social environments were used. Data collectors and supervisors were trained with respect to the objectives of the study; confidentiality of information, respondent's rights, and interviewing technique prior to the actual data collection.

Wealth quintile information was by asking about the presence or absence of durable assets and services at the house hold level. Different indicators were used for urban and rural areas to measure wealth quintiles. The index was constructed for each household via principal components analysis. Indicators having ≥50 % rescaled communalities were used to construct wealth index and further categorized into five wealth quintiles (as lowest, second, third, fourth and highest based on the Ethiopian demographic and health survey classification [18].

Data were entered to Epi Info version 7 and transferred to SPSS 20 for further statistical analysis. Descriptive and summary statistics were computed. Both bivariable and multivariable logistic regression models were used to identify associated factors. Variables having p value less than 0.2 in the bivariable analysis were remained in the multivariable model to control the effect of confounders. The Hosmer–Lemeshow goodness-of-fit statistic was used to assess the fitness of the model. Odds ratios (OR) with their 95 % confidence intervals (95 % CI) were calculated to measure the strength of association. P value less than 0.05 were considered to be significant determinants for cases and controls.

Qualitative data were collected by the principal investigator through FGD parallel to quantitative data collection. The recorded data were transcribed, translated and analyzed using thematic analysis under the sub headings of the quantitative findings and new themes for new findings.

Ethical consideration

This study was carried out after receiving ethical approval from the Institutional Review Committee of University of Gondar. Prior to approval, the proposal was provided to reviewers to assure the ethical issues. Permission letter was also obtained from the respective health institutions (medical director or persons in charge of institutions) to identify cases and controls through chart review by authorized ART case managers or ART nurses. Before interviewing or recording, the data collector fully explained the purpose of the study to each participant and obtained written informed consent from each participant. To ensure confidentiality, names were not mentioned in the questionnaire and result report. In addition, the collected data were locked.

Result

A total of 413 HIV positive individuals (147 cases and 266 controls) participated in this study. The median age (IQR) at time of presentation was 30 (±13) years. The median age (IQR) at time of presentation for cases and controls were 30 (±11) and 30 (±13), respectively (Table 1).

Determinants of late presentation

Age group, having had multiple sexual partners, poor socioeconomic status, non-disclosure status to partner, presentation before 2011, low household social support, desire to protect family, severity of illness, fear of stigma and fear of losing job were all found to be independent risk factors for late presentation to HIV/AIDS care (Table 2).

Participants in the age group of 25–29 years [AOR 3, 95 % CI (1.15–8.12)] and those 35–39 years [AOR 4.1, 95 % CI (0.35–12.46)] were 3 and 4.1 times more likely to present late, respectively, as compared to those 18–24 years of age.

Year of presentation was associated with likelihood of late presentation. Those study participates who were visiting the HIV care before 2008 were presenting lately. The risk of late presentation to HIV care among PLWHA who presented in the years 2011–2012 [AOR 0.31, 95 % CI (0.12–0.77)] and 2013–2014 [AOR 0.14, 95 % CI (0.05–0.37)] was decreased by 69 and 86 %, respectively, as compared to those presenting before the year 2008.

Presence of more than one lifetime sexual partner was also associated with late presentation to HIV care. HIV-positive individuals with two lifetime sexual partners were six times [AOR 6, 95 % CI (1.28–28.02)] more likely to present late as compared with participants with none. Those with more than two life time sexual partners were also 5.2 times [AOR 5.2, 95 % CI (1.08–24.76)] more likely to present late compared to those with none.

The second (next to lowest) wealth quintile of HIV-positive individuals was 3.3 times [AOR 3.3, 95 % CI (1.31–8.46)] more likely to present late as compared to the highest wealth quintile group.

Partner or spousal HIV status disclosure was found to deter presentation. Married participants who did not disclose their HIV status to their partner were two times more likely to present late [AOR 2, 95 % CI (1.05–4.14)] compared to those who did.

HIV positive individuals who had poor house hold social support were 2.3 times more likely to present late as compared to those who had good social support at home [AOR 2.3, 95 % CI (1.26–4.30)].

Barriers perceived by PLWHA were also associated with late presentation. Participants who reported fear of stigma were 4.4 times more likely to present late as compared to those who did not [AOR 4.4, 95 % CI (2.23–8.27)]. Participants who reported fear of losing their source of income were 6.8 more likely to present late as compared to those who did not [AOR 6.8, 95 % CI (1.8–24.54)].

The way participants perceived the benefits of HIV care also contributed to discrepancy in stage at presentation. Participants who responded that "protecting family" was their reason for initiating care were 81 % less likely to present late, as compared to those who did not [AOR 0.19, 95 % CI (0.09–0.37)]. By contrast, participants who responded that "severe illness" was a reason for initiating care were 4.3 times more likely to present late as compared to those who did not [AOR 4.3, 95 % CI (2.26–8.0)].

The qualitative results revealed that fear of stigma, fear of losing income source/former job, use of alternative

Table 1 Socio-demographic characteristics at first presentation of cases and controls, Southern Tigray zone, Northern Ethiopia, 2014

Variables	Categories	Cases, N (%)	Controls, N (%)
Sex	Male	55 (37.4)	86 (32.3)
	Female	92 (62.6)	180 (67.7)
Marital status at first presentation	Married	73 (49.7)	122 (45.9)
	Widowed	22 (14.9)	37 (13.9)
	Divorced	34 (23.1)	67 (25.2)
	Never married	18 (12.2)	40 (15)
Pregnancy (18–49)	Yes	11 (12.4)	29 (17)
	No	78 (87.6)	141 (82.9)
Education at first presentation	Can't read and write	87 (59.2)	167 (62.8)
	Primary (1–8)	40 (27.2)	74 (27.8)
	Secondary and above	20 (13.6)	25 (9.4)
Residence	Urban	93 (63.3)	154 (57.9)
	Rural	54 (36.7)	112 (42.1)
Occupation	Farmer	34 (23)	79 (29.7)
	Professional/business occ.	37 (25)	49 (18.4)
	Unemployed	25 (17)	45 (16.9)
	House wife	27 (18.4)	53 (19.9)
	Daily laborer	24 (16.3)	40 (15)
Age category	18–24	19 (12.9)	63 (23.7)
	25–29	35 (23.8)	48 (18)
	30–34	36 (24.5)	58 (21.8)
	35–39	28 (19)	32 (12)
	40–44	16 (10.88)	32 (12)
	45+	13 (8.8)	33 (12.4)
Wealth quintiles (SES)	Lowest	40 (27.2)	42 (15.8)
	Second	39 (20.4)	47 (17.7)
	Third	24 (16.3)	57 (21.4)
	Fourth	26 (17.7)	59 (22.2)
	Highest	18 (12.2)	61 (22.9)

therapies, lack of familial pressure to initiate care, inadequacy of social support (spouse, friends and religious leaders) and inadequate knowledge about delay to care were the barriers reported by people living with HIV/AIDS in the study area (Table 3).

Discussion

This study identified determinants of late presentation to HIV/AIDS care in ART services are accessible at primary health care units. Although different studies reported various risk factors for late presentation, the present study assessed people's perceived need for care, perceived barriers to HIV care, socioeconomic status, and the role of social support.

Consistent with previous studies in Europe and Africa [11, 19–22, 29] HIV-positive participants were present late for care when their age gets old. It has been posited that when age increase adults are more likely to have a moral or ethical reason for presenting earlier to care. However, a study in India reported young adults present late [23]. This could be explained by differences in method and project design, as well as varying social and cultural issues. In countries like Ethiopia, old peoples considered as immaculate. In the context of the study setting elder individuals are a pronounced in the milieu.

Participants with a history of multiple sexual partners were more likely to present late to care. This was also reported in previous study in Ethiopia [17]. However, in Uganda [11] and Venezuela [24] HIV-positive individuals with more than one sexual partner presented early. One factor for this different finding might be the emphasis of taboo on sexually active behaviors in Ethiopian society, and an increased propensity to feel embarrassment regarding this behavior [25]. Although having legal multiple sexual partners are practiced in Islamic religions of

Table 2 Binary and multiple logistic regressions showing determinants of late presentation to HIV/AIDS care, among PLWHA receiving HIV care, Southern Tigray zone, Northern Ethiopia, 2014

Determinants/factors	Presentation to HIV care		COR (95 % CI)	AOR (95 % CI)
	Cases (%)	Control (%)		
Year of presentation				
Before 2008	37 (25.2)	46 (17.3)	1	1
2009–2010	62 (42.2)	65 (24.4)	1.2 (0.681–2.06)	0.76 (0.33–1.73)
2011–2012	27 (18.4)	65 (24.4)	0.51 (0.277–0.963)	0.31 (0.12–0.77)**
2013–2014	21 (14.3)	90 (33.8)	0.29 (0.153–0.552)	0.14 (0.05–0.37)**
Age category				
18–24	19 (12.9)	63 (23.7)	1	1
25–29	35 (23.8)	48 (18)	2.4 (1.23–4.73)	3.0 (1.15–8.12)*
30–34	36 (24.5)	58 (21.8)	2.0 (1.06–3.98)	1.4 (0.52–3.65)
35–39	28 (19)	32 (12)	2.9 (1.41–5.96)	4.1 (1.35–12.46)*
40–44	16 (10.88)	32 (12)	1.7 (0.75–3.65)	1.1 (0.34–3.71)
45+	13 (8.8)	33 (12.4)	1.3 (0.62–3.29)	1.3 (0.37–4.23)
No. of life time sexual partners				
None	4 (2.7)	28 (10.5)	1	1
One	49 (33.3)	77 (28.9)	4.4 (1.47–13.47)	4.0 (0.86–18.59)
Two	46 (31.3)	98 (36.8)	3.3 (1.08–9.9)	6.0 (1.28–28.02)*
More than two	48 (32.7)	61 (22.9)	5.5 (1.80–16.7)	5.2 (1.08–24.76)*
Presence of HIV infected HH member				
Yes	16 (10.9)	51 (34.7)	1	
No	131 (89.1)	215 (65.3)	1.9 (1.06–3.54)	
Presence of HIV care attendee				
Yes	14 (9.5)	44 (16.5)	1	
No	133 (90.5)	222 (83.5)	1.8 (1.1–3.56)	
Witnessed stigma				
Low stigma	91 (61.9)	184 (69.2)		
High stigma	56 (38.1)	82 (30.8)	1.4 (0.90–2.10)	
Depression				
Not depressed	56 (38.1)	154 (57.9)	1	
Depressed	91 (61.9)	112 (42.1)	2.2 (1.47–3.37)	
Level of social support				
Poor social support	103 (70)	95 (35.7)	4.2 (2.73–6.49)	2.3 (1.26–4.30)*
Good social support	44 (30)	171 (64.3)	1	1
Wealth quintile (SES)				
Lowest	40 (27.2)	42 (15.8)	3.2 (1.63–6.37)	1.05 (0.38–2.83)
Second	39 (20.4)	47 (17.7)	2.8 (1.43–5.52)	3.3 (1.31–8.46)*
Third	24 (16.3)	57 (21.4)	1.4 (0.70–2.90)	0.8 (0.27–2.31)
Fourth	26 (17.7)	59 (22.2)	1.5 (0.74–3.0)	1.1 (0.44–2.82)
Highest	18 (12.2)	61 (22.9)	1	1
Disclosure to partner				
Yes	26 (35.6)	72 (59)	1	1
No	47 (64.4)	50 (41)	2.6 (1.43–4.74)	2.0 (1.05–4.14)*
HIV support groups in community				
Yes	70 (47.6)	150 (56.4)	0.70 (0.47–1.05)	
No	77 (52.4)	116 (43.6)	1	

Table 2 continued

Determinants/factors	Presentation to HIV care		COR (95 % CI)	AOR (95 % CI)
	Cases (%)	Control (%)		
Diet and life style change for positive result				
Yes	49 (33.3)	122 (45.9)	0.59 (0.39–0.89)	0.45 (0.24–0.87)*
No	98 (66.6)	144 (54.1)	1	1
Desire to protect family				
Yes	23 (15.6)	126 (43.4)	0.20 (0.12–0.34)	0.19 (0.09–0.37)**
No	124 (84.4)	140 (52.6)	1	1
To know CD4 count				
Yes	5 (3.4)	33 (12.4)	0.25 (0.095–0.65)	0.37 (0.09–1.43)
No	142 (96.6)	233 (87.6)	1	1
Severity of illness				
Yes	89 (60.5)	66 (24.8)	4.7 (3.01–7.16)	4.3 (2.26–8.0)**
No	58 (39.5)	200 (75.2)	1	1
Fear of stigma				
Yes	94 (63)	65 (24.5)	5.5 (3.5–8.5)	4.4 (2.2–8.3)**
No	53 (37)	201 (75.5)	1	1
Fear of disclosure				
Yes	60 (40.8)	40 (15)	3.9 (2.43–6.23)	2.0 (0.99–4.32)
No	87 (59.2)	226 (84.9)	1	1
Fear of losing job/income source				
Yes	27 (18.4)	6(2.3)	9.8 (3.92–24.2)	6.8 (1.8–24.54)*
No	120 (81.6)	260 (97.7)	1	1

* Significant ($p \leq 0.05$)

** Highly significantly ($p < 0.001$)

Ethiopia, seeking treatment related to sexual transmitted disease is still lack.

Socioeconomic positions of the study participants were also the determinant factors to present late for HIV care. Participants in the second (next to the lowest) wealth quintile were statistically associated with late presentation. This was also consistent with previous systematic review of three indicators of socio economic status (education, income and occupation) [26]. Despite the difference in measurement of socioeconomic positions of HIV positive individuals, some studies also describe income as a determinant factor for late presentation [6, 14, 17]. In the context of Ethiopian health care delivery system voluntary counseling and testing, diagnosis and ART services are exempted.

In Ethiopia peoples are most of the time living together; shares the same dish and chalice in different occasions. Participants with poor social support were more likely present late, consistent with studies done in Durban, South Africa [14] and Houston, Texas [27]. Here we believe that social stigma and lack of social support can contribute towards people feeling inhibited in seeking HIV/AIDS care. The qualitative data also support this finding. Behavioral change and communication concerned with social stigma and poor social support needs to be done using key informants, religious person and mother supporting groups.

Poor partner's communication on reproductive health matters has an impact for health status of the family. Partners who did not disclose their status to their partner were more likely to present late. Similarly, studies done in Uganda [6], Kenya [28] and Ethiopia [17], revealed that disclosure to partners can initiate timely HIV/AIDS care. HIV/AIDS related stigma and discrimination has declined dramatically in Ethiopia and support following disclosure has improved.

The current study reported that participants who had been visiting health facilities in recent years were more likely to present early as compared to those visited health facilities before 2008. This finding is consistent with studies done in Nigeria [29], Belgium and France [22], New York City [30] and India [23]. This could be due to the increased access to care, overall awareness of HIV, media accessibility and a reduction in stigma over time [31–33].

Fear of stigma and losing one's job were determinant factors for late presentation consistent with previous studies in Sub-Saharan Africa [34] and Zimbabwe [35]. This is also supported by the qualitative FGD report that

Table 3 FGD results extracted from HIV positive individuals works on mothers supporting groups concerning barriers to early HIV/AIDS care, Southern Tigray Zone, April 2014

Barriers to HIV/AIDS care	HIV/AIDS positive individuals working on Mother Supporting Group
Fear of stigma	"... I was worried that people will talk about me if they hear I tested positive"... Male-32 "When I became aware of my HIV status my challenge was fear of health professionals and seeing other individuals I know while attending the ART clinic", Female-27.
Fear of losing income source/former job	"People seem supportive towards HIV positives at first, but the pain is that they gradually change their feeling and treat you as 'too weak' to accomplish your duty ...HIV positives will be shifted to lower status/position", Male-55 "Although they are HIV positive, numerous commercial sex workers in the town continue their commercial sex work", Female-27
Use of non-medical treatment	"...then she ate a dried Wild boar's meat and Wild boar's bile", Female-30 "...he told me a very bitter plant called 'Oure' or 'Eret' is medicine for HIV and he had been drinking it until he ended up dying", Female-30 "I went to a local traditional healer called 'Tonqualli' or magician and spent around 3000 Ethiopian Birr then he told to my wife wash my body using sheep's blood and dung added together ....", Male-38 "There was one HIV-positive neighbor with symptoms of diarrhea, she bought drugs from the pharmacy, was relieved of her symptoms for some time and then went to other pharmacy a few days later....", Female-30 "My husband and were severely diseased and confined to bed for around 6 months. He had been telling that his illness was due to other diseases like malaria, and he has been getting medicines from drug stores", Female-34
Low families driving force for initiation care	"We should let peoples think for the next generation...If my children are healthy.....", Male -32 ... "My child is negative", Female-27, "My wife and children are negative", Males-32, 55
Inadequacy of social support (spouse, friends and religious leaders)	"... I show him my ART drugs that I am taking and he became persuaded to take his treatment too", Female-55 "I become angry and decided not to take any treatment for 1 year. Later on my friends were taking HIV treatment and they encouraged me to take treatment." Male-28 "Males say that we are healthy even though we have the HIV and nothing bad is going on us, but, females become ill and suffer from headache and they come to ART clinics saying I tested positive for HIV ...", Female-27 "....later on my wife went to the health center and tested positive after that she encouraged me to be tested ...", Male-38 ".....I then persuaded my husband to be tested for HIV and avoided taking other drugs from outside the treatment center", Female-34 "My brother shouts at me, you should be tested and know the cause for your illness today; I will help every expense that follows .....", Female-35 "...she was severely ill and her family said that they didn't want to take care of the dead", Female-27
Inadequate knowledge	"The HIV testing sites that are conducted in the shade in town are always crowded with people being tested, especially males. But they don't come to care once they have tested positive [F-55] and they can only be accessed after they become diseased, arriving on a stretcher or by ambulance, or when found during house-to-house tracing by volunteer HIV support groups. ...", Female-34

showed fear of stigma and losing job/customers were barriers. This is could be common problem of female participant's sex worker.

Our study also showed that participants who perceived HIV as a sever disease were more likely to seek care early. This is demonstrated in the qualitative data in which protecting family members was a driver to initiate HIV care early.

In this study the use of traditional medicine and a holy water as a treatment and sex of respondents were not statistically significant with late presentation to HIV/AIDS care. However, data from the FGD indicates that male's patients who had visited traditional medicine and/or holy water sites were more likely to present late for HIV/AIDS care. This discrepancy could be due to that HIV positive individuals might fear to disclose the utilization of these services. It could be also due to the rareness of such traditional treatments.

The potential limitations of this study were that the study may have been prone to recall biases and that there may have been misclassification of presentation or diseases do to social pressure.

Conclusion

Age older than 25, having multiple sexual partners, poor socioeconomic status, non-disclosure to partner, presentation before 2011 for care, low house hold social support, desire to protect family, severity of illness, fear of stigma and fear of losing job were all found to be independent risk factors for late presentation to HIV/AIDS care.

Authors' contributions

GHS designed the study, performed the statistical analysis, and drafted the paper. YAG and AAA participated in the paper writing. YAG, AAA and KAA participated in manuscript drafting and editing. All authors contributed to the data analysis. All authors read and approved the final manuscript.

Author details

[1] College of Medicine and Health Sciences, Wollo University, Dessie, Ethiopia.
[2] Department of Epidemiology and Biostatistics, College of Medicine and Health Sciences, University of Gondar, Gondar, Ethiopia.

Acknowledgements
The Southern Tigre zonal Health Department, hospitals' and Health centers' staff, study participants, and data collectors deserve appreciation for their cooperation and assistance.

Competing interests
The authors declare that they have no competing interests.

References
1. World Health Organization. HIV and adolescents: guidance for HIV testing and counselling and care for adolescents living with HIV: recommendations for a public health approach and considerations for policy-makers and managers. 2013.http://www.who.int/iris/bitstream/10665/94334/1/9789241506168_eng.pdf.
2. Antinori A, et al. Late presentation of HIV infection: a consensus definition. HIV Med. 2011;12(1):61–4.
3. Lahuerta M, et al. The problem of late ART initiation in Sub-Saharan Africa: a transient aspect of scale-up or a long-term phenomenon? J Health Care Poor Underserved. 2013;24(1):359–83.
4. Ford N, et al. Getting to zero HIV deaths: progress, challenges and ways forward. J Int AIDS Soc. 2013;16(1):18927.
5. World Health Organization. Global update on HIV treatment: results, impact and opportunities. 2013. Available: http://www.who.int/hiv/pub/progressreports/update2013/en/.
6. David HS. CROI: cardiovascular disease and co-morbidities in HIV. 20th conference on retroviruses and opportunistic infections. March 3–6. Atlanta, GA. 2013.
7. Geng EH, et al. Trends in the clinical characteristics of HIV-infected patients initiating antiretroviral therapy in Kenya, Uganda and Tanzania between 2002 and 2009. J Int AIDS Soc. 2011;14:46.
8. Mulissa Z, Jerene D, Lindtjorn B. Patients present earlier and survival has improved, but pre-ART attrition is high in a six-year HIV cohort data from Ethiopia. PLoS One. 2010;5(10):e13268.
9. Lahuerta M, et al. Factors associated with late antiretroviral therapy initiation among adults in Mozambique. PLoS One. 2012;7(5):e37125.
10. Nash D, et al. Program-level and contextual-level determinants of low-median CD4+ cell count in cohorts of persons initiating ART in eight Sub-Saharan African countries. AIDS. 2011;25(12):1523–33.
11. Abaynew Y, Deribew A, Deribe K. Factors associated with late presentation to HIV/AIDS care in South Wollo ZoneEthiopia: a case–control study. AIDS Res Ther. 2011;8(8):8.
12. Mocroft A, et al. Risk factors and outcomes for late presentation for HIV-positive persons in Europe: results from the collaboration of observational HIV epidemiological research Europe study (COHERE). PLoS Med. 2013;10(9):e1001510.
13. CSA. Ethiopia Demographic and Health Survey 2011. Addis Ababa. Central Statistical Agency [Ethiopia] and ICF International; 2012.
14. Gupta A, et al. Early mortality in adults initiating antiretroviral therapy (ART) in low- and middle-income countries (LMIC): a systematic review and meta-analysis. PLoS One. 2011;6(12):e28691.
15. Kigozi IM, et al. Late-disease stage at presentation to an HIV clinic in the era of free antiretroviral therapy in Sub-Saharan Africa.
16. Wanyenze RK, et al. Missed opportunities for HIV testing and late-stage diagnosis among HIV-infected patients in Uganda. PLoS One. 2011;6(7):e21794.
17. Camoni L, et al. Late presenters among persons with a new HIV diagnosis in Italy, 2010–2011. BMC Public Health. 2013;13(1):281.
18. Zoufaly A, et al. Late presentation for HIV diagnosis and care in Germany. HIV Med. 2012;13(3):172–81.
19. Mojumdar K, et al. Late presenters to HIV care and treatment, identification of associated risk factors in HIV-1 infected Indian population. BMC Public Health. 2010;10:416.
20. Ndiaye B, et al. Factors associated with presentation to care with advanced HIV disease in Brussels and Northern France: 1997–2007. BMC Infect Dis. 2011;11:11.
21. Agaba PA, et al. Patients who present late to HIV care and associated risk factors in Nigeria. HIV Med. 2014;15(7):396–405.
22. Alvarez-Uria G. Factors associated with delayed entry into HIV medical care after HIV diagnosis in a resource-limited setting: data from a cohort study in India. PeerJ. 2013;1:e90.
23. Nyblade L, et al. Disentangling HIV and AIDS stigma in Ethiopia, Tanzania and Zambia; 2003.
24. Peltzer K, Pengpid S. Socioeconomic factors in adherence to HIV therapy in low- and middle-income countries. J Health Popul Nutr. 2013;31(2):150–70.
25. Kelly JD, Hartman C, Graham J, Kallen MA, Giordano TP. Social support as a predictor of early diagnosis, linkage, retention, and adherence to HIV care: results from the steps study. J Assoc Nurses AIDS Care. 2014;25(5):405–13.
26. Medley AA, et al. Early uptake of HIV clinical care after testing HIV-positive during home-based testing and counseling in western Kenya. Curr HIV/AIDS Rep. 2011;8(3):172–80.
27. Jenness SM, et al. Delayed entry into HIV medical care after HIV diagnosis: Risk factors and research methods. AIDS Care. 2012;24(10):1240–8.
28. Getnet MK, Damen HM. Level of stigma among female sex workers: comparison of two surveys of HIV behavioral data, Ethiopia. Afr Health Sci. 2011;11(4):543–9.
29. Bonjour MA, Montagne M, Zambrano M, Molina G, Lippuner C, Wadskier FG, et al. Determinants of late disease-stage presentation at diagnosis of HIV infection in Venezuela: a case–case comparison. AIDS Res Ther. 2008;5:6.
30. Sidibé M, Goosby EP. Global action to reduce HIV stigma and discrimination. J Int AIDS Soc. 2013;16(3Suppl 2):18893.
31. Alemu T, et al. Experience of stigma and discrimination and the implications for healthcare seeking behavior among people living with HIV/AIDS in resource-limited setting. SAHARA J. 2013;10(1):1–7.
32. Govindasamy D, Ford N, Kranzer K. Risk factors, barriers and facilitators for linkage to antiretroviral therapy care: a systematic review. AIDS. 2012;26(16):2059–67.
33. Seyoum E, et al. ART scale-up in Ethiopia: success and challenges; 2009.
34. Waters L, Sabin CA. Late HIV presentation: epidemiology, clinical implications and management. Expert Rev Anti Infect Ther. 2011;9(10):877–89.
35. Makasi T, Modiba L. Factors associated with delayed entry into HIV medical care among HIV positive people who are aware of their status in Bulawayo, Zimbabwe. Online J Med Med Sci Res. 2012;1(4):55–62.

Permissions

All chapters in this book were first published in AIDS R&T, by BioMed Central; hereby published with permission under the Creative Commons Attribution License or equivalent. Every chapter published in this book has been scrutinized by our experts. Their significance has been extensively debated. The topics covered herein carry significant findings which will fuel the growth of the discipline. They may even be implemented as practical applications or may be referred to as a beginning point for another development.

The contributors of this book come from diverse backgrounds, making this book a truly international effort. This book will bring forth new frontiers with its revolutionizing research information and detailed analysis of the nascent developments around the world.

We would like to thank all the contributing authors for lending their expertise to make the book truly unique. They have played a crucial role in the development of this book. Without their invaluable contributions this book wouldn't have been possible. They have made vital efforts to compile up to date information on the varied aspects of this subject to make this book a valuable addition to the collection of many professionals and students.

This book was conceptualized with the vision of imparting up-to-date information and advanced data in this field. To ensure the same, a matchless editorial board was set up. Every individual on the board went through rigorous rounds of assessment to prove their worth. After which they invested a large part of their time researching and compiling the most relevant data for our readers.

The editorial board has been involved in producing this book since its inception. They have spent rigorous hours researching and exploring the diverse topics which have resulted in the successful publishing of this book. They have passed on their knowledge of decades through this book. To expedite this challenging task, the publisher supported the team at every step. A small team of assistant editors was also appointed to further simplify the editing procedure and attain best results for the readers.

Apart from the editorial board, the designing team has also invested a significant amount of their time in understanding the subject and creating the most relevant covers. They scrutinized every image to scout for the most suitable representation of the subject and create an appropriate cover for the book.

The publishing team has been an ardent support to the editorial, designing and production team. Their endless efforts to recruit the best for this project, has resulted in the accomplishment of this book. They are a veteran in the field of academics and their pool of knowledge is as vast as their experience in printing. Their expertise and guidance has proved useful at every step. Their uncompromising quality standards have made this book an exceptional effort. Their encouragement from time to time has been an inspiration for everyone.

The publisher and the editorial board hope that this book will prove to be a valuable piece of knowledge for researchers, students, practitioners and scholars across the globe.

List of Contributors

M Scott Killian
Department of Medicine, University of California San Francisco, Parnassus Avenue, San Francisco, CA 94143-1270, USA

Chenglong Liu, Cuiwei Wang and Mary Young
Department of Medicine, Georgetown University, 2115 Wisconsin Avenue NW, Suite 130, Washington, DC 20007, USA

Marshall J Glesby
Division of Infectious Diseases, Weill Cornell Medical College, New York, NY, USA

Gypsyamber D'souza
Department of Epidemiology, Johns Hopkins School of Public Health, Baltimore, MD, USA

Audrey French
Division of Infectious Diseases, Cook County Hospital, Chicago, IL, USA

Howard Minkoff
Department of Obstetrics and Gynecology, Maimonides Medical Center, Brooklyn, NY, USA

Toby Maurer
Department of Dermatology, University of California at San Francisco, San Francisco, CA, USA

Roksana Karim
Departments of Pediatrics and Preventive Medicine, University of Southern California, Los Angeles, CA, USA

Stephen Brown
AIDS Research Alliance, Los Angeles, CA, USA

David M Simpson
Mount Sinai School of Medicine, New York, NY, USA

Graeme Moyle
Chelsea and Westminster Hospital, London, United Kingdom

Bruce J Brew
St Vincent's Hospital, Darlinghurst, Australia

Giovanni Schifitto
University of Rochester, Rochester, NY, USA

Nicholas Larbalestier
St Thomas' Hospital, London, United Kingdom

Chloe Orkin
Andrews Out Patients Unit, London, United Kingdom

Martin Fisher
HIV/GUM Research, Elton John Centre, Brighton, United Kingdom

Geertrui F Vanhove and Jeffrey K Tobias
NeurogesX, Inc, San Mateo, CA, USA

Thep Chalermchai and Narin Hiransuthikul
Department of Preventive and Social Medicine, Faculty of Medicine, Chulalongkorn University, Bangkok, Thailand

Thep Chalermchai and Jintanat Ananworanich
SEARCH, The Thai Red Cross AIDS Research Center, Bangkok, Thailand

Pisit Tangkijvanich
Department of Biochemistry, Faculty of Medicine, Chulalongkorn University, Bangkok, Thailand

Suteeraporn Pinyakorn, Anchalee Avihingsanon and Jintanat Ananworanich
HIV-NAT, The Thai Red Cross AIDS Research Center, Bangkok, Thailand

Anchalee Avihingsanon and Jintanat Ananworanich
Department of Medicine, Faculty of Medicine, Chulalongkorn University, Bangkok, Thailand

Denise C Hsu
The Kirby Institute for Infection and Immunity in Society, University of New South Wales, Sydney, Australia

Irini Sereti
HIV Pathogenesis Unit, Laboratory of Immunoregulation, NIAID/NIH, Bethesda, MD, USA

Jintanat Ananworanich
HIV Netherlands Australia Thailand Research Collaboration and SEARCH, Thai Red Cross AIDS Research Centre, Bangkok, Thailand

Dibesh Karmacharya, Sameer Dixit, Rajesh Rajbhandari, Bhawana Subedi, Sonu Shrestha and Sulochana Manandhar
Center for Molecular Dynamics Nepal, Sawraj Sadan, Thapathali-11, Kathmandu, Nepal

Dongmei Yu
Massachusetts General Hospital, Psychiatric and Neurodevelopmental Genetics Unit, Center for Human Genetic Research, Boston, MA, USA

Susan L Santangelo
Harvard Medical School, Psychiatry, Harvard School of Public Health, Epidemiology, and Massachusetts General Hospital, Psychiatric and Neurodevelopmental Genetics Unit, Center for Human Genetic Research, Boston, MA, USA.

Vicky Jocelyne Ama Moor and Jeanne Ngogang Yonkeu
Laboratory of Biochemistry, Yaounde University Teaching Hospital, Yaounde, Cameroon

Vicky Jocelyne Ama Moor, Constant Anatole Pieme and Jeanne Ngogang Yonkeu
Department of Biochemistry and Physiological Sciences, University of Yaounde I, Yaounde, Cameroon

Corinne Tchoula Mamiafo
Department of Biochemistry, Faculty of Sciences, University of Yaounde I, Yaounde, Cameroon

Jobert Richie N Nansseu
Intensive Care Unit, Mother and Child Centre, Chantal Biya Foundation, Yaounde, Cameroon

Claude Tayou
Laboratory of Hematology, Yaounde University Teaching Hospital, Yaounde, Cameroon

Robert Sebunya, Victor Musiime, Sabrina Bakeera Kitaka and Grace Ndeezi
Department of Paediatrics and child Health Makerere, University college of Health Sciences, Kampala, Uganda

Victor Musiime
Joint Clinical Research Centre, Kampala, Uganda

Sureshnee Pillay, Ruth M Bland, Richard J Lessells, Justen Manasa, Tulio de Oliveira and Sivapragashini Danaviah
Africa Centre for Health and Population Studies, College of Health Sciences, University of KwaZulu-Natal, Durban, South Africa

Ruth M Bland
Royal Hospital for Sick Children, Glasgow, UK

Richard J Lessells
Department of Clinical Research, London School of Hygiene and Tropical Medicine, London, UK

Tulio de Oliveira
Research Department of Infection, University College of London (UCL), London, UK

Sivapragashini Danaviah
Rm 135, 1st Floor, DDMRI, 719 Umbilo Road, Congella 4013, South Africa

Edward R Cachay, Francesca Torriani, David Wyles and William C Mathews
Department of Medicine, Owen Clinic, University of California at San Diego, 200 W. Arbor Drive, San Diego, CA 92103-8681, USA

Lucas Hill, Craig Ballard and Bradford Colwell
Skaggs School of Pharmacy and Pharmaceutical Sciences, University of California at San Diego, San Diego, CA, USA

Edward R Cachay, Francesca Torriani and David Wyles
Department of Medicine, Division of Infectious Diseases, University of California at San Diego, San Diego, CA, USA

Alain Lafeuillade
Department of Infectious Diseases, General Hospital, Toulon, France

Vicente Soriano
Department of Infectious Diseases Hospital Carlos III, Madrid, Spain

Marie Suzan-Monti
INSERM, U912 (SESSTIM), Marseille, France
Aix Marseille Université, IRD, UMR_S912, Marseille, France

ORS PACA, Observatoire Régional de la Santé Provence Alpes Côte d›Azur, Marseille, France

Mario Stevenson
Miller MedicalSchool, University of Miami, Miami, FL, USA

Jacques Izopet
Laboratoire de Virologie, Institut Fédératif de Biologie, Hôpital Purpan, Toulouse, France

Hans-Jürgen Stellbrink
Infektions Medizinisches Centrum Hamburg Study Center, Hamburg, Germany

Rachel A Bender Ignacio
Division of Allergy and Infectious Diseases, University of Washington, 1959 NE Pacific St, BB545, 98195 Seattle, WA, USA

Jacqueline Chu
Department of Medicine, Massachusetts General Hospital, Grey/Bigelow 740, 55 Fruit St, 02114 Boston, MA, USA

Melinda C Power
Johns Hopkins Bloomberg School of Public Health, Department of Epidemiology, 615 North Wolfe Street, W6508, 21205 Baltimore, MD, USA

Jeffrey Douaiher
Department of Surgery, Johns Hopkins Hospital, 600 N Wolfe St, 21287 Baltimore, MD, USA

Jordan D Lane
Harvard Medical School, Tosteson Medical Education Center, 260 Longwood Ave, 02115 Boston, MA, USA

Jeffrey P Collins
Department of Medicine, CHC Urgent Care, Massachusetts General Hospital Chelsea Healthcare Center, 151 Everett Ave, 02150 Chelsea, MA, USA

Valerie E Stone
Department of Medicine, Harvard Medical School, 25 Shattuck St, 02115 Boston, MA, USA
Department of Medicine, Mount Auburn Hospital, 330 Mount Auburn Street, 02138 Cambridge, MA, USA

Rachel A Bender Ignacio
Fred Hutchinson Cancer Research Center, M1B-140 1100 Fairview Ave N, Seattle, WA 98109, USA

Nicholas C Obitte
Department of Pharmaceutical Technology and Industrial Pharmacy, Faculty of Pharmaceutical Sciences, University of Nigeria, Nsukka, Nigeria

Lisa C Rohan
Department of Pharmaceutical Sciences, School of Pharmacy, Magee Womens Research Institute, University of Pittsburgh, Pittsburgh, PA, USA

Christianah M Adeyeye
Department of Biopharmaceutical Sciences, College of Pharmacy, Roosevelt University Schaumburg, Shaumburgh, IL, USA

Michael A Parniak
Department of Microbiology and Molecular Genetics, School of Medicine, University of Pittsburgh, Pittsburgh, PA, USA

Charles O Esimone
Department of Pharmaceutical Microbiology and Biotechnology, Faculty of Pharmaceutical Sciences, Nnamdi Azikiwe university, Awka, Anambra, Nigeria

Madhuri Thakar, Bharati Mahajan, Nawaj Shaikh, Salman Bagwan, Suvarna Sane and Ramesh Paranjape
Department of Immunology, National AIDS Research Institute, G-73, MIDC, Bhosari, Pune 411 026, India

Sandhya Kabra, Bharat Rewari and Mohamad Shaukat
National AIDS Control Organization, New Delhi, India

Namita Singh and Peter Trevor
Clinton Health Access Initiative, New Delhi, India

Amit C Achhra and Mark A Boyd
The Kirby Institute, University of New South Wales, Sydney, Australia

Agnes Meybeck, Lydie Lecomte, Nicolas Van Grunderbeeck, Nicolas Boussekey, Arnaud Chiche, Hugues Georges and Olivier Leroy
Service de Réanimation et Maladies Infectieuses, Hôpital de Tourcoing, 135 rue du Président Coty, Tourcoing BP 619, France

Michel Valette and Yazdan Yazdanpanah
Service des Maladies Infectieuses et du Voyageur, Hôpital de Tourcoing, 135 rue du Président Coty, Tourcoing BP 619, France

Agnes Meybeck
Service de Réanimation et Maladies Infectieuses, Centre Hospitalier Dron, 128 rue du Président Coty, Tourcoing 59200, France

Stephen J Penney, Maureen E Gallant and Michael D Grant
Immunology and Infectious Diseases Program, Division of BioMedical Sciences, Faculty of Medicine, Memorial University of Newfoundland, St. John's, NL A1B 3 V6, Canada

Michael D Grant
H1803-Immunology, Faculty of Medicine, Memorial University of Newfoundland, 300 Prince Philip Drive, St. John's, NL A1B 3 V6, Canada

Jean Joel R. Bigna
Department of Epidemiology and Public Health, Pasteur Center of Cameroon Member of International Network of the Pasteur Institutes, Yaoundé, Cameroon

Paule Sandra D. Sime and Sinata Koulla-Shiro
Faculty of Medicine and Biomedical Sciences, University of Yaoundé 1, Yaoundé, Cameroon

Sinata Koulla-Shiro
Infectious Diseases Unit, Yaoundé Central Hospital, Yaoundé, Cameroon

Valentine Budambula
Department of Environment and Health Sciences, Technical University of Mombasa, Mombasa, Kenya

Francis O. Musumba, Mark K. Webale and Collins Ouma
Department of Biomedical Science and Technology, Maseno University, Maseno, Kenya

Francis O. Musumba
Centre for Virus Research, Kenya Medical Research Institute, Nairobi, Kenya

Titus M. Kahiga
Department of Pharmacy and Complementary Medicine, Kenyatta University, Nairobi, Kenya

Francisca Ongecha-Owuor
Department of Medicine, Therapeutics, Dermatology and Psychiatry, Kenyatta University, Nairobi, Kenya

James N. Kiarie
Department of Obstetrics and Gynecology, University of Nairobi, Nairobi, Kenya

George A. Sowayi
Department of Medical Laboratory Sciences, Masinde Muliro University of Science and Technology, Kakamega, Kenya

Aabid A. Ahmed
Bomu Hospital, Mombasa, Kenya

Collins Ouma
Health Challenges and Systems Program, African Population and Health Research Centre, Nairobi, Kenya

Tom Were
Department of Medical Laboratory Sciences, Masinde Muliro University of Science and Technology, Kakamega 50100, Kenya

Lin Chen, Jiezhe Yangs, Renjie Zhang, Yun Xu, Jinlei Zheng, Jianmin Jiang, Jun Jiang, Lin He and Ning Wang
Zhejiang Provincial Center for Diseases Control and Prevention, Hangzhou, China

Ning Wang
National Center for AIDS/STD Control and Prevention, China CDC, Beijing, China

Philip Chun Yeung
Department of Surgery, Faculty of Medicine, The Chinese University of Hong Kong, Shatin, Hong Kong

Xiaohong Pan
Department of HIV/AIDS Prevention and Control, Zhejiang Provincial Center for Diseases Control and Prevention, 3399 Binsheng Road, Hangzhou, Zhejiang, People's Republic of China

Stephen Okoboi, Jonathan Wangisi, Josephine Birungi, Darius Kato, Maureen Nyonyintono, Aggrey Egessa and Celestin Bakanda
Mulago Hospital Complex, The AIDS Support Organization (TASO), Kampala, Uganda

Erin Ding, Susan Shurgold and David M. Moore
The BC Centre for Excellence in HIV/AIDS, Vancouver, Canada

Steven Persuad and David M. Moore
Faculty of Medicine, University of British Columbia, Vancouver, Canada

Paula Munderi and Pontiano Kaleebu
MRC/UVRI Uganda Research Unit on AIDS, Entebbe, Uganda

Elizabeth Gathoni Kibaru
Department of Paediatrics and Child Health, Egerton University, Egerton, Kenya

Ruth Nduati, Dalton Wamalwa and Nyambura Kariuki
Department of Paediatrics and Child Health, University of Nairobi, Nairobi, Kenya

Nyambura Kariuki
Paediatric Hematology and Oncology, University of London, London, UK

Elizabeth Gathoni Kibaru
Nakuru, Kenya

Goitom Halefom Senbete
College of Medicine and Health Sciences, Wollo University, Dessie, Ethiopia

Yalemzewod Assefa Gelaw, Akelew Awoke Adane and Kefyalew Addis Alene
Department of Epidemiology and Biostatistics, College of Medicine and Health Sciences, University of Gondar, Gondar, Ethiopia

Index